TRANSFUSION MEDICINE: QUO VADIS?
WHAT HAS BEEN ACHIEVED, WHAT IS TO BE EXPECTED

DEVELOPMENTS IN HEMATOLOGY AND IMMUNOLOGY

Volume 36

The titles published in this series are listed at the end of this volume.

Transfusion Medicine: Quo Vadis? What Has Been Achieved, What Is to Be Expected

Proceedings of the jubilee Twenty-Fifth International Symposium on Blood Transfusion, Groningen, 2000,
Organized by the Sanquin Division Blood Bank Noord Nederland

edited by

C. TH. SMIT SIBINGA
Blood Bank Noord Nederland,
Groningen, The Netherlands

and

J. D. CASH
Edinburgh, Scotland, U.K.

SPRINGER-SCIENCE+BUSINESS MEDIA, B.V.

Library of Congress Cataloging-in-Publication Data

ISBN 978-1-4613-5700-1   ISBN 978-1-4615-1735-1 (eBook)
DOI 10.1007/978-1-4615-1735-1

Printed on acid-free paper

ISBT SITS

COUNCIL OF EUROPE CONSEIL DE L'EUROPE

This jubilee 25th International Symposium was co-sponsored by WHO and conducted under the auspices of the Secretary General of the Council of Europe, Mr. Walter Schwimmer and the International Society of Blood Transfusion.

25

Baxter

Acknowledgement

This publication has been made possible through the support of Baxter, which is gratefully acknowledged.

CONTENTS

III. QUALITY PRINCIPLES AND RISK MANAGEMENT

IV. TRANSFUSION MEDICINE AT THE BEDSIDE

MODERATORS AND SPEAKERS

Moderators

J.D. Cash (chairman)	–	Edinburgh, Scotland, UK
W.G. van Aken	–	Sanquin Blood Supply Foundation, Division CLB, Amsterdam, NL
D.H. Buchholz	–	Baxter Healthcare Corporation, Round Lake, IL, USA
F. Canal	–	Fenwal Europe, Madrid, E
S. Poppema	–	University of Groningen, Faculty of Medical Sciences, Groningen, NL
C.Th. Smit Sibinga	–	Sanquin Blood Supply Foundation, Division Blood Bank Noord Nederland, Groningen, NL
H.J.C. de Wit	–	Sanquin Blood Supply Foundation, Amsterdam, NL

Speakers

J-P. Allain	–	East Anglian Blood Centre, Cambridge, UK
J.P. AuBuchon	–	Dartmouth-Hitchcock Medical Center, Lebanon, NH, USA
A. Brand	–	Sanquin Blood Supply Foundation, Division Blood Bank Leiden-Haaglanden, Leiden, NL
K-F Bopp	–	Directorate III – Social Cohesion, Health and Social Policy Division, Council of Europe, Strasbourg, F
M. Bruce	–	SNBTS Headquarters, Edinburgh, Scotland, UK
L. Corash	–	Cerus Corporation, Concord, CA, USA
N. Drouet	–	University Centre of Grenoble, Grenoble, F
J.C. Emmanuel	–	Department of Blood Safety and Clinical Technology, WHO, Geneva, CH

P.R. Foster	–	Protein Fractionation Centre, Edinburgh, Scotland, UK
J.F. Harrison	–	National Blood Service, London, UK
M. Kavanagh	–	Medicines Control Agency, London, UK
J. Koistinen	–	Finnish Red Cross BTS, Helsinki, SF
A.P.M. Los	–	Sanquin Blood Supply Foundation, Division Blood Bank Noord Nederland, Groningen, NL
Th.E.P. Lotgerink	–	Science & Business Connection, Groningen, NL
D.B.L. McClelland	–	Scottish National Blood Transfusion Service, Edinburgh, Scotland, UK
J. McCullough	–	Center for Molecular and Cellular Therapy, Minneapolis, MN, USA
H.T. Meryman	–	Naval Medical Research Institute, Bethesda, MD, USA
P.M. Ness	–	John Hopkins Hospital, Baltimore, MD, USA
K. Sazama	–	U.T. M.D. Anderson Cancer Center, Houston, TX, USA
M.L. Turner	–	Edinburgh & S.E. Scotland BTS, Edinburgh, Scotland, UK
E.C. Vamvakas	–	Blood Bank, New York University Medical Center, New York, NY, USA

Prepared Discussant

M.J. Postma	–	Groningen University Institute for Drug Exploration, Groningen, NL

FOREWORD

It is a great pleasure for me to open the jubilee 25th International Symposium on Blood Transfusion here in Groningen.

This symposium is co-sponsored by the World Health Organization and is being held under the auspices of the ISBT and the Secretary General of the Council of Europe, Mr Walter Schwimmer. The patronage was granted with great pleasure for several reasons. First of all, Dutch experts are very active in our Committees and have largely contributed in developing the Council of Europe principles in the blood area. Secondly, the Council of Europe is active today in the area of blood transfusion due to a tragic event, which occurred in 1953 in the Netherlands; following a flooding many of the blood products given for assistance could not be used due to incompatibilities and differences in labelling.

Some words to present the Council of Europe since the organisation is sometimes confused with institutions of the European Union:
The organisation has been founded in 1949 to establish the principles of democracy and rule of law all over Europe. Since 1989, the year of the fall of the Berlin wall and the opening up of the iron curtain, these principles could be extended to the countries of Central and Eastern Europe. Today this makes the Council of Europe the only pan-European organisation with 41 Member States thus representing more than 750 million people.

Why, as an organisation promoting and protecting human rights, do we deal with issues related to blood transfusion? The reason is that the human body and its parts should not, as such, give rise to financial gain or comparable advantage.
Ladies and Gentlemen, in the first part of this symposium you are reviewing achievements made in the blood transfusion over the last 25 years. I would like to use this occasion to recall the role and the contribution of the Council of Europe in this field over the last 50 years.

Activities before 1989

In the beginning of the 50ties, the work of the Council of Europe in the blood transfusion area has been built around three major principles; voluntary and non-remunerated donation, the goal to achieve self-sufficiency and the protection of both the donors and the recipients.

With these objectives in mind, the Council of Europe concentrated on studying the ethical, legal and organisational aspects of blood transfusion with a view to ensuring quality, increasing availability of blood, ensuring optimal use and analysing the possible ethical and organisational impact of new scientific developments.

The first Agreement on the exchange of substances of human origin was adopted in 1958. It was followed by Agreements on the exchange of blood grouping reagents and tissue-typing reagents in 1962 and 1976 respectively. All three European Agreements (No 26, 39 and 84) ensured at that time free movement throughout Europe of blood and blood products, as well as of blood grouping and tissue-typing reagents in cases of emergency.

In 1968 a European bank of frozen blood of rare groups was set up in Amsterdam, the Netherlands to provide for the storage of extremely rare blood where the quantities collected at national level were insufficient.

Activities After 1989

With the opening up of the iron curtain, the new challenge was to extend the Council of Europe principles to the new Member States from Central and Eastern Europe. In 1993, a survey on « Blood transfusion services of central and eastern European countries and their co-operation with Western transfusion services » was published [1]. The special concern of the Council of Europe in sponsoring this study was to ensure within « Greater Europe » :

- Harmonisation of policies
- Promotion of voluntary, non-remunerated donation
- Stability and self-sufficiency of blood transfusion services
- Introduction of quality standards for both blood and plasma products

A Pan-European Conference followed in 1994 on the Restructuring of Blood Transfusion and Plasma Fractionation in Central and Eastern Europe. As an immediate result, a Task Force on Blood Transfusion has been created with the aim of helping in restructuring the countries' blood transfusion services.

Since then, Task Force missions have taken place in Estonia, Lithuania, Latvia, Slovak Republic, Bulgaria and Romania.

Recently, budgetary provisions have been made available to carry out a Task Force mission to Albania in 2000.

Task Force missions have always been prepared by a Group, which included Dr. Emmanuel from WHO. The excellent co-operation with WHO in this field is highly appreciated.

A specific programme called ADACS (Activities for the Development and Consolidation of Democratic Stability) had been set up, which included in 1998 a training course on blood transfusion organised in Sofia with participants from Bulgaria, Romania and FYROM (Former Yugoslav Republic of Macedonia).

In 1999, a workshop in Corfu, hosted by the Greek Authorities on "Quality management and organisation of blood transfusion services" bringing together transfusion specialists from Albania, FYROM, Russia and Ukraine. Dr. Smit Sibinga was one of the main speakers at this workshop.

A major success story started in 1995, when the Council of Europe adopted a *Guide to the preparation, use and quality assurance of blood components as technical appendix to Recommendation No R (95) 15*, on which many countries base formal national blood transfusion guidelines. It has been translated into numerous languages including Spanish, Russian and Japanese. Updated annually, the 6th edition was published in January 2000 and preparations for the 7th edition are in a very advanced stage.

The "Guide", as it is called, is of great interest to blood transfusion centres, legislators, health personnel and all those working in the field of blood transfusion.

Reference to its chapter on selection of donors is made in the European Pharmacopoeia monograph on *Human Plasma for Fractionation* as well as in the relevant notes for guidance on plasma-derived products issued by the European Medicines Evaluation Agency (EMEA). I am pleased to announce that the complete 6th edition has just now been put on our web site, which should foster its use to an even wider audience.

Current activities of the Council of Europe in the area of blood transfusion include the elaboration of Recommendations on the prevention of the possible transmission of variant Creutzfeldt-Jakob disease (vCJD) by blood transfusion and on the hospital's and clinician's role in the optimal use of blood. A study on pathogen inactivation of labile blood components is nearly finalised.

Outlook

I am glad to learn from the programme, that you are also looking into what is to be expected in the future.

New techniques may become daily practice soon;

- inactivation/elimination of bio-burden;
- alternatives to human blood resources;
- the development of gene therapy.

We thus approach a zero risk for the greater safety of the public. However, the question of cost/benefit ratio has then to be addressed.

Health Authorities are depending on your advice.

Thank you again for the invitation. I wish you a good symposium with fruitful discussions.

Gabriella Battaini-Dragoni,
Director of Social Affairs and Health
Council of Europe

I. BLOOD SUPPLY SYSTEMS AND ORGANISATION

BLOOD TRANSFUSION: QUO VADIS? CUSTOMER ORIENTATION AS THE LEADING PRINCIPAL FOR BLOOD BANKS IN THE FUTURE

Th.E.P. Lotgerink[1], J.C.Hoekstra[2]

Introduction

Several developments in the environment of organisations demand for a different approach to customers. A large number of studies have come to the conclusion that, unless an organisation embraces a concept of customer orientation, it will not be able to compete in its market in the near future. Most studies concerning customer orientation are focussed on organisations that need to make profit. There is little or no research done to establish the need for customer orientation in the public sector. Recent studies show that the changes in the environment of public organisations are the same as in the private sector, and that public organisations, such as blood supply organisations, need to adapt in more or less the same way to those changes as private organisations. For most of the organisations the implementation of a customer orientation requires dramatic changes in management. There are several strategies for change management. An organisation needs to choose that strategy that best fits the requirements of a customer orientation. Commitment to the change process of every stakeholder within the system is essential. Constant monitoring of the effectiveness of improvements is of vital importance.

The objective of this paper is to present a scientific paradigm as well as a managerial concept that enables blood supply organisations to become customer oriented. The so-called Customer Concept is introduced, which is complemented with both psychological concepts and concepts from change management literature. The Market Orientation Barometer is introduced, that is meant to help small and medium-sized enterprises to become more competitive. It is useful for public organisations as well, no matter what the size of the organisation. The potential of this Barometer for blood transfusion organisations is discussed.

In section 2 we discuss the need for a customer orientation. Section 3 offers a description of the Customer Concept and defines a customer orientation. In section 4 the question is discussed whether using the Customer Concept and embracing a customer orientation might be the way to lead blood supply organisations successfully into the 21st century. Different ways of changing organisations are presented in section 5, each with its limitations and advantages for the

1. Science and Business Connection, Groningen, NL.
2. Faculty of Economics, University of Groningen, Groningen, NL.

change process that is needed to become a customer oriented organi-sation. In section 6 the Market Orientation Barometer is discussed. Section 7 offers implications for blood supply organisations.

The Need for a Customer Orientation

"Change is business as usual". This quote (that was used by the former HRM director of Robeco, chairman of the Dutch Organisation of HRM-managers P. Peppelenbosch) is the shortest and clearest description of the situation organisations are facing nowadays. The world is changing more rapid then ever, and more radical then ever. Changes occur in the social, economical, political and technical environment of organisations:

- Customer demands are increasing. Customers are being spoiled up to a level were it becomes almost impossible to satisfy them, let alone deliver service to the level of customer delight.
- Society demands more attention for the protection of environment. The Brent Spar affair dramatically changed the strategy of oil companies.
- The legislation that regulates the rights of employees and employers is changing.
- Privatising of public organisations, the withdrawal of government leads to more freedom in one field and less freedom in other areas. The influence of the State nowadays is perhaps less important than that of multinational organisations like Shell or Philips.
- The costs of collecting, storing and analysing data have decreased drastically in comparison to a couple of years ago [1].
- Interactive media such as Internet and WAP change the communication between suppliers and customers.
- It has become very easy for customers to order products in another part of the world, see Amazon.com.
- Because of individualisation of customers, segmentation becomes less effective. Customers might buy there suits from Hugo Boss and drive a Jaguar, but buy their groceries at a discount supermarket.
- The buying pattern of customers is changing rapidly [2].
- The lifecycle of products has become very short, innovations happen in rapid succession [3]. Investment made for the development of new products and services need to be regained in a shorter period of time.
- New technologies are being copied more rapidly by competitors. An illegal version of Windows97 was introduced to the market before the legal version had been introduced.
- Products become more similar and competing on price has become more difficult.

These developments result in a changing relationship between suppliers and customers. The initiative and the power in supplier-customer relationships are shifting from the supplier to the customer. Since product specifications and price are no longer effective tools for a supplier to create sustainable advantages, organisations focus more on service. Instead of selling products, organisations try to add customer value. Customer value is defined as the value a customer receives from buying, possessing and/or using a product or service [4]. Buying a

Volvo might be buying safety, buying a Mercedes might be buying reliability and buying a BMW might be buying status. Suppliers more and more shift their focus from transaction-oriented to relationship-oriented. Research shows that retaining customers is more beneficial then trying to attract new ones [5]. Thus, an increasing number of organisations recognise the need for a customer orientation. Most organisations even claim in one form or another to be customer oriented [6]. Yet, from our own experiences as a customer, we all know that many organisations seem unable to meet our expectations.

In order to bridge the gap between the scientific progress that has resulted in paradigms such as the Customer Concept (see section 3 and Hoekstra et al., 1999 [1]) and our own disappointing experiences as a customer, management of organisations has to be facilitated to make the necessary changes. Implementing customer orientation using a specific combination of change management strategies, enables organisations to meet customers needs.

The Customer Concept and Customer Orientation

The Customer Concept

Hoekstra, Leeflang and Wittink show in their paper [1] that the existing paradigms in marketing are no longer capable of describing the current relationships between suppliers and customers. Therefore, they introduce a new paradigm. Following the market developments as described above, as well as the changing relations between parties, they recommend that the new marketing paradigm:

- be directed to the realisation of individual customer values and the redefinition of these values; delivering customer value is the target of the customer oriented organisation [4];
- encompass the intimacy between partners in the marketing system and, as a consequence, focus on relationships instead of transactions;
- match customers' preferences and the firm's capabilities;
- force the fit between customer values and the firm's capabilities to be based on a market feedback system which measures the behaviour, the satisfaction, and unmet needs of individual customers continuously;
- reflect the idea that marketing is a state of mind which is not restricted to one functional area;
- stimulate the internal organisation to be constantly monitored and adapted to changing needs and preferences of customers, and always take the customer as the focal point [1].

In their view a marketing paradigm consists of three elements (Figure 1): (1) a concept (idea, philosophy, vision, orientation), which is the core of the paradigm, (2) a set of activities (decisions; marketing management: the implications of the concept), and (3) a domain (area, field of research where the concept and its implications are applied).

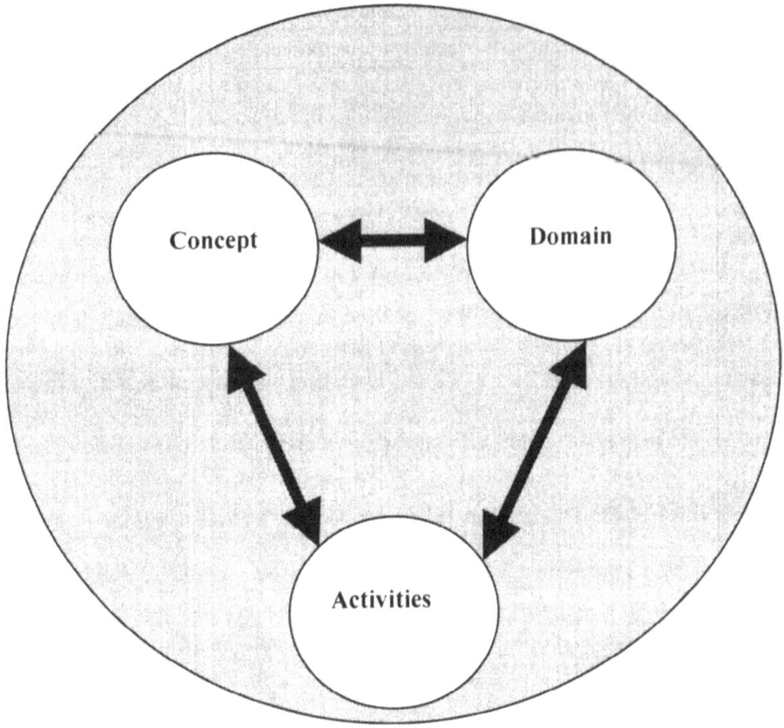

Figure 1. A new marketing paradigma [1].

The new marketing paradigm is based on the Customer Concept. Traditionally under the old paradigms the relationship between a supplier and a customer is not based on mutual interest. A customer is someone to whom a product is sold. In the Customer Concept the customer is the focal point. The Customer Concept maintains that "organisations establish relationships with selected individual target customers with whom superior customer values are designed, offered, redefined and realised in close coorperation with other parties in the marketing system such as suppliers and intermediaries, in order to realise long-term profits through customer-, partner- and employee-satisfaction" [1].

The *new marketing activities* will focus on customers instead of products, and therefore on developing relationships instead of developing products. New marketing activities include decisions with regard to vision, mission, targets, organisational strategy, allocation of manpower and money, organisational structure and culture, HRM, knowledge management and ICT systems, and the redesign of business processes.

The *domain of the new marketing* is changing as well. The role and function of marketing in the organisation is changing. Marketing is not just a department that supports other decision makers in the organisation by supplying the necessary customer information, marketing has to be a state of mind. Not just for marketeers, but for everyone in the organisation. Marketing becomes the central concept in the behaviour of every employee and manager. Part of the domain is the internal organisation. The marketing domain includes relationships with all stakeholders of the organisation, not only with the customers.

Customer Orientation: Philosophy, Strategy and Methodology

Customer orientation is defined as the desire of an organisation to build and maintain lasting and mutual beneficial relationships with carefully selected customers [7a,b]. Customer orientation is a three-dimensional managerial concept. It contains a way of thinking (philosophy), a way of doing business (strategy) and a complex of coherent actions (methodology). The confidence of organisations that state to be customer oriented, is funded mostly on the first dimension: having a philosophy that might be called customer oriented. The customers of the organisation, when coming into contact, of course do not experience the philosophy but the third dimension: the actions of the organisation. More specific, they experience the actions of the employees [8].

This discrepancy becomes more and more visible, since we change from a production society into a service delivery society. Buying a service is very different from buying a product. For instance, buying a car does not imply close contact with the employees that built the car and who therefore are responsible for the overall quality of the vehicle. In most cases the customer in this buying process comes into contact with a salesperson only, and perhaps later on with a service engineer. The customer does not come into contact with the production process. How different is the service delivery process. The one who delivers the service is also responsible for the quality of the service. The service is not produced in a factory somewhere in the Far East, but it is made here and now. The quality of the relationship and interaction between the supplier and the customer is very relevant for the perceived quality of the service delivery process. This indicates that customer value is not only derived from the buying, possessing and using of products and services, as defined above, but also from experiencing a respectful relationship. The customer being a part of the service delivery process makes the quality of the relationship and of the interaction key factors in the attempts of organisations to realise customer satisfaction.

It is necessary for organisations to recognise that not only customer values in terms of buying, processing and using products or services are important. Values that form the foundation of healthy relationships are the cornerstones of customer satisfaction. Core values that are important in service delivery organisation are [9]:

- Excellence;
- Fun;
- Renewal;
- Respect;
- Teamwork;
- Social benefit;
- Integrity.

Each and everyone of us that has been involved in a personal relationship will recognise most of these values as being important for maintaining relationships. It seems that the core competencies that are needed to build and maintain relationships are very similar to those that are important in the delivery process of services. In other words, the more customers come into very close contact with the delivery process, the more important the quality of the relationship with customers becomes. The customer changes into a co-producer. Whenever the organisation has not succeeded in making a good translation from philosophy into strategy, and from strategy into action (based on a congruent set of values), there is bound to be a discrepancy between the believes of the organisation and the experiences of customers. The more intimate a relationship with a customer becomes, the more important the values become which form the basis of a mutual beneficial relationship. Also, the more he/she will be disappointed when expectations are not met (product/service expectations but most of all relational expectations), and the greater the impact of customer (dis)satisfaction. It is essential that relationships with each and every stakeholder are based on the same set of values. The organisation has to be congruent in its relations.

The Customer Concept can be used to determine the customer value as defined by Webster [10] and Hoekstra et al. [1]. However, we need a more comprehensive understanding of customer value, including the quality of the relationship. Being congruent in building relationships with all stakeholders, congruent in the relational values that form the foundation of those relationships, lies within the heart of the customer orientation. Psychological concepts such as the Social Dilemma Theory [11, 12] can be used to gain a better understanding of the needs of both the customer and the organisation in the field of relationship quality. Social dilemmas (such as the prisoner's dilemma) may occur in the relationship with the customers, but also with other stake holders [13]. Also, the interests of one stakeholder might conflict with the interests of others. Managing social dilemmas in such a way that they result in a mutual win-win situation for all stakeholders might be essential for organisations that want to embrace a customer orientation. Thus, customer orientation adds an-other dimension to the concept of customer value, being the value that a customer derives from having a beneficial, fulfilling relationship with the supplier.

Implementing a customer orientation means integrating a thorough understanding of the Customer Concept and the psychological knowledge in the field of inter-human relationships. Just as marketing includes concepts, strategies, tools and skills, the same is true for psychology. Combining marketing and psychological concepts such as the Customer Concept and the Social Dilemma Theory, and bringing together tools and skills from those disciplines, are prerequisites for managing a customer orientation (Figure 2). It enables organisations to formulate a vision that is focussed on building and maintaining relationships, to translate that vision into a mission, targets and strategies, and most of all facilitates everybody within the organisation to turn thinking and talking into action.

Turning Talk Into Action

In general a vision is the answer to the question "what future do we want to create"? [14]. Ford had the vision of the man in the street owning his own car. "What role do we want to play in that future?" is the question that, when answered, gives the mission of an organisation. This role has to be operationalised

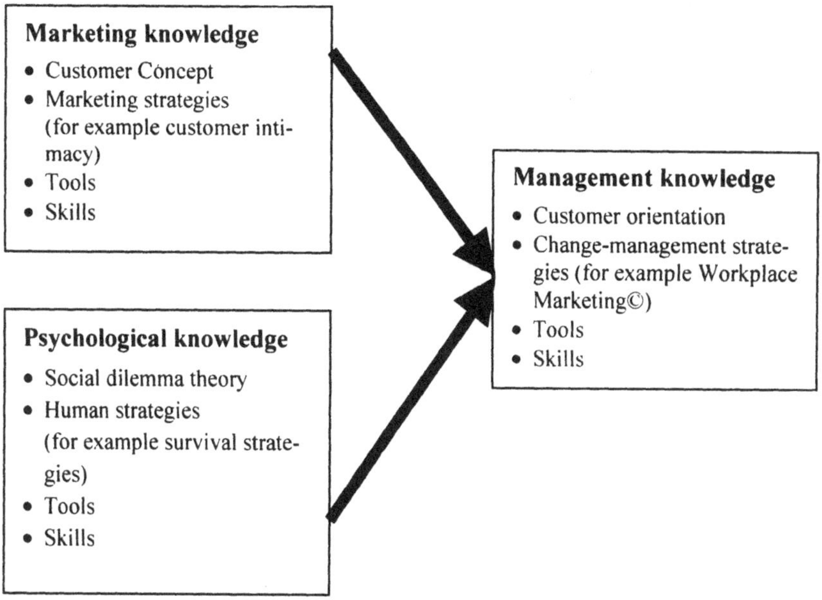

Figure 2. Requirements for implementing a customer orientation.

into measurable targets. Delivering customer value is the target of the customer oriented organisation. As stated above customer value not only is the value a customer gets from buying, possessing and/or using a product or service. It also is the value a customer derives from having a mutual beneficial relationship with a supplier. Determining the desired customer values (for instance by using a marketing research technique called 'laddering') is an essential step in the process of choosing a value delivery strategy [15]. This has to be done for both the relational dimension of customer value as well as for the product dimension. Only then it can be decided which road to travel, which strategy to use in order to deliver the desired customer values. The choice of a strategy is based on the needs and desires of the customer and on the capabilities of the organisation on both value dimensions. Treacy and Wiersema [16] state that in order to become leading in their market, organisations need to choose one of three possible strategies:

- Operational excellence: offer products or services at competitive prices, with a competitive quality, in the most convenient way;
- Product leadership: develop a stream of state of the art products and realise the shortest possible time to market;
- Customer intimacy: create individual relationships with carefully selected customers in order to create a win-win situation, by offering customised products and services to the right customer, at the right moment and at the right price.

In accordance with the chosen strategy, means and manpower have to be assigned to different processes (tactics). Most important, the organisation has to turn thinking, talking and planning into action [17]. The translation from vision into operations has to supply each and every employee with the knowledge, skills and attitude to deliver the right values to the customer. Internal communication is essential for this translation to be effective.

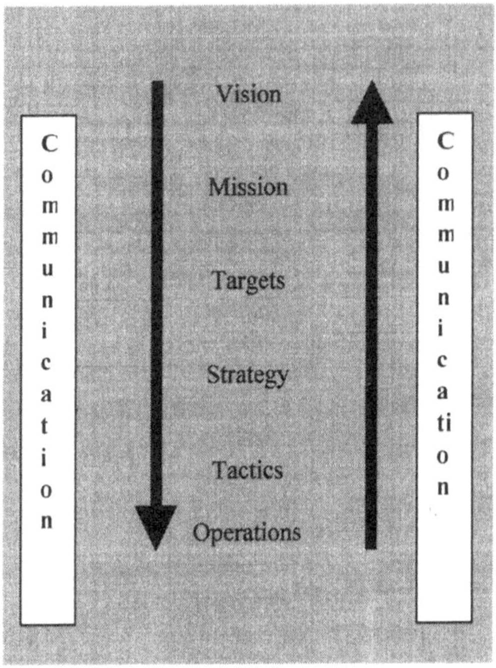

Figure 3. Translating vision into operation and vice versa [6a].

To become a customer oriented organisation, it is absolutely insufficient to communicate in the annual business plan, that 'from now on the customer comes first'. One has to perform the whole exercise: formulate the vision, define the mission, operationalise the mission into targets, choose a strategy and tactics, and do the right things. It is absolutely insufficient just to organise a vision session with the board of directors and the management team. It is absolutely insufficient just to build a customer database, and it is absolutely insufficient just to train the front-office employees to act more customer friendly. The only way to become customer oriented is by rethinking each and every complex process that might have to be redesigned, including production, billing, communication, marketing, R&D and HRM, etc. This means the transition of an organisation into a customer oriented organisation is very radical and very difficult. The whole system has to be changed. For every process new knowledge, new skills and, most of all, new attitudes are necessary. This requires an integral change approach [17b, 18]. Most important is that every-body (every manager but also every employee) has to be able to make the translation from philosophy into action. The key question for everyone is: "Given this line of thinking and planning, what would be the consequences for my acting?".

Private Sectors Only?

The most prevalent trends in the private sector are towards continuous change and increasing interdependencies [19]. Organisations evidently face a turbulent environment, characterised by increasing uncertainties [20]. This is true for public organisations as well. Since the environmental changes that one has to respond to are very similar for both private and public organisations, close parallels can be drawn between the private and the public sectors [21, 22]. Public sector organisations are confronted with demands such as a higher efficiency and effectiveness [23, 24], accountability, entrepreneurial behaviour [25], competition among public sector organisations and adopting a private-sector management style [21]. With issues to deal with such as unemployment, health, poverty care for the elderly and youth crime, the challenges that the public sector is facing are enormous [26]. Because these problems are interconnected, no single organisation has the capacities to tackle them adequately [27]. Furthermore, the role of private and voluntary organisations will increase, asking for new ways for delivery and new kinds of services. Therefore, according to Lowdnes and Skelcher [28], new expectations for public organisations are:

- form new relationships and partnerships;
- think and act strategically;
- network with other agencies;
- effectively manage resources;
- redefine boundaries of systems;
- govern for accountability and transparency.

In order to respond to the environmental changes as described in section 2, and in order to meet these new expectations, organisations in the public sectors need to review or revise their ways of working. This can be done by implementing new systems, reorganising and/or adopting new methods of working [29]. Therefore, management of change is needed, not only in the private sector but in the public sector as well [30]. It has been suggested that a stronger focus on the consumer, involving users of services and improving accountability, would enhance the ability of public organisations to adapt to change [31]. This indicates that a customer orientation is applicable to and beneficial for public organisations in general, and therefore for blood supply organisations. Donors will be more inclined to keep their appointments, and will be more committed to the needs of the blood transfusion organisation. This will improve the continuity of the blood supply.

Customer orientation provides an integral guideline for management and employees in blood transfusion organisations to become a customer oriented organisation. In meeting the new expectations, public institutions such as blood supply organisations (form new relationships and partnerships, think and act strategically, network with other agencies, effectively manage resources, redefine boundaries of systems and govern for accountability and transparency) will be facilitated by embracing a customer orientation. This implies significant changes in the existing blood supply organisations. Managing this change process is a major challenge that these organisations will have to face in the nearest future.

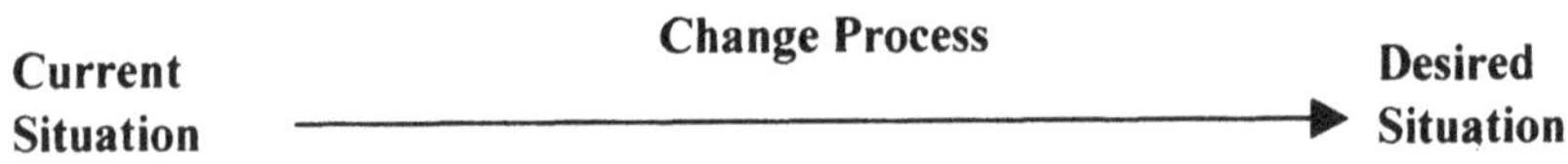

Figure 4. Planned chage [32].

Change Management

Organisational change invariably follows Lewin's three-step process [32], consisting of un-freeze, change and re-freeze. This model suggests a designed, linear change process and is characterised by a top-down approach to change. This model has been dominant in change management for decades. It has proven to be very successful for organisations working in an environment that does not change dramatically. As stated earlier, this is no longer the case: the world is changing, and it is changing fast. As the desired situation is changing during the change process, planned change is no longer the answer to organisational challenges.

Society has become more democratic, and this also influences the way in witch labour is organised [33]. Strategic planning, developing vision and mission no longer is the privilege of top management. Employees want to be involved in decision making. Organisational design by top management is joined by organisational development, including white- and blue-collar workers in the decision making process [34, 35]. Top-down or bottom-up, that is the question. In order to be effective in change processes, organisations need to make a choice between the design approach and the development approach. Boonstra et al. [34] state a number of criteria to be important in making this decision, as shown in Figure 5. The upper half of Figure 5 shows the criteria needed for making the right decision, the lower half shows characteristics of both design and development approaches to change.

There is a way of bringing together the best of both worlds, by commuting between design and development of organisations [34]. This way of changing, commuting change management, enables management to give direction to the change process (Figure 6). It also allows for employees to participate in the decision making process. Furthermore, it enables the organisation to adjust the change process to changes in the environment of the organisation.

This change management strategy allows for employees to become more involved in the change process. Though commuting change management is an improvement as compared to the design and the development approach, additional methods of change are required. If an organisation is part of a larger system, being an open system itself, it is not sufficient to involve employees only.

Design	*Development*
– Limited time for change	– Sufficient time for change
– Radical change needed	– Minor change needed
– Uniform large scale implementation	– Differentiated, small-scale implementation
– Need for control	– Need for flexibility
– Existing knowledge not important	– Existing knowledge has to be used
– No consensus on goals of change process can be achieved	– Consensus
– Fierce resistance to change	– Little resistance
– Bad relationship between management and works council	– Mutual trust between management and works council
– Dramatic lay off needed	– Limited lay off needed
Design	*Development*
– Organisation as source of shortcomings	– Sufficient time for change
– New design with blueprint	– Minor change needed
– Top-down	– Differentiated, small-scale implementation
– Focus on solution	– Need for flexibility
– Stable end-situation	– Existing knowledge has to be used
– Non-recurring linear process	– Consensus
– Tight schedule and planning	– Little resistance
– Economic-technical process rationality	– Mutual trust between management and works council
– From abstract models to concrete process	– Limited lay off needed
– Separation between design and implementation	

Figure 5. Design or Development [34].

It then becomes necessary to bring in all the stakeholders, to involve the whole system. In this respect, the most popular methods are:
- future search [36];
- search conferences [37];
- open space [38];
- team syntegrity [39],

which are applicable for the private sector as well as for the public sector [18].

These methods have in common that they assemble all the members of the whole system at one moment in time. In organisational terms, all the stakeholders get together and decide on topics as vision and strategy, and come to a common understanding of the consequences for management and operation. By allowing every stakeholder (see Figure 7) to be involved in the decision-making process, these methods create a large amount of support. Managing this process is not possible while having a stake in the outcome of the process; it therefore has to be done by outside facilitators.

Methods such as 'open space', 'search conferences' etc. result in a shared vision, strategy and commitment to change. They therefore provide an effective starting-point for the necessary change process aimed at implementing a customer orientation.

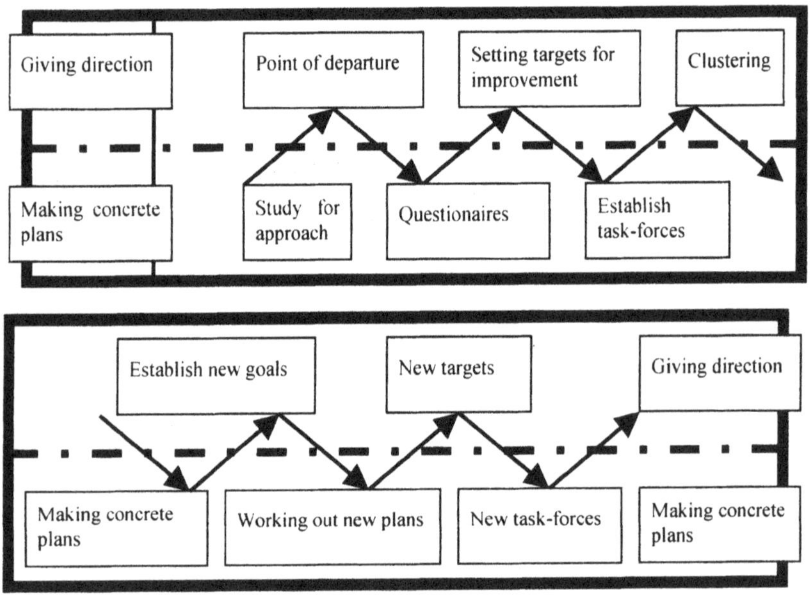

Figure 6. Commuting change management [34].

Next, the use of commuting change management best facilitates the process of implementing the necessary changes in the organisation itself. Management and employees transform vision and strategy into concrete plans of change. A taskforce including representatives of all stakeholders (resulting from the open space meeting) takes the role of monitoring and redirecting the change process.

Using a combination of an open space-like method and commuting change management, blood supply organisations should be able to make the transition into customer oriented organisations. In order to assess the success of the change process, an instrument for measuring the improvements is needed. The Market Orientation Barometer, which is described in the next section, is such a measurement instrument.

Market Orientation Barometer

As mentioned before, the importance of customer satisfaction is broadly documented. The research that has taken place in this area has been particularly con-

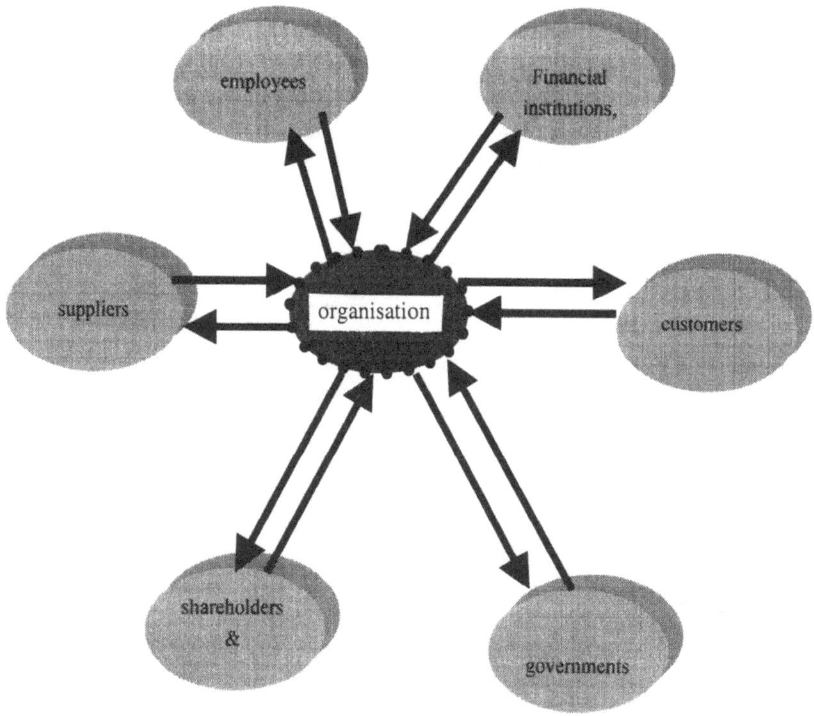

Figure 7. The organisation and stakeholders [7].

cerned with the development of measurement methods [40-47]. However, it is frequently a measurement of satisfaction coupled with an end result (how satisfied are you with the product?) and there is little or no attention paid to the individual processes that have led to the end result.

Improving internal management has been the subject of several studies as well. Several instruments have been developed for continuously monitoring organisational performance, and in doing so facilitating organisations in improving their performance [48-50]. Both increasing customer satisfaction [5] as well as improving internal processes have proven to be beneficial for organisations. Yet, no research has been done aimed at combining customer satisfaction measurement with management of improvements within the organi-sation.

In order to solve this problem, a research project will be performed by the RijksUniversiteit Groningen. Its objective is to develop an instrument that enables organisations to combine insights into customer satisfaction and management of change. Although this instrument is developed for the private sector and for small and medium-sized enterprises, it is also useful for public organisations. The instrument, the Market Orientation Barometer, consists of two measurements, a customer satisfaction measurement and an internal measurement (Figure 8). Combining these two measurements indicates which improvements have to be made in order to increase customer satisfaction. A number of aspects of management that will be measured are: owner-director influence, customers, market, competitors, resources, products, delivery and follow-up service, culture, employees, leadership, personnel management, information and communication. Customer satisfaction aspects that will be measured are for instance: quality of managerial aspects, including the price-quality relationship, frequency of the representative's visits, response to complaints and clarity of brochures. Measuring customer satisfaction in a way that informs the organisation about the nature of change that is needed in order to increase customer satisfaction is important for blood supply organisations.

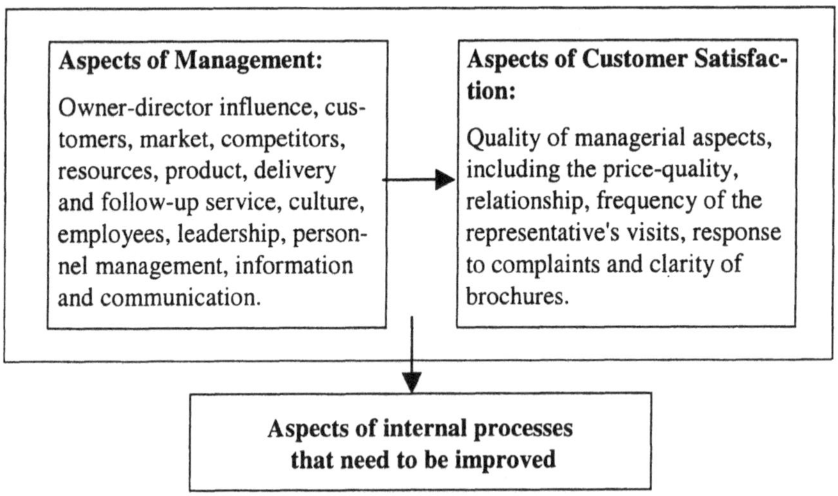

Figure 8. Research model, based on Hoekstra and Zwart [51].

Implications for Blood Supply Organisations

The relationship between a blood supply organisation and its stakeholders is rather particular. It is in some aspects similar to the relationships of stakeholders with other public organisations. But there are some differences as well. First of all, none of the parties in the relationship is seeking for profit: the relationship is based on idealism and altruism. This is true for some other public organisations, but not for all. Secondly, the relationship between a donor and a blood supply organisation involves the delivery of services. Again this is true for some other public organisations, but not for all. The far most specific aspect of the relationship between a donor and a blood supply organisation is the fact that the donor is paying for whatever customer value with his own blood. All of the above implies that concepts developed for private organisations are not automatically applicable for blood supply organisations. The same is true for concepts that are developed for other public organisation. Nevertheless, combining the Customer Concept and the Social Dilemma Theory might provide for the right questions that make it possible to gain an understanding of the complex relationship between a donor and a blood supply organisation. Using methods that involve the whole system in the change process, and directing the change process by using commuting change management, blood supply organisations should be able to develop a customer orientation. Having a customer orientation will enable them to adapt to changes in their environments more effectively. Using the Market Orientation Barometer enables them to monitor customer satisfaction. It also provides for insight into the improvements that need to be made in order to increase customer satisfaction. Furthermore, by using the same instrument for monitoring customer satisfaction and managing improvements, blood supply organisations will be able to learn from each other through benchmarking and exchange of knowledge and experiences.

References

1. Hoekstra JC, Leeflang PSH, Wittink D. The customer concept: The basis for a new marketing paradigm. J Market Focused Management 1999;4:43-76.
2. Buttle F. Relationship marketing; Theory and practice. Paul Chapman Publishing Ltd., London, 1996.
3. Hamel G, Prahalad CK. Competing for the future. Harvard Business School Press, Boston, Massachusetts, 1994.
4. Webster FE. Defining the new marketing concept; Forget about being market-driven! The future belongs to companies that are customer value-driven. Marketing Management 1993;2.
5. Reichheld FF, Sasser WE. Zero Defections: Quality Comes to Services. Harvard Business Review 1990;Sept.-Oct.:105-11.
6. Alsem KJ, Hoekstra JC, van der Heide B. "Marketing orientation and strategies in The Netherlands", Research Report Graduate School/Research Institute Systems, Organisations and Management, No. 96B02, Groningen, 1996.

7a. Lotgerink ThEP. De klantgerichte organisatie doorgelicht. Customer Base 2000;1: 18-20.

7b. Lotgerink ThEP, De klantgerichte organisatie doorgelicht (2). Customer Base 2000; 2:18-20.

8. Williams J. Workplace marketing: A 1990s Business imperative. J Direct Marketing 1994;8:66-74.
9. Berry, L. Excellente dienstverlening: de 9 elementen voor duurzaam succes. Samson, Alphen aan den Rijn, 1999.
10. Webster FE Jr. Market-driven management. John Wiley, New York, 1994.
11. Luce RD, Raiffa H. Games and decisions. John Wiley, New York, NY, 1957.
12. Van Lange PAM, Liebrand WBG, Messick DM, Wilke HAM. Social Dilemmas: The state of the art, introduction and literature review. In: Liebrand WBG, Messick DM, Wilke HAM (eds). Social dilemmas: Theoretical issues and research findings. Pergamon Press, Oxford, 1992:3-28.
13. Willenborg GBW. Relationship marketing and consumers: A social dilemma approach. In: Grover R (ed). Special issue on customer-based marketing, University of Groningen. J Market-Focused Management 1998;3: 223-55.
14. Senge PM. De vijfde discipline; de kunst & praktijk van de lerende organisatie. Scriptum Books, Schiedam, 1992.
15. Woodruff RB, Gardial SF. Know your customer. Blackwell, 1996.
16. Treacy M, Wiersema F. Customer intimacy and other value disciplines. Harvard Business Review 1993;71:84-93.

17a.Lotgerink ThEP, Hoekstra JC. Klantgerichtheid: marketing of management? Direct Marketing Gids. Beerens Business Press bv, Woerden, 1997:13-24.

17b.Lotgerink ThEP, Hoekstra JC. Putting the customer first. Tijdschrift voor Marketing 1997;3:13-15.

17c.Lotgerink ThEP, Hoekstra JC. Klantgerichtheid centraal in bedrijfsvoering. Tijdschrift voor Marketing 1997;4:30-33.
18. White L. Changing the 'whole system' in the public sector. J Organisational Change Management 2000;13:162-77.
19. Beckhard R, Pritchard W. Changing the essence: The art of creating and leading fundamental change in organisations. Jossey-Bass, San Francisco, CA. 1992.
20. Emery F, Trist . The causal texture of organisational environments. Human Relations 1965;18:21-32.
21. Hood C. A public management for all seasons? Public Administration 1991;69:3-19.
22. Lovell R. Managing change in the new public sector. Longmann, London, 1995.
23. Hood C. Contemporary public management: a new global paradigm? Public Policy and Administration 1995;10:104-07.
24. Walsh K. Public services and market mechanism. Macmillan, Basingstoke, 1995.
25. Leadbetter C. The rise of the social entrepreneur. Demos, London, 1997.
26. Department of Health. Partnership in action: New opportunities for joint working between health and social services. Department of Health, London, 1998.
27. Cadbury R. The partnership challenge. Public Policy Review 1993;1:11-12.
28. Lowdnes V, Skelcher C. The dynamics of multi-organisational partnerships. Public Administration. 1998;76:313-34.
29. Stewart J, Kimber M. The transformation of bureaucracy, Austr J Public Administration 1996;55:235-50.
30. Stewart J, Walsh K. Change in the management of public services. Public Administration 1992;70:499-518.
31. Lupton C, Peckman S, Taylor P. Managing public involvement in healthcare purchasing. Open University Press, Buckingham, 1998.
32. Lewin K. Field theory in social science. Harper & Row, New York, NY, 1951.
33. Ackoff RL.The democratic corporation. Oxford University Press, New York, 1994.
34. Boonstra JJ, Steensma HO, Demenint MI. Ontwerpen en ontwikkelen van organisaties. Elsevier/De Tijdstroom, Maarssen, 1996.
35. Mastenbroek W. (1997), Verandermanagement. Holland Business Publications, Heemstede, 1997.
36. Weisbord M, Janoff S. Future search. Barret-Koehler, San Francisco, CA, 1995.
37. Emery F, Purser R. The search conference. Jossey-Bass, San Francisco, CA. 1996.
38.Owen H. Open space technology. Abbott, Potomac, MD, 1992.
39. Beer S. Beyond dispute: The invention of team syntegrity. Wiley, Chichester, 1995.
40. Anderson EW, Sullivan MW. The Antecendents and consequences of customer satisfaction for firms. Marketing Science. 1993;12:125-43.
41. Anderson EW, Fornell C, Lehmann DR. Customer satisfaction, market share, and profitability: Findings from Sweden. J Marketing 1994;58:53-66.
42. Cadotte ER, Woodruff RB, Jenkins RL. Expectations and norms in models of consumer satisfaction. J Marketing Research 1987;24:305-14.
43. Edgett S, Snow K. Benchmarking measures of customer satisfaction, quality and performance for new financial service products. J Services Marketing 1996;10:6-17.
44. Fornell C. A national customer satisfaction barometer: The Swedish Experience. J Marketing 1992;56:6-21.
45. Fornell C, Johnson MD, Anderson EW, Cha J, Everitt Bryant B. The American customer satisfaction index: Nature, purpose and findings. J Marketing (1996;60:7-18.
46. Patterson PG, Johnson LW, Spreng RA. Modeling the determinants of customer satisfaction for business-to-business professional services. J Acad Marketing Science 1997;25:4-17.
47. Ryan MJ, Buzas Th, Ramaswamy V. Making CSM a power tool. Marketing Research 1995;7:11-16.
48. George S. The Baldrige quality system. John Wiley & Sons, Inc. New York, 1992.
49. Kaper AM de, Knaapen RAG. Praktische kwaliteitsanalyse, Deventer-Antwerpen: Kluwer, 1991.

50. Parasuraman A, Zeithaml VA, Berry LL. SERVQUAL: A multi-item scale for measuring customer perceptions of the service quality. J Retailing, 1988;64:12-40.
51. Hoekstra JC, Lotgerink TEP, Zwart PS. Verbetering van de advisering aan het MKB: een klantgerichtheidsbarometer. In: Alsem KJ, Leeflang PSH and Willenborg GBW, eds. Ten dienste, recente ontwikkelingen in de marketing van diensten, Vriendenboek voor prof.dr. J.C. Reuijl, Wolters-Noordhoff, Groningen, 1998:96-107.

COMMUNITY INVOLVEMENT: THE DEVELOPMENT – THE PAST, THE PRESENT AND THE FUTURE OF BLOOD DONATION AS A FORM OF COMMUNITY INVOLVEMENT

A.P.M. Los[1], C.Th. Smit Sibinga

The Past, Early 20th Century: The Development of Community Involvement

Since 1900, blood transfusion therapy has become an increasingly important factor in health care. Two major discoveries were responsible for this development: First the discovery of the blood group (ABO) system by Karl Landsteiner (Figure 1) in the year 1900, and second in 1914 the introduction of sodium citrate for anti-coagulation, as developed by Albert Hustin (Figure 2) [1].

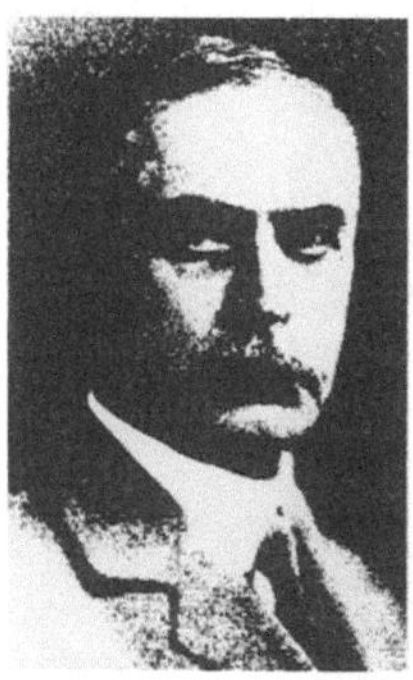

Figure 1. Karl Landsteiner

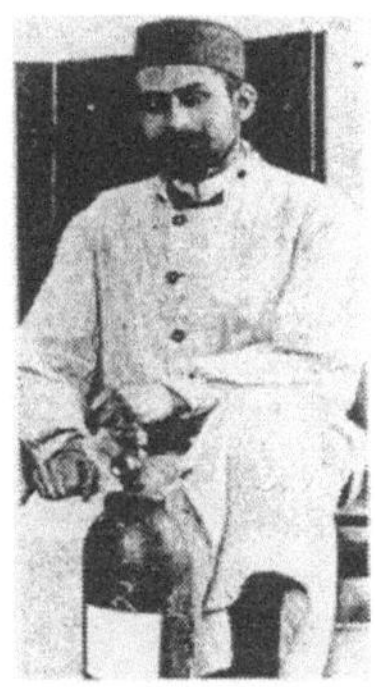

Figure 2. Albert Hustin

From that moment on there was a growing demand for human donor blood, implicating an appeal to the altruistic characteristics of the general population.

Altruism is a concept derived from the term 'alter' (L), which means 'the other'. Altruistic behaviour is behaviour which is unselfish, selfless. Altruism can be defined as "doing something for the benefit of others at some cost to oneself [2]."

Altruistic behaviour in general and in various forms is found in all times and in all cultures. Voluntary, non-remunerated, blood donation is a form of altruistic behaviour.

1. Sanquin Divison Blood Bank Noord Nederland, Groningen, NL.

The majority of the early blood donors were males. Donors were recruited from police and fire brigade. Also women who worked in health care belonged to the group of early blood donors

In 1921 the first Blood Transfusion Service was established by Percy L. Oliver, secretary of a department of the London Red Cross. It was already emphasized in that time that blood donation should be voluntary and unselfish, without any obligations or remuneration i.e. payment.

In 1936 The Board of Governors of the League of Red Cross Societies passed a resolution "observing that the development of blood transfusion enables the Red Cross to render noteworthy additional service to the public" and recommended that "the League Secretariat continue to place all available information on this subject at the disposal of National Societies".

Throughout the 1950's, 1960's and 1970's the Red Cross blood transfusion services continued to grow. In 1988 it was estimated that the Red Cross and Red Crescent Societies were responsible for the collection of one-third of the blood collected in the world [3].

Recruitment of volunteer blood donors in general was worldwide supported by Red Cross and Red Crescent Societies, endorsing the principle of voluntar-ism and non-remuneration. Symbol for volunteer donorship was the pelican feeding her young with her own blood (Figure 3).

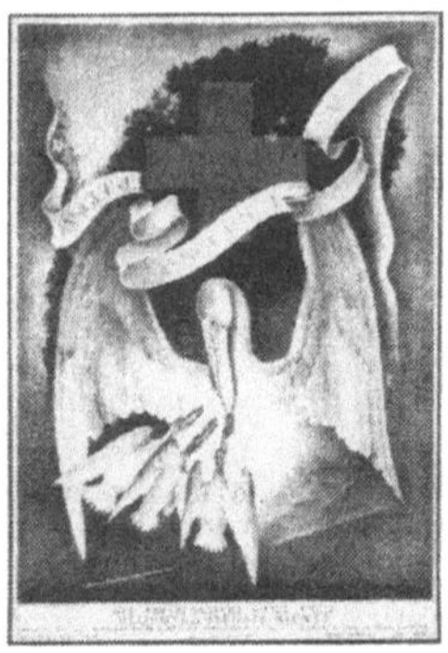

Figure 3. The Red Cross symbol of altruism.

It resulted in the (enthusiastic) work of many local organisations and volunteer donor recruiters: It was the field of 'welfare'. In that time the immediate result of recruitment efforts counted. There was no long term policy, with systematic evaluation of the recruitment efforts.

The demand for human donor blood resulted worldwide in various systems to meet the demand. Variation in systems originated from social, organizational and political structure, and the level of economy and health care of the countries involved.

Although the principle of voluntary blood donation was preached worldwide, the reality shows us another picture. Non-remuneration is not always realised.

Remuneration in the form of food, facilities, and often but not always, under severely restricted economic circumstances even payment for blood can be observed, for example in certain parts of Eastern- and Western Europe, the United States, South America and the developing countries [4-9]. In 1976, the London social scientist Richard M. Titmuss (Figure 4) in his book "The Gift Relationship", described a typology of blood donors / blood donation, covering the total range from complete and true non-remunerated voluntarism to professional and paid blood 'donation', with a number of in-between categories, such as family credit or replacement, and fringe benefit donors. (Table 1) [10].

Table 1. R.M. Titmuss typology of donors.

– Paid Donor
– Professional Donor
– Paid Induced Voluntary Donor
– Responsibility Fee Donor
– Family Credit Donor
– Captive Voluntary Donor
– Fringe Benefit Voluntary Donor
Voluntary Community Donor

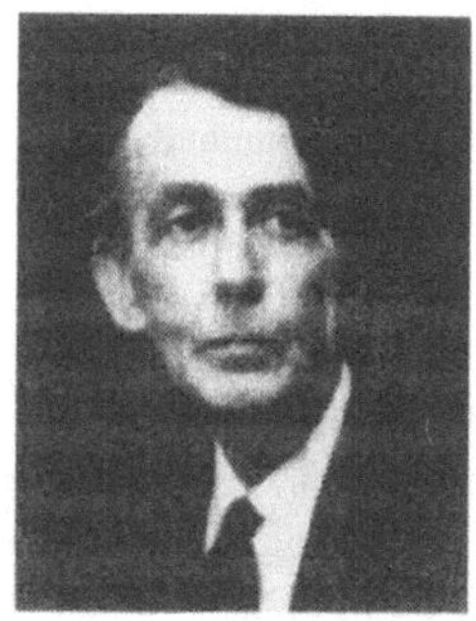

Fig. 4 R.M. Titmuss.

Family credit or replacement implies that the family of the patient should give blood in return for the blood needed. Under certain circumstances this may lead to 'hidden payment', when no family is available and people 'from the street'are paid for their donation. Fringe benefit implies blood donation in return for a day off: a practice for example used in the army in the Netherlands.

This typology can be regarded as still up-to-date. Only the last category 'Volunteer' blood donation can be regarded as the category which is to be striven for worldwide and actively promoted by WHO in their Global Blood Safety Program [11].

To summarize: In the more developed countries donors are mostly volunteers. In developing or restricted economy countries we often face a system of 'family replacement' and 'paid' blood donation.

Motivation of volunteer blood donors was subject of investigation in many research projects since 1952, although in an overview of the literature, Oswalt concluded in 1979 that "essentially the same information (on donor motivation) has been forthcoming for the last twenty years or so", Boe and Ponder came to the same conclusion in 1981, and Piliavin, in 1990, confirmed their statement [12-14]. Reasons for giving blood and not-giving blood are summarized in table 2 and table 3.

From Knowledge Towards Action

Donation of blood by volunteer donors implicates the agreement of the general population with this form of behaviour. People have to know about blood donation. They must have heard from it through various media like family, friends, or public media.

Table 2. Reasons for giving blood (Oswalt, Boe & Ponder, Piliavin).

- Altruism / humanitarian
- Personal or family credit
- Social pressure
- Replacement
- Reward
- Perceived community needs and community support

Table 3. Reasons for not-giving blood (Oswalt, Boe & Ponder, Piliavin).

- Medical ineligibility
- Medial (poor?) excuses
- Fear (fainting, needle, pain, sight of blood, infection – AIDS)
- Time constraints
- Inconvenience of opportunity
- Apathy

Common agreement in the general population on the rightness and significance/whether it is meaningful, will result in a development of community involvement. The crucial question therefor is 'how to reach the community' and 'how to establish and develop community involvement'.

A fundamental theoretical basis for this approach can be found in early American sociology, especially in the thoughts of the sociologist William I. Thomas (1863-1947) (Figure 5). The famous theorem of Thomas reads: "If men define situations as real, they are real in their consequences" [15]

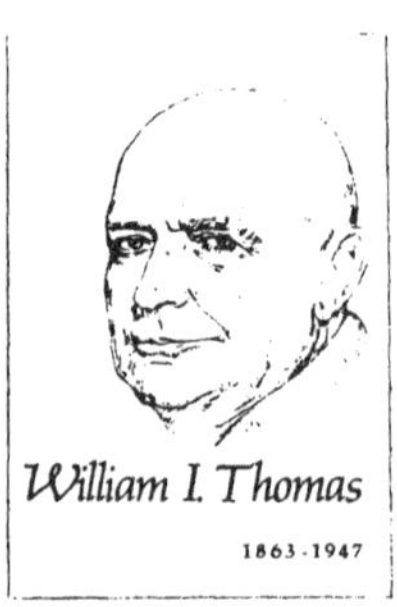

Figure 5. W.I. Thomas.

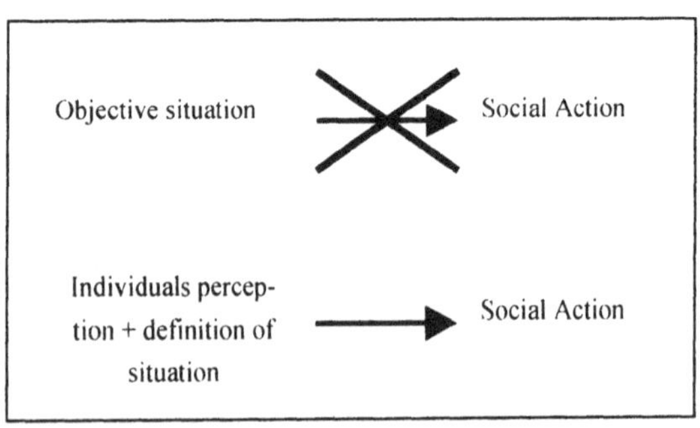

Figure 6. The principle of social action

Thomas emphasized the fact that in human behaviour it is not the objective situation that leads to social action but the individuals' perception and definition of situation (Figure 6).

Applied to blood donation as a form of altruistic human behaviour based on a perception of the situation, we get the following (Figure 7).

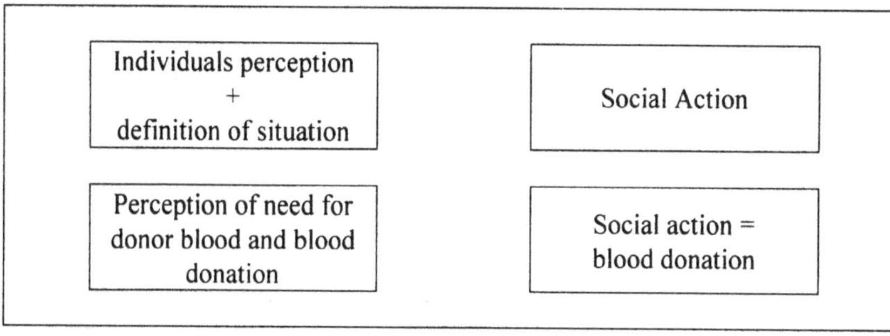

Figure 7. Social action and altruistic behaviour.

The individuals' perception and definition of the situation leads to social action i.e. blood donation. As a prerequisite for being able to develop a perception of a defined situ-ation, the individual must know i.e. have heard about the situation (Figure 8).

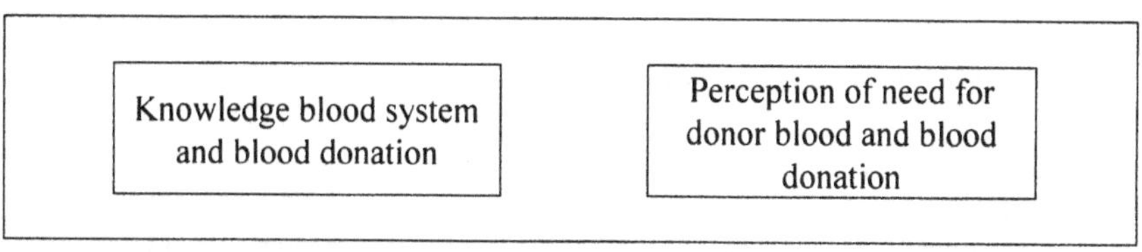

Figure 8. From knowledge towards perception.

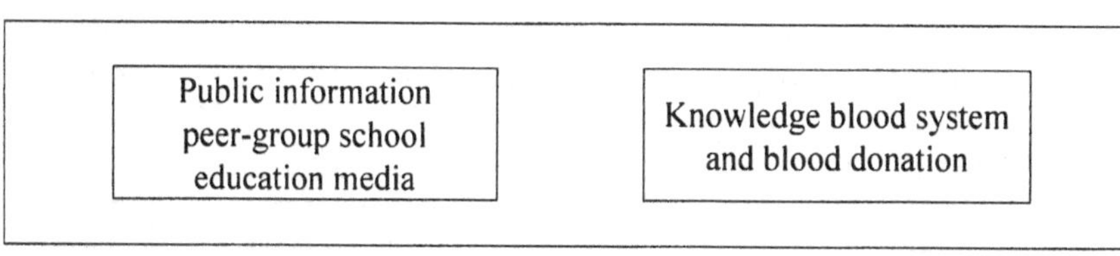

Figure 9. From information towards knowledge.

Knowledge of the blood system (need for donor blood) and blood donation can be derived from various sources (Figure 9). One of the most important sources, concluded in many studies on blood donation, is the peer-group of the individual. Peer-group includes: family, friends, colleagues. It is the first reference-group of the individual, where it derives and mirrors its opinion. Another important source is school education.

A last but not least important sources are public information through the relevant channels (pamphlets, posters, billboards) and the public media.

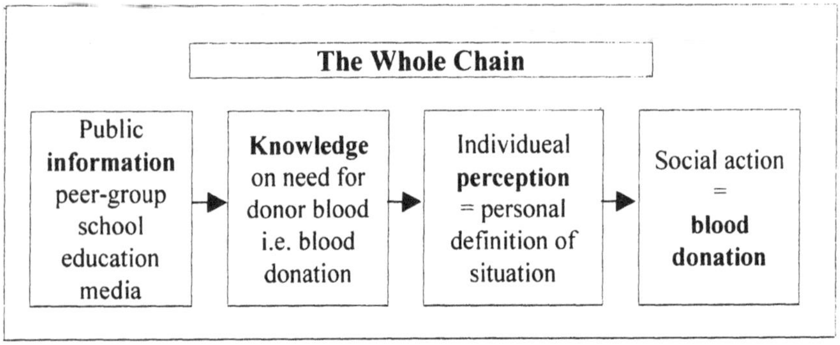

Figure 10. The social action chain.

The complete chain from (public) information to social action i.e. blood donation gives an idea at what items we should address in the future to continue the system of voluntary blood donation where it already exists, and to implement the system where it is needed. It starts with the implementation or improving public information through the available media, to implement or improve knowledge. This knowledge forms the basis for an individual per-ception of the situation, i.e. the need for donor blood.. The ultimate action is to register as a voluntary non-remunerated blood donor.

Future

Donor recruitment never was professionalised, until the last two decades, coinciding with an increasing number of publications on 'donor management' [16-20].

A common believe, and acceptance in the society of the need for blood and voluntary blood donation, should be realized through thoroughly designed, monitored and evaluated programs on donor management [21]. This will effectuate a sufficient, reliable, and sustainable blood supply for the future. A necessary condition is profound research on the efficacy and impact of the instruments of communication that play an important role in the fundamental aspects of donor management: Motivation and selection of first-time donors (reaching the general population), motivation and retention of active donors, and prevention of unnecessary resignations and lapse.

Despite the technical advances, blood products from human donor material will not become obsolete. A professional approach to donor management (recruitment) will further gain field, with emphasis on marketing research techniques [22, 23]. Requirements of GMP, ISO-9001, and finally TQM will be applied to donor management to effectuate proof of the effectiveness of techniques and proper evaluation.

Fundament for these requirements are sophisticated information systems with characteristics of donors. To meet this demand in developing countries, characteristics of the actual donor population, whether family replacement, paid or volunteer, should be documented into data bases, to permit access for motivation purpose and further analysis. In the developed world, these already existing data bases of volunteer donors should be the starting point for analysis and 'evidence based' policies.

WHO's plea for recruitment of voluntary donors worldwide will demand tremendous efforts to change from family replacement and paid donors into true volunteers. Additional efforts will include sufficient attention to public information and school education to the younger [11].

The demand for safety will make donor selection even more crucial, and increase costs further [24-28]. Furthermore there will be an increased attention to the risks of blood donation and transfusion, i.e. risk perception. "Communicating the nature and consequences of environmental and health risks to the public is now a days one of the most problematic areas for policy makers. Given the perceived risks associated with the food we eat, chemicals in the environment, and modern technologies (i.e. blood transfusion), consumers more and more need clear and timely explanations of the nature of those risks – but they rarely get them." [29-31]

Increasing demand for specific types of blood donation (apheresis techniques, processing on the donor), will require well motivated donors, although the specific need on itself has already proved to be a strongly motivating factor [32, 33].

To the range of recruitment techniques and media (brochures, pamphlets, newspaper, radio, TV) the new medium internet will be added, becoming more and more important. The scope will change from local and national to international and global.

Apart from all sophisticated technical developments and changes to come, it could be questioned whether the findings of Oswalt c.s. (almost the same motivating factors over the last decades) would become untrue for the decades to come.

In other words: Is it likely that something fundamental in the willingness of human beings to give blood voluntarily as a form of basic altruistic behavior, should sudden change in the near future?

To the opinion of the authors this is not likely, and basic altruistic behaviour remains to be the fundament of blood transfusion therapy, as it has been in the past century.

References

1. Aken P van, Strengers PFW, et al. Bloed. Van magie tot wetenschap. 1994. Natuur &Techniek. Maastricht, Brussel (in Dutch).
2. Piliavin JA, Callero PL. Giving blood. The development of an altruistic identity. 1991. John Hopkins University Press, Baltimore, Maryland, USA.
3. Leikola J. How much blood for the world? Vox Sang 1988;54:1-5.
4. Von Auer F. Payment for blood donations in Germany. BMJ 1995;310:399.
5. Cash JD. Payment proposed for blood donations in Germany. BMJ 1994;309:1160.

6. Oakley A. Blood donation – altruïsm of profit? BMJ 1996;312:1114.
7. Howden-Chapman P, Carter J, Woods N. Blood money: blood donors' attitudes to changes in the New Zealand blood transfusion service. BMJ 1996;312:1131-32.
8. Von Schubert H. Donated blood – gift or commodity? Some economic and ethical considerations on voluntary versus comercial donation of blood. Social Science and Medicine 1994;39:201-06.
9. Prozo PR. Paying donors and the ethics of blood supply. Journal of Medical Ethics 1994;20:31-35.
10. Titmuss RM. The gift relationship. 1970. Allen and Unwin, UK
11. WHO Global Blood Safety Initiative. WHO/LBS/92.1, p.2
12. Oswalt RM. A review of blood donor motivation and recruitment. Transfusion 1977;17:123-35.
13. Boe GP, Ponder LD. Blood donors and non-donors: a review of the research. Am J Med Technol 1981;47:248-53.
14. Piliavin JA. Why do they give the gift of life? A review of the research on blood donors since 1977. Transfusion 1990;30:444-59.
15. Thomas WI, Thomas DS. The child in America. Alfred Knopf, New York 1928.
16. Los APM, Smit Sibinga CTh. Donor management information system: An investment in the future. Transfusion Today: Quarterly news letter of the International Society of Blood Transfusion 1994;18:4-6.
17. Los APM, Lumey LH, Smit Sibinga CTh. Demographic characteristics of a donor and non-donor population in the north of the Netherlands. In: Third International Colloquium on the Recruitment of Voluntary Blood Donors. LRCS/ISBT/FIODS Geneva 1991:48-52.
18. Los APM, Smit Sibinga CTh. Managing the blood donor base. IFRCS Transfusion International 1998:74:3-4.
19. Halperin D, Baetens J, Newman B, The effect of short-term, temporary deferral on future blood donation. Transfusion 1998;38:181-83.
20. Ownby HE, Kong F, Wataneby K, Tu Y, Nass C, for the Retrovirus Epidemiology Donor Study. Analysis of donor return behavior. Transfusion 1999; 39:1128-35.
21. Los APM, Smit Sibinga CTh. Transfusion medicine, education and the community: donor motivation and community oriented aspects. In: Smit Sibinga CTh, Das PC, Cash JD (eds). Transfusion Medicine: Fact and Fiction. Proc 16th International Symposium on Blood transfusion. Kluwer Academic Publ Dordrecht/Boston/London, 1992:97-109.
22. Los APM, Achterhof L, vd Veen D, de Wit HJC, Smit Sibinga CTh. Internal audit for donor management and policy: a survey of donor opinion on treatment and communication in the North of the Netherlands. Proc Vth European Regional Congress, Venice, 1995:581-85.
23. Puylaert CENM, Los APM. Internal audit for donor management and policy: a survey of donor opinion on treatment and communication in a regional blood bank in the Netherlands. Abstract book ISBT 25th Congress, Oslo, Norway 1998:#59.
24. Glynn SA, Schreiber GB, Busch MP, et al. Demographic characteristics, un-reported risk behaviors, and the prevalence and incidence of viral infections: a comparison of apheresis and whole-blood donors. Transfusion 1998;38: 350-358.
25. Thomson RA, Bethel J, Lo AY, et al. Retention of 'safe' blood donors. Transfusion 1998;38:359-67.
26. Liu TC, Kuperand P, Tan C, Lin TK, Lee SH. Structuring a safer do nor-replacement program. Transfusion 1998;38:368-72.
27. Mahl MA, Hirsch M. Sugg U. Verification of the drug history given by potential blood donors: results of drug screening that combines hair and urine analysis. Transfusion 2000;40:637-41.
28. Orton SL, Virvos VJ, Williams AE. Validation of selected donor-screening questions: structure, content, and comprehensionTransfusion 2000;40:1407-13.

29. Powell D, Leiss W. Mad cows and mother 's milk. The Perils of Poor Risk Communication. McGill-Queen's University Press. Montreal & Kingston, London, Buffalo 1997.
30. Ratzan SC (ed). The Mad Cow Crisis. Health and the Public Good. 1998 UCL Press, London, UK.
31. Finucane ML, Slovic P, Mertz CK. Public perception of the risk of blood transfusion. Transfusion 2000;40:1017-22.
32. Los APM, Tijmstra T, Achterhof L, Smit Sibinga CTh. A volunteer bone marrow donor program: Social, psychological and ethical information need-ed for the organization on a regional basis. Abstracts 18th Congress ISBT, Karger S Basel. 1984:150
33. Los APM, Tijmstra T, Achterhof L. Smit Sibinga CTh. Social, psychological and ethical information needed for a volunteer bone marrow donor program. Transfusion 1984;24:420.

STRUCTURE AND COMMITMENTS BLOOD SUPPLY SYSTEMS AND ORGANIZATION

J.C. Emmanuel[1]

Background

The dramatic life-saving properties of blood transfusions cannot be more forcefully emphasised than in those situations that arise as a result of conflicts and trauma. The two world wars served as potent forces in promoting blood transfusion services, first as a military necessity and then as a public need as an important part of clinical medicine. Blood and its constituent components were identified and put to good use as technologies emerged not only in the area of immunohaematology, diagnostic testing and component production but in the collection systems. With the advent of plastic blood bag systems and additive solutions as well as technologies for apheresis blood and components utilization increased dramatically. Sterility, storage, transport and pharmaceutically prepared products all were improved. Voluntarism for blood donation was easily promoted during years of conflict and recognition of the benefits of voluntary non-remunerated blood donation were quickly recognised and strengthened in subsequent years of post-war hardships in the period of reconstruction.

How then did the national health authorities respond to this need for blood?

Structure

How then did the national health authorities respond to this need for blood? The conventional wisdom of applying good management practice for organisation and running of blood transfusion services is now well established and many countries have reduced, the large number of fragmented services into a rationalised and co-ordinated body that is answerable to the national health authority.

Well-run, efficient and cost-effective blood transfusion services (BTSs) are characterised by the key ingredients of good organisation and management. BTSs can ensure their financial viability through an annual fiscal budget, or cost recovery system on a fee for service basis. BTSs run along these lines can attract and retain the necessary medical, technical and administrative skills essential to maintaining the standards required for a high quality service.

Successful BTS programmes are organised and managed following established business practices. However, these principles are tempered by medical

---

1. Director WHO Department Blood Safety and Clinical Technology, Geneva, CH.

and ethical considerations and the correct balance of non-profit motive. The principles of a non-profit organisation must be realistic and dependent on the prevailing circumstances in each country. Costing of the BTS must take into consideration inflation, devaluation of local currency, depreciation and replacement of capital expenditure items, recurrent expenditure and the training and retention of skilled staff.

A number of successful BTSs in developed and developing countries are non-profit organisations (i.e. National Red Cross or charitable/voluntary). They must, however, be run efficiently with careful accounting and cost containment to ensure that the BTS is sustainable. This aspect is often overlooked by many countries, particularly in economically restricted or developing countries. Cost analysis will provide the BTS with the necessary information to identify costs of service, provision and expansion to develop the budget plan and ensure a sustainable service, allow for monitoring of BTS activities and to support an evaluation process. In this way, cost-effectiveness can be assessed and compared with other services in the health care structure.

Too often humanitarian sentiments to assist economically restricted countries lead to development projects which concentrate on assisting BTS programmes with short-term capital and recurrent expenditure only without making plans to ensure that the services will be sustainable. In developing countries BTSs are often based on the same lines as BTSs in developed countries, which have clearly identified programmes, recognised and supported by the health authority with appropriate structure and budgets. The programme structure in developing countries is often neither appropriate for the needs of a developing country nor sustainable without the continued assistance of external financial aid and manpower.

A BTS is a complex and organisationally difficult service area. It requires professional, technical and administrative staff who are efficient and well trained. The structure and functions of the national blood programme (NBTS) is dependent on effective and efficient leadership and management. However, the BTS should develop policies in accordance with those of the national health authority to meet the needs for blood and blood products at all levels of the community. There are several layers of organisation which overlap but provide the necessary information and skills for the NBTS to carry out its functions.

There should be an executive board which is a fully functioning body to efficiently and effectively assume the responsibility of managing the BTS in conformity with the national health plan, take executive decisions within the mandate of a national blood policy and have the overall responsibility for the BTS. An example of the executive board, will include membership of BTS leadership management (medical director, manager and departmental senior staff members) and an advisory committee (a small number of people with specialist skills to assist the direction of the blood programme and to add credibility to the decision-making process). Members of the board may also be nominated by the National Blood Transfusion Committee (NBTC).

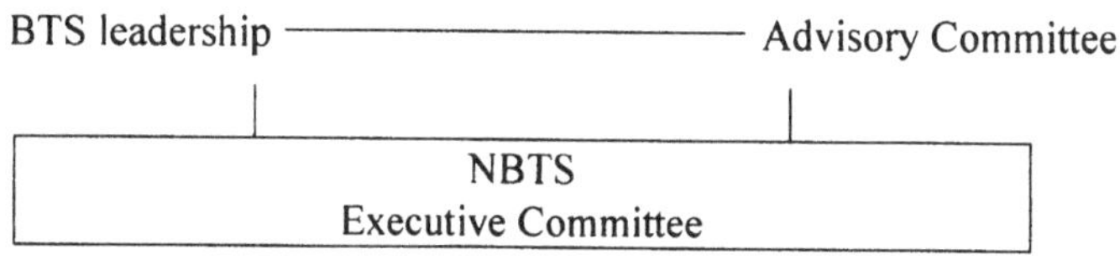

Figure 1.

Commitment

Establishing and maintaining a system that will ensure the safety and adequacy of the blood supply is ultimately the responsibility of government through the health authority. This responsibility may be delegated to a non-profit organisation or be government-run but must have official support and commitment. With the ability to detect infectious agents such as syphilis, Hepatitis B, the human immunodeficiency virus (HIV), Hepatitis C, Chagas and other infectious agents and the recognition of the need for quality assurance and Good Manufacturing Practices (GMP) including pharmaceutical manufacturing practices for plasma-derived medicinal products, there has come a need to implement policies and plans under nationally-organised or co-ordinated bodies. The adoption of the World Health Assembly resolution WHA28.72 of 1975, in which the Ministers of Health requested the WHO Director-General to urge Member States to promote the development of national blood transfusion services (BTSs) based on voluntary non-remunerated blood donation. After nearly a quarter of a century this has become a meaningful reality in many developed countries. This movement is recognised world wide with the need for a safe and adequate blood supply a priority for all countries in the new millennium.

However, commitment is without meaning unless there is appropriate support to ensure sustainable blood programmes. Up until the beginning of the 1990s, the surprising fact was that there were very few true nationally organised and co-ordinated blood transfusiòn services responsible for the provision of blood and blood products based on voluntary non-remunerated blood donation. This made the collection of accurate data from countries difficult in most cases and impossible in many. Apart from the two city states of Hong Kong and Singapore, two developing countries in Africa were examples of a nationally co-ordinated BTS and a nationally co-ordinated service. Finland served as an example of a developed country with a nationally organised blood transfusion service.

In 1995, WHO began collecting data using the Global Database on Blood Safety from all Member States in order to:

- Accurately assess the global situation on blood safety
- Obtain accurate information regarding each member state's situation
- Identify areas of need with the view to provide necessary technical assistance

The data was collected by submission of a checklist that was based on the four key WHO strategies for blood transfusion services (BTS):

Government commitment and support for organisation and management of the BTS
- Safe blood donors
- Screening of all donated blood
- Appropriate clinical use of blood

The current analysis covers period 1997-1999 and available for 167 countries of the 191 WHO Member States. The analysis used the four key WHO strategies as identified in the 'Aide-Memoire for Blood Safety'. In order to provide uniformly acceptable data, reference was made to the United Nations Development Programme Human Development Index (HDI) which classifies countries as having a low, medium or high HDI based on the following criteria:
- Life expectancy
- Educational Attainment
- Adjusted income

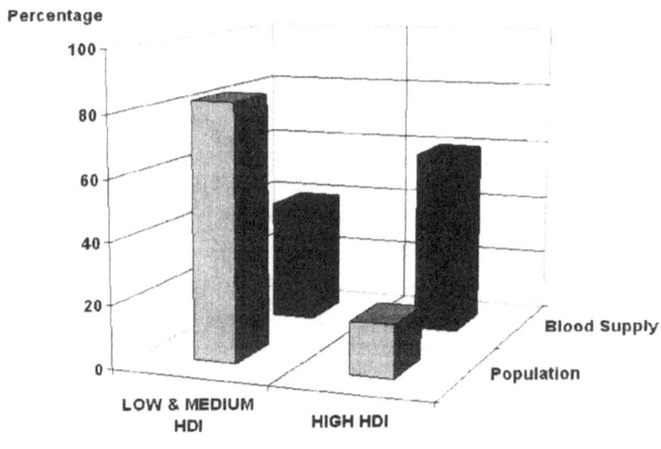

Figure 2. Global population and global blood supply.

Government commitment and support as has been stated is essential for an efficient Blood Transfusion Service (BTS) which should be nationally co-ordinated with policies and plans, and an appropriate legal framework in place to cover its activities. Data showed that only 59% of countries have the basic requirements for a nationally co-ordinated service or a single organisation responsible for the BTS. However, due to fragmentation of services, the reporting countries showed that only 35% of countries had all three of the following elements: one specific co-ordinating organisation; a blood policy; and national regulation. Only 21% of countries reported all three of the following: a national executive body, advisory groups and a medical director/manager. Only 34% of countries were able to report that there was a quality system in place and of those only 23% had a trained quality manager/officer was in place. A total of 46% of countries had a specific budget and 60% of countries did not have costing procedures in place.

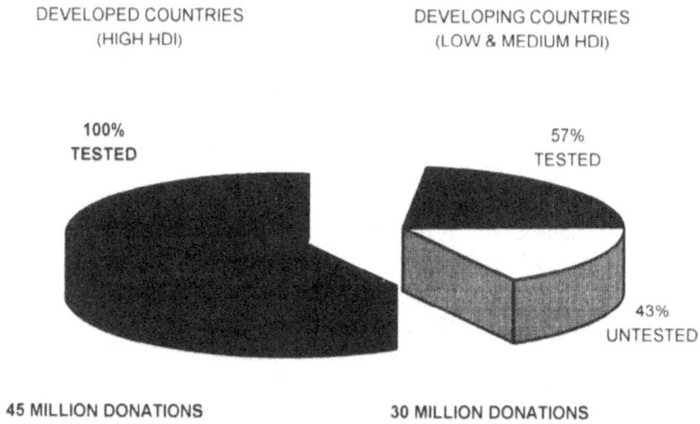

Figure 3. Blood safety.

17% of the global population has access to 60% of the global blood supply
80% of the global population has access to only 20% of the global supply of safe blood

The global estimate for the number of donations per annum is 75 million. It is worth noting that 17% of the world's population live in countries with a high HDI and they have access to 60% of the global blood supply.

Of the 75 million donated units, 6 million were from paid donations and 14 million from family/replacement donations, which is a large source of a hidden paid donor system. More than 13 million of the total 75 million units of blood collected annually are not tested for HIV, HBsAg and HCV. This is 43% of blood collected in the developing world that is not adequately tested (Figure 3).

Safe blood starts with me
Blood Saves lives

Governments need to share the decision-making process and agree with the actions taken by blood transfusion services. This is necessary to ensure that where costs and risks are involved that there is support at the highest level. Blood Transfusion Services need the confidence, support and commitment of the public. It is essential that the services educate and communicate with the public in an open and transparent manner. Commitment is required from the prescribers of blood products to ensure that this vital commodity is utilised correctly and with respect for the donor and the recipient. Only a well organised, co-ordinated and managed blood transfusion service, with the commitment and support of government, can the efficiency and effectiveness of the service be monitored and evaluated. This is essential for continuing improvement of the safety, adequacy and affordability of blood products.

References

1. World Health Organization: Twenty-eighth World Health Assembly resolution, WHA28.72, Geneva, 29 May 1975.
2. Hollán SR, Wagstaff W, Leikola J, Lothe F. Management of Blood Transfusion Services. World Health Organization, Geneva, 1990.
3. Gibbs WN, Britten AFH: Guidelines for the Organization of a Blood Transfusion Service. WHO/LBS/92.9. Geneva, World Health Organization, 1992.
4. Guidelines for Quality Assurance Programmes for Blood Transfusion Services. Geneva, World Health Organization, 1993.
5. Establishment and Organization of a Blood Transfusion Service. Vox Sang, 1994, 67(suppl 5): 4-7.
6. Leikola, J. Organisation of Quality Management of Blood Transfusion Services (Blood Transfusion Services in Europe), ESTM.
7. Human Development Report, UNDP, Geneva,1999.
8. WHO Report on Global Database for Blood Safety. Geneva, 1997.

APPLYING DECISION ANALYSIS TO TRANSFUSION MEDICINE IN THE REAL WORLD TO IMPROVE TRANSFUSION SAFETY

J.P. AuBuchon[1]

Introduction

When faced with a direct threat, the appropriate response is usually fairly clear. One can learn a pattern of response from such an experience, of course, and that learning may or not be adaptive. When applied to a situation that is truly different from the initial threat, the response may no longer be appropriate and the outcome may not be truly what is desired.

Transfusion recipients, potential transfusion recipients and thus society as a whole, learned in the 1980's that transfusion could be life-threatening and have very serious, unintended consequences. From the time of its origins, transfusion was never free of risk, of course; however, the menace of a new, poorly understood and seemingly uncontrollable deadly agent in the blood supply shook the public's confidence in the ability of technology to overcome all obstacles. Furthermore, it undermined the public's confidence in those entrusted with ensuring the safety of a common blood supply. Since recognition of the transmission of HIV through transfusion and its catastrophic consequences, the public has been clamoring for a 'zero-risk' blood supply, or as close to that goal as can be achieved.

From a psychological analysis, this may indeed be a reasonable response. A transfusion recipient does not wish to be faced with the prospect of certain death from a complication of the transfusion [1]. However, blood safety decisions cannot be made in a vacuum. Almost all steps to improve safety in some way restrict supply and consume resources that could be used to improve some other aspect of health care. As the population in developed nations continues to age in the era after World War II, and medical therapies become more and more complex, increasing demands will be placed on the blood supply [2]. In addition, burgeoning healthcare budgets have forced many industrialized societies to attempt to place caps on healthcare spending; this economic concern may impose limits on improvements in many fields of medicine, including the provision of a safer blood supply. At the same time, the expansion of safety measures instituted in developed nations widen the gulf of safety between them and the meager and under-tested blood supplies of developing nations, some of which

1. Professor of Pathology and Medicine, Dartmouth-Hitchcock Medical Center, Lebanon, NH, USA.

have even more to fear because of a higher prevalence of infectious disease in their donor population [3].

Therefore, the quest for a safer blood supply often runs into competing claims for limited resources from other parts of the healthcare system or even from the competing claim for resources to maintain blood supply adequacy. Furthermore, when risks become very low, the risks inherent in a new intervention deserve close scrutiny to ensure that they do not outweigh the potential benefits. These kinds of situations are those where decision analysis techniques could be used to optimize the health of the treated population [4]. However, tools such as cost-effectiveness analysis have been successful recently primarily in delineating just how little can be accomplished further in blood safety for incredibly large sums of money [5]. These resources, when applied to other fields of medicine, might be predicted to yield much greater health benefits for society. So what value is decision analysis in transfusion medicine, and how can we use this analytic tool to guide our research and development efforts?

Current Status of Transfusion Safety

The improvements in pathogen detection techniques over the last decade have produced phenomenal capabilities to rapidly and reliably detect minuscule levels of contamination directly without having to depend on the donor's immune system response. For those assays where antibody detection is still the format, these assays, too, are increasingly sensitive. As a result, transmission of the feared viruses are so infrequent that special modeling techniques have had to be developed to determine the likelihood of viral transmission, and these risks are now best expressed as cases *per ten million* units transfused. In comparison to a time when the risks of HIV and HCV transmission were in the range of 1% in some locales of developed nations, this is an astounding achievement [6-8].

Complicated formulas are not necessary, in a situation such as this, to demonstrate that achievement of a high level of safety precludes a new intervention from preventing many additional transmissions of these agents. This is both the good news of our efforts and the challenge that we face as a field dedicated to making transfusion safer. Once most of a risk has been removed, there is much less to remove at a later time with additional interventions! While this observation is intuitive, it is not so profound as to redirect our attention and that of the public away from what they have feared the most over the last two decades.

While people remain focused on the diseases they know and fear, vanquishing the HIV and HCV threats leaves other challenges relatively more important. These include the risks of bacterial contamination of platelets and mistransfusion and acute haemolysis after red cell transfusion. The relative health benefits to be obtained by moving the discussion from *blood* safety to *transfusion* safety can be quantified, and cost-effectiveness analyses could be performed to quantify how much better spent resources would be if directed toward eradication of these problems. We will return to this subject later in the chapter.

Why have the public, the media and governmental regulators continued to focus on HIV and HCV risks in transfusion to the point of almost ignoring much greater risks to recipients' health and longevity emanating from other sources?

Transfusion risks are often regarded with great dread because of their perceived inequity and randomness [9]. A person who dies bungy jumping is assumed to have accepted the risk and the potential of an adverse outcome; as good health is presumed to be 'due' to all, however, a complication of transfusion is perceived as impinging on one's right to (continued) health. When the transmitted disease, such as HIV, has come to be associated with certain activities that many people do not accept (such as drug use and homosexuality), the feelings of inequity deepen. Furthermore, the certainty of death associated with HIV transmission (at least before highly active anti-retroviral therapies) can have a profound effect on people's choices [1]. Avoidance of certain death as an outcome can galvanize action even if the probability of ending up with that outcome is extremely low. The veiled nature of viral transmission through transfusion serves to heighten these fears.[9] Although one could argue that it would be better to live for several years after being infected by HIV than to die immediately of an acute transfusion reaction, the fact that transmission of an infection is not generally known – but may be feared – for a considerable time after transfusion makes avoidance of viral infection even more important. These are some of the reasons that have resulted in the safety of transfusions continuing to be framed in terms of HIV and HCV to the ignoring of other, larger threats.

Options to Improve Transfusion safety

As an example of the relative magnitude of the risks involved, let's compare the health benefit yields achievable by reducing the risks of HIV transmission, fatal bacterial contamination and fatal acute haemolysis each by 50% (Table 1).

Table 1. Comparison of alternatives in transfusion safety improvement

Threat	HIV transmission	Bacterial contamination of platelets		Mistransfusion/ Acute hemolysis
Approximate current risk (per million units)	1	7		1
Intervention	MP→ID NAT	Routine culture	Observation for swirling	Barrier system
New risk (per million units)	0.5	<1	2	(<)0.1
Estimated cost (per unit, in US dollars)	15	17	(negligible)	3.25

MP: Mini-pool; ID: Individual donation; NAT: Nucleic Acid Testing.

The risk of HIV transmission with the use of third generation enzyme immunoassay antibody detection techniques coupled with minipool (MP) nucleic acid testing (NAT) is approximately 1 per million units transfused; this (already small) risk might be reduced by moving from MP NAT to individual donation (ID) NAT. In this example, let's assume (somewhat of an overestimate) that this change in the testing protocol would decrease the risk by half, to 0.5/million units [8,10]. Further, let's assume the cost of this improvement would add USD15 to the cost of each unit. If the availability of resources were no limitation, this intervention would be overwhelmingly adopted because of the continued concern about the possibility of HIV transmission. While the health benefit yield would be very small, the presence of sufficient resources to accomplish this without diminishing the potential implementation of other blood safety or health care improvement measures would preclude antagonistic arguments.

Of course, resources are not unlimited. Therefore, let us compare this potential intervention to improve transfusion safety with another that has received increasing attention lately. The risk of a fatality from a bacterially contaminated single donor platelet unit is approximately 7 per million units, or 7 times the HIV risk [11]. (Since HIV transmission may not substantially reduce the post-transfusion longevity of patients, on average, because of their underlying illnesses while a fatal bacterial contamination would, almost by definition, shorten a patient's life span to some extent, the relative magnitude of the fatality risk imposed by bacterial contamination of platelets is actually *more* than 7 times greater than that posed by HIV risk.) A number of research and development efforts are underway to create means to detect bacterial contamination simply, reliably and quickly in a transfusion service laboratory. Addressing this problem, however, need not await development of nucleic acid-based amplification schemes or other yet-to-be-developed methods. A simple bacterial culture *could* be used to detect contamination with a high degree of reliability for a cost that is far less than 7 times the cost of decreasing HIV risk by half. For example, culturing platelet units on their second day of storage will detect almost all – if not indeed all – contaminated units for approximately USD16.50/unit [12,13]. Thus for about the same cost as converting from MP to ID HIV NAT, the number of (immediate) deaths that could be prevented would be at least *7-fold greater*. One need not create a formal cost-effectiveness analysis model to determine which of these two expenditures of money would yield a greater net health benefit!

Alternatively, training technologists to detect loss of swirling in platelet units (as bacterial growth causes pH to fall) would be even less expensive, indeed, probably of negligible cost. Although this technique could detect perhaps only 50-75% of bacterially contaminated units [14], its cost-effectiveness would appear far better than that of a larger expenditure (such as conversion of NAT from MP to ID format) that prevented fewer adverse outcomes.

Consider also mistransfusion and the potential for acute haemolysis. Even with well-developed systems of patient identification and quality assurance, fatalities due to mistransfusion occur at least once each million units of red cells transfused [15-17]. These occurrences are beginning to be recognized widely as failures of the system in which samples are collected, labeled, and tested and units are designated, delivered and transfused to patients [18]. Human error, being inevitable, must be blocked by process controls that prevent our frailties from creating problems for others. Prevention of most of these mistransfusion events could be achieved using a mechanical barrier system or a computerized tracking device [19,20]. Formal costing of the former has shown that a system utilizing this concept costs approximately USD 3.25 per unit [21]. While the cost-effectiveness of a mechanical barrier system from a societal perspective is above the usual threshold of acceptability (at about USD 200,000/quality-adjusted life year), it is far better than most other blood safety interventions that have occurred recently, most of which have cost-effectiveness estimates in the *millions* of dollar per QALY range [5]. Furthermore, from a hospital perspective, this 'additional expense' is actually *cheaper* than taking care of the subsequent morbidity and paying to defend oneself in a liability lawsuit (the filing of which would be a foregone conclusion in the U.S. medical/legal system) [21].

Let us 'scale up' these estimates to the entire U.S. blood system. If we had an additional USD 200 million to spend on transfusion safety improvements, these resources could be put into MP→ID NAT conversion to prevent perhaps as many as 8 transmissions annually (assuming 1.6 components transfused per donation). (This model obviously overstates the risk of HIV considerably, but this erroneous assumption serves only to highlight the point that other risks are today much greater.) That same amount of resources could prevent approximately 30 deaths annually from bacterial contamination of platelets – for *three entire years*. Or it could be spent over *five years* to prevent about a dozen mistransfusion-related deaths in *each* of those years.

Even without additional resource availability, comparisons such as this can trigger consideration of ways to make improvements. For example, swirling may not be as sensitive a means to detect contamination as culturing, but it has almost no cost yet 50+% sensitivity [14]. Thus, assessing units for swirling before issuance represents a simple, inexpensive means of making a substantial improvement in transfusion safety. To invest additional resources, culturing to ensure bacterial sterility might allow extension of the storage time of platelet units [22,23]. This could reduce outdating and, therefore, costs of providing platelets to patients. In some circumstances, the savings associated with this might entirely offset the cost of culturing [12] in the same manner that considering all the costs of a mistransfusion for a hospital make implementation of a mechanical barrier system for prevention a cost-saving endeavor [21].

Moving Forward with Circumspection

Analyses such as those illustrated above can help guide our attention to those areas of transfusion where additional resources can improve recipient safety to the greatest extent or focus efforts on incomplete yet inexpensive measures that may have considerable health impact. In deciding to augment our armamentarium of safeguards to reduce risks for transfusion recipients, care should be taken that we do not inadvertently take a step in the wrong direction.

The concept of *competing risks* becomes applicable in transfusion medicine as the safety of allogeneic transfusion reaches a point where even a small risk associated with a further intervention could negate the intent of the effort. Several examples have already been published that highlight the small latitude for increased risk created by low viral transmission risks. Collection of autologous units before coronary artery bypass grafting (CABG) surgery could prevent transmission of viral agents, but if such patients (with obvious cardiovascular disease) suffered peri-donation mortalities at a rate of just 1/101,000 donations, all the benefit of avoiding the feared viruses would be overwhelmed [24]. Given that collection of autologous units may force the postponement of surgery by several weeks and that the death rate for patients awaiting CABG is approximately 0.5%/month, is delaying surgery to collect autologous units really a safer approach? Noting that severe reactions after a donation cannot be readily predicted [25] the potential health benefit for these patients in collecting their own blood may well be lacking. The risks of dissemination of non-enveloped viruses by the solvent-detergent viral inactivation technique that requires pooling have received considerable attention; based on a pool size of 1000L, a non-enveloped virus that had clinical effects similar to HIV would need to be present in an undetectably low frequency of 1 in 71 million donors before the benefits of avoiding enveloped viruses such as HIV, HCV and HBV were negated [26]. The small size of this window for improvement is further narrowed by realizing that the risks of viral transmission on which these calculations were based are (at least for HIV and HCV) an *order of magnitude* lower currently than when the calculations were performed.

The next approach to be applied to reduce viral transmission risk of cellular components is likely to be a viral inactivation step that involves the addition of a chemical that interacts with the genome of a contaminating virus. While such a process may be highly successful in achieving its intended outcome, the compounds to be added also have the potential to interact with the genome of cells of the recipient and be carcinogenic and/or teratogenic. Developers of these techniques are applying methods to inactivate or remove the chemicals after they have achieved their viral inactivation purpose. However, when the risk of HIV or HCV has been reduced to below 1 in 1 million units (such as with the introduction of NAT), the level of security that will have to be provided by toxicologic testing will require tests of incredible stringency and projections of extremely low likelihoods of adverse outcome for viral inactivation techniques just to achieve health benefit *neutrality*, let alone cost-effectiveness.

NAT already poses questions about a safety improvement that may have unintended consequences. In most centers in the U.S., the addition of NAT to the testing protocol has delayed the availability of platelets units by about a day. One might then presume that the average age of a unit at transfusion has increased by a similar amount. Since bacterial contamination is initially at a very low level in platelet units but the inoculum increases with the 'incubation' time [27] the risk of infectious morbidity or mortality is believed to increase with the age of the unit. Therefore, excitement about the advantage of reducing the risk of HCV or HIV from 1 per million units to something slightly less through ID NAT must be tempered by the realization that the risk of bacterial contamination has been increased at the same time. Available data do not allow determination of the precise trade-offs being made in this situation, but the potential for a *decrement* in safety attributable to NAT should prompt efforts to minimize the potentially negative aspects of a promising technology.

Can We Move in a Sensible Direction?

A dispassionate analysis of the risks facing an allogeneic transfusion recipient in a developed country today might lead to the conclusion that current efforts toward improving transfusion safety are not directed toward the most important risks. Why, then, do we in the field of transfusion medicine and those in commercial concerns that supply us with technology seemingly persist in focusing our attention in such a narrow area of viral transmission? If this is to satisfy the public's concern about threats that have truly been vanquished already, how can we redirect the public's interest in order to capture their support (and society's resources) so that we can actually make transfusion substantially safer?

We first must acknowledge the depth of fear that HIV (and HCV, to a lesser extent) has created in the public's consciousness. HIV remains a major health concern – because of its consequences and its correlations – even for those who are at no risk of exposure to the virus. Blood transfusion represents a potential exposure to a feared agent over which the recipient has no control. To say that the risk is minimal is not enough. We will have to take the unusual step of seeking out opportunities to demonstrate graphically and comparatively the level of transfusion safety our societies now enjoy while we accumulate additional years of transmission-free transfusions to bolster our claims further.

At the same time, we will have to take the unusual step of highlighting the significant residual risks in order to focus attention on them and garner support. Absent the unfortunate death of a celebrity through an acute hemolytic transfusion reaction or a bacterially contaminated unit, we will have to create our own opportunities to demonstrate that the focus of transfusion safety must be realigned. This may mean bringing up in conversations with the media, regulators, elected officials and the public that there are risks to transfusion they may not have previously considered. This may mean that we need to answer questions about the safety of the blood supply by claiming that it is so safe (with respect to HIV and HCV, for example), that we can now redirect our attention to older problems that are actually much greater in magnitude.

Blood transfusion has become a much more visible part of modern healthcare than it was two decades ago. Some of this attention has brought unwanted focus on problems that have already be relegated to risks estimated to be so small they cannot be easily quantified. Our next task is to focus the public's attention, society's resources and our interest on the remaining issues that truly represent the greatest risks to transfusion recipients.

References

1. Publ Health 1992:82:584-86.
2. U.S. Department of Health and Human Services. The nation's blood resource. NIH publication 85-2028. Washington, DC, 1985.
3. World Health Organization, Geneva, 2000. http://www.who.int/inf-pr-2000/en/r2000-25.html.
4. Gold ME, Siegel JE, Russell LB, Weinstein MC. Cost-effectiveness in health and medicine. New York: Oxford University Press, 1996.
5. AuBuchon JP, Birkmeyer JD, Busch MP. Blood safety: Challenges and opportunities. Ann Int Med 1997:127:904-09.
6. Busch MP, Korelitz JJ, Kleinman SH, Lee SR, AuBuchon JP, Schreiber GB and the Retrovirus Epidemiology in Donors Study (REDS). Declining yield of alanine aminotransferase for screening of blood donors for prevention of post-transfusion hepatitis B and C virus infection. Transfusion 1995:35:903-10.

7. Busch M, Giachetti C, Conrad A, et al. Dynamics of HCV viremia during early HCV infection: implications for minipool (MP) vs individual donation (ID) nucleic acid amplification testing (NAT). (abstract) Transfusion 2000;40(suppl):25-6S.
8. Fiebig E, Heldebrant C, Smith R, et al. HIV viremia preceding antibody (Ab) seroconversion (SC): detection by p24 Antigen (Ag), minipool nucleic acid amplification tests (MP-NAT) and individual donation (ID) NAT. (abstract) Transfusion 2000;40(suppl):25S.
9. Morgan MG. Risk analysis and management. Sci Am 1993; 269:32-5, 38-41.
10. Jackson BR, AuBuchon JP, Busch MP. Cost-effectiveness of nucleic acid testing for HIV and HCV in donated blood. (abstract) Transfusion 2000;40(suppl):138S.
11. Perez P, Bruneau C, Chassaigne M, et al. Multivariate analysis of determinants of whole blood donation bacterial contamination. (abstract) Transfusion 1999;39(suppl): 116-17S.
12. Cooper L, Leach MF, Tracy JE, Zuaro DE, Schwartzman JD, AuBuchon JP. Application of a universal culturing approach to reduce the risk of bacterial contamination of platelet units. (abstract) Transfusion 1999;39:119-20S.
13. Brecher ME, Holland PV, Pineda A, Tegtmeier G, Yomtovian R. Bacterial growth in inoculated platelets: Implications for bacterial detection and the extension of platelet storage. Transfusion 2001:41:(in press)
14. Leach MF, Pickard CA, Herschel LH, et al. Evaluation of glucose and pH test strips for detection of microbial contaminants in apheresis platelets. (abstract). Transfusion 1998;38(suppl):89S.
15. Linden JV, Paul B, Dressler KP. A report of 104 transfusion errors in New York State. Transfusion 1992;32:601-06.
16. Linden JV, Tourault MA, Scribner CL. Decrease in frequency of transfusion fatalities. (letter) Transfusion 1997;37:243-44.
17. Sazama K. Reports of 355 transfusion-associated deaths: 1976 through 1985. Transfusion 1990;30:583-90.
18. Myrhe BA, McRuer D. Human error-a significant cause of transfusion mortality. Transfusion 2000;40:879-85.
19. Wenz B, Burns ER. Improvement in transfusion safety using a new blood unit and patient identification system as part of safe transfusion practice. Transfusion 1991; 31:401-03.
20. Jensen NJ, Crosson JT. An automated system for bedside verification of the match between patient identification and blood unit identification. Transfusion 1996;36: 216-21.
21. AuBuchon JP, Littenberg B. A cost-effectiveness analysis of the use of a barrier system to reduce the risk of mistransfusion. Transfusion 1996;36:222-26.
22. McDonald CP, Roy A, Lowe P, et al. The first experience in the United Kingdom of the bacteriologic screening of platelets to increase the shelf life to 7 days. Vox Sang 2000;78(suppl 1):375.
23. Vucetic D, Taseski J, Balint B, Mirovic V. Use of BacT/Alert system for bacterial screening of platelet concentrates. (abstract) Vox Sang 2000;78(suppl 1):371.
24. Birkmeyer JD, AuBuchon JP, Littenberg B, et al. The cost-effectiveness of preoperative autologous donation in coronary bypass surgery. Ann Thoracic Surg 1994;57: 161-69.
25. AuBuchon JP, Popovsky MA. The safety of preoperative autologous blood donation in the non-hospital setting. Transfusion 1991; 31:513-17.
26. AuBuchon JP, Birkmeyer JD. Safety and cost-effectiveness of solvent-detergent treated plasma. In search of a zero-risk blood supply. JAMA 1994;272:1210-14
27. Morrow JF, Braine HG, Kickler TS, et al. Septic reactions to platelet transfusions. A persistent problem. JAMA 1991;266:555-58.

COST-EFFECTIVENESS OF HIV NAT SCREENING FOR DUTCH DONORS

M.J. Postma[1], A.P.M. Los[2], EJ Ruitenberg[3], C.Th. Smit Sibinga[2]

Introduction

Up to today, safety for transfusion of blood and blood products has been determined by supply of available technology. The goal of public health authorities in this field has been to achieve maximum transfusion safety. For example, newer, better and more expensive tests for blood-borne viruses were rapidly introduced in screening procedures for blood donors without full consideration of costs, benefits and health gains [1]. In recent years, nucleic acid testing (NAT) was introduced in the Netherlands for screening blood donors on hepatitis C virus (HCV) and Human Immunodeficiency Virus (HIV), without any prior pharmaco-economic evaluation.

We argue that pharmaco-economic factors provide yet another point of view on transfusion safety, in particular as standardised methodology is becoming available. The latter is illustrated by the emergence of guidelines for pharmaco-economic research in several countries, amongst which the Netherlands. In this paper, we review the Dutch guidelines for pharmaco-economic research and illustrate the pharmaco-economic approach by an ex-post estimation of cost-effectiveness for HIV NAT in Dutch blood donors.

Dutch Guidelines for Pharmaco-Economic Research

As resources for health care are scarce and become scarcer with medical technology progressing, the question arises whether specific utilisation of health-care resources is justifiable when compared to other health-care interventions that compete for the same budget. Pharmaco-economic analysis enables to weigh the costs, benefits and health gains for specific interventions and to compare these different interventions using a similar outcome ratio. Obviously, fair comparisons between interventions can only be made if pharmaco-economic analyses are all done according to the same methodology. For that purpose the Dutch guidelines for pharmaco-economic research were developed [2].

---

1. University of Groningen Research Institute for Drug Exploration (GUIDE/GRIP), Groningen, NL.
2. Sanquin Division Blood Bank Noord Nederland, Groningen, NL.
3. Sanquin Division CLB, Amsterdam, NL.

Often used outcome ratios for pharmaco-economic research are: net costs per infection averted, net costs per life-year gained and net costs per quality-adjusted life-year (QALY) gained. Net costs are the costs of the intervention – investment and follow-up – minus the benefits related to averted health care utilisation. For the Netherlands, the guidelines indicate that net costs per life-year gained present a suitable outcome ratio. For example, recently threshold cholesterol levels for treatment with lipid-lowering agents were derived based on an acceptable cut-off for net costs per life-year gained at EUR 15,000 [3].

An ongoing discussion has been on discounting of life-years gained. Discounting relates to economic growth and should be applied to monetary costs and benefits next to appropriate deflators. The value of the discount rate should be chosen in accordance with national marginal rates on investment and market interest. The Dutch guidelines indicate a discounting percentage of 4% per year [2]. Furthermore and referring to the so-called Keeler & Scretin paradox, the guidelines suggest discounting of life-years gained at the same rate [4]. Some authors do however still claim that life-years gained should not be discounted [5].

Specific attention is given in the Dutch guidelines to the adequate time horizon of a pharmaco-economic study [2]. The adequate time horizon should encompass all the relevant costs and effects. For example, for HIV-infection the long-term most costly stage of AIDS should fall within the chosen time horizon for disease progression follow-up. Also, the time horizon should allow for modelling the relevant externalities of an intervention. For example, if HIV-infection is averted in an index person, we should allow for secondary infections averted in partners through averting the index infection. One could even consider aversion of tertiary infections and beyond.

According to the Dutch guidelines, indirect costs of production losses should be included in the analysis [2]. These costs reflect the loss in welfare of society due to the fact that patients are not able to produce while ill or after death. Indirect costs of production losses may be estimated using the human capital or friction costing approach [6]. The Dutch guidelines favour the friction costing approach, with valuations as published by Koopmanschap et al. [7].

Presentation of the analysis should be done distinguishing in the baseline analysis and sensitivity analysis [2,8]. The baseline analysis comprises parameter value estimations that are considered to be most likely. In sensitivity analysis, the analyst varies on these baseline parameter values in plausible ranges.

In the next section HIV NAT of blood donors will be evaluated according to the specific criteria of the Dutch guidelines mentioned above.

Pharmaco-Economics Analysis of HIV NAT for Blood Donors

Introduction

Towards the end of 2000 HIV NAT was introduced in Dutch Blood Banks for all donations, in addition to the ELISA[1]. Given that during the years prior to HIV NAT approximately four HIV-infected donations per year by ELISA were

1. p-24 test was never applied in the Netherlands for donors.

detected, expectations on extra detection by HIV NAT are 1-2 per year at maximum. HIV NAT costs approximately EUR 75 according to health-care tariffs. In the framework of a large-scale screening of donations the costs per donation are EUR 50, due to scale effects. HIV NAT can be done single donor or pooled. Single donor HIV NAT is very expensive and obviously not cost-effective in western settings. For example, for the USA single donor HIV NAT was estimated to net cost more than USD 2 million per life-year gained [9]. USA Blood Banks recommend to perform HIV NAT in pools of 24 donors. In the Netherlands, Blood Banking authorities decided for pooling by 48, lowering costs per donation to approximately EUR 1. In the next two sections we present assumptions for cost-effectiveness analysis. Cost-effectiveness was estimated in the baseline analysis and in sensitivity analysis. In the baseline analysis we assumed 1 donor detected by HIV NAT (0.5 and 2 in sensitivity analysis). All costs, benefits and health gains were discounted at 4% (non-discounting of life-years gained in sensitivity analysis) and monetary costs were expressed in EURs (price level 2000).

Health Gains

For HIV NAT health gains relate to the extra (compared to ELISA alone) HIV-infections detected in donors:

- Discounted life-years gained for detecting HIV more early in the donor than would otherwise have been the case;
- Discounted life-years gained for HIV-infection averted in the transfused patient; and
- Discounted life-years gained for HIV-infection averted in partners of the transfused patient and the donor.

We assumed that early detection of HIV in the donor prolongs survival by one life-year [10]. During this year Highly Active Antiretroviral Therapy (HAART) will be given. If HIV remains undetected in the absence of NAT, we assumed that two recipients of donor's blood products become infected.

For our current analysis we assumed that HIV-infections detected by NAT would avert two transmissions of HIV to transfused patients undergoing cardiac surgery, such as coronary artery bypass grafting (CABG). Distribution of cardiac-surgery patients over age and gender were from Van de Watering et al (majority is male) [11]. For survival, we developed a Markov-model with annual cycles, specifying gender- and age-specific annual risk of dying due to all causes, excess risks for persons who underwent CABG and for HIV-infection (Figure 1). For HIV-infection, we assumed average survival of 16 years (8 in sensitivity analysis), corresponding with annual excess risk of death of 6.25% [10]. For estimating probabilities of actually surviving until year 16 after transfusion, gender- and age-specific general mortality rates were used and 1% extra annual mortality for persons who underwent cardiac surgery [12]. In sensitivity analysis we investigated 10% extra annual mortality to reflect cost-effectiveness in non-CABG patient groups confronted with higher mortality risks due to, for example, certain forms of cancer. General mortality data were derived from the national registration by the Dutch Central Bureau of Statistics (Rijswijk), as were age- and gender-specific estimates of life-years lost per death.

We assumed that per detected donor by HIV NAT one transmission to partners was averted (two in sensitivity analysis). This refers both to partners of the donor due to behavioural change by the donor and to partners of the transfused patient due to aversion of transmission. For calculating life-years gained, we assumed similar age-distribution and inverse gender distribution (majority women) and general mortality as referred to above.

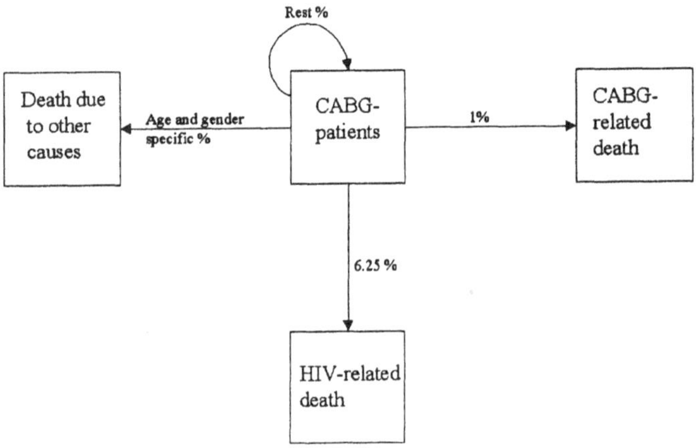

Figure 1. Markov-model for survival of persons who underwent CABG and were infected with HIV during transfusion, including excess death risks due to post-CABG and HIV and risk of death due to other causes. The Markov model applies an annual cycle.

Monetary Benefits

Next to the costs of EUR 1 for the test per donor, HIV NAT has monetary consequences that relate to:

- Benefits of *direct medical* costs averted for lifetime treatment and care for HIV-infection in the transfused patient and partners;
- *Net indirect medical* costs, reflecting the monetary consequences of detecting HIV in the donor a few years earlier than would have been the case if the donor would not have been tested; and
- *Indirect non-medical* costs of production losses.

Discounted lifetime costs for HIV were previously estimated at EUR 59,000 [13]. These costs were assumed to reflect the benefits of averting HIV-infection by preventing transmission through HIV NAT.

Detection of HIV in a donor by HIV NAT involves early diagnosis, around one year before the time infection would have been diagnosed in the absence of HIV NAT (detection by ELISA at next donation). During this year HAART is prescribed with costs of EUR 4800. Due to discounting relatively small monetary benefits are acquired by shifting the expensive last stage of HIV-infection (AIDS) further into the future (benefit of approximately EUR 1000) [10].

Production losses were assumed to occur on average halfway the simulated period between HIV-infection and HIV/AIDS-related death. This point in time may reflect the onset of serious symptoms. Production losses were quantitatively valued using the friction costing approach if the time of onset of serious symptoms is before the age of retirement at 65 years. Most recent age- and gender-specific production losses were derived a pulication by Rutten - van Mölken et al. [14].

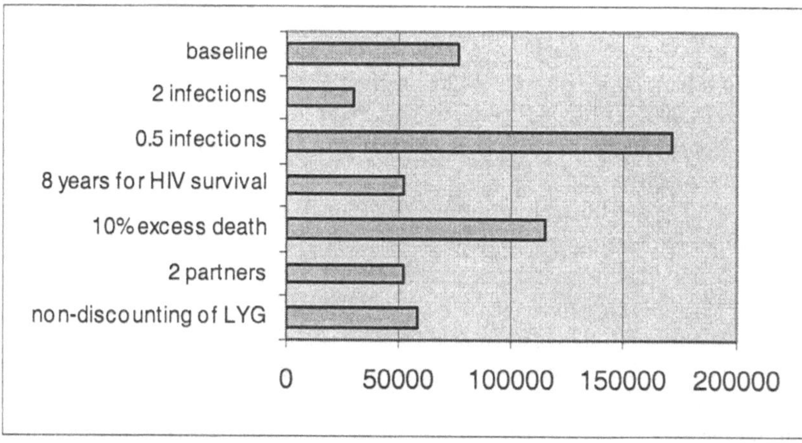

Figure 2: Cost-effectiveness in net costs per discounted life-year gained for the baseline (one infection detected by HIV NAT per year; average survival after HIV-infection of 16 years; excess death rate for CABG-patients at 1%; HIV-infection averted in one partner; discounting of costs, benefits and life-years gained at 4%) and in sensitivity analysis:

- 2 infections instead of 1 infection detected by HIV NAT per year;
- 1 infection detected per 2 years;
- average survival after HIV-infection of 8 years;
- excess death rate at 10% reflecting non-CABG patient groups; and
- HIV-infection averted in 2 partners; and non-discounting of life-years gained (LYG)

Results and Discussion

Life-years gained by averting HIV-infection in the recipient were 2.92 years in the baseline. The range in sensitivity analysis goes from 1.16 for non-CABG patient groups with a 10%-annual excess risk of death to 4.40 if average survival after HIV-infection is only 8 years. Baseline life-years gained for partners were 3.80 in the baseline and up to 5.89 in sensitivity analysis. Indirect benefits of production losses averted were EUR 1219 per HIV-infection averted for the recipient and EUR 710 for the partner. Ranges in sensitivity analysis were: EUR 619-1701 for recipients and EUR 361-992 for the partner. The deviating figures for partners reflect the different gender-distribution of partners than of recipients. The majority of partners is female with better remaining life expectancy and lower production than the majority of male recipients.

Figure 2 shows estimated cost-effectiveness of HIV NAT in Dutch blood donors. In the baseline net costs are EUR 77,500 per life-year gained. If two infections instead of one were detected annually by HIV NAT, cost-effectiveness more than halves. If however only one infection were detected per two year, cost-effectiveness increases up to EUR 171,000. Obviously, further lowering of the number of annual detections by HIV NAT worsens cost-effectiveness further beyond EUR 200,000.

For average HIV-survival at 8 instead of 16 years, for two HIV-infections averted in partners instead of one and for non-discounted life-years gained, cost-effectiveness is in the range of EUR 50,000-60,000. Finally, a 10%-excess death rate related to the causing factor for transfusion raises cost-effectiveness to EUR 116,000 per life-year gained. This might reflect cost-effectiveness for non-CABG patient groups, such as leukaemia patients with worse survival prospects than CABG-patients.

International literature provides one other analysis of HIV NAT in donors. Aubuchon et al investigated single-donor HIV NAT. Extra costs for HIV NAT and extra infected transfusions prevented rendered a net cost of more than USD 2 million per life-year gained. If we insert single donor HIV NAT in our model net costs per life-year gained approach EUR 5 million per life-year gained.

The cut-off point for acceptable net cost per life-year gained differs over time and between societies. Such a cut-off point has not yet been officially defined for the Netherlands. The above mentioned cut-off for cholesterol treatment of EUR 15,000 may however be indicative. In the USA cost-effectiveness below USD 50,000 is considered reflect favourable cost-effective-ness among pharmaco-economists and warrants adoption of the health-care technology under consideration [15]. Given our above analyses HIV NAT for donors is above both thresholds. Adoption of more costly programmes than the threshold would depend on societies' preferences and abilities to pay the additional costs. Of course, pharmaco-economics do not provide the only relevant viewpoint, since budgetary, legal and ethical aspects are also involved.

Conclusion

Estimated cost-effectiveness of HIV NAT for Dutch donors ranges from EUR 30,500 to 171,000, with EUR 77,500 per life-year gained as baseline estimate. Pharmaco-economics present the potential for rational analysis of risks and safety in transfusion. With health-care costs rising and the necessity to make choices in allocating budgets available for health-care, pharmaco-economics provide advanced techniques for rational decision. Guidelines for pharmaco-economic research enhance comparability and plausibility of pharmaco-economic analyses, for example in transfusion medicine.

Acknowledgement

The authors acknowledge the assistance of Rogier Klok (GUIDE/GRIP) in preparing this manuscript.

References

1. Postma MJ, Jager JC, Heeg BMS, Ruitenberg EJ: Pharmaco-economics of Transfusions Safety. Vox Sang 2000;78(S1):736.
2. ollege voor Zorgverzekeringen (CvZ). Guidelines for Pharmaco-economic Research (Richtlijnen voor Farmacoeconomisch Onderzoek: in Dutch). Amstelveen: CvZ 1999.
3. Centraal Begeleidingsorgaan voor de Intercollegiale Toetsting (CBO). Treatment and prevention of coronary heart disease by lowering cholesterol-levels (Behandeling en Preventie van Coronaire Hartziekten door Verlaging van de Plasmacholesterolconcentratie; in Dutch). Utrecht: CBO 1998.
4. Keeler EB, Scretin S. Discounting of life-saving and other nonmonetary effects. Management Science 1983;29:300-06.
5. Parsonage M, Neuburger H. Discounting and health benefits. Health Econ 1992;1:72-76.
6. Drummond MF, O'Brien B, Stoddart GL, Torrance GW. Methods for the Economic Evaluation of Health Care Programmes. Oxford: Oxford University Press 1997.
7. Koopmanschap MA, Rutten FFH, van Ineveld BM, van Roijen L. The friction cost method for measuring indirect costs of disease. J Health Econ 1994;14:171-89.
8. Gold MR, Siegel JE, Russel LB, Weinstein MC (eds.) Cost-effectiveness in Health and Medicine. New York: Oxford University Press 1996.
9. AuBuchon JP, Birkmeyer JD, Bush MP. Cost-effectiveness of expanded human immunodeficieny virus testing protocols for donated blood. Transfusion 1997;37:45-51.
10. Bos JM, Fennema JSA, Postma MJ. Cost-effectiveness of HIV-screening for Persons attending Clinics for Sexually Transmitted Diseases in Amsterdam (the Netherlands). AIDS 2001; accepted.
11. Van de Watering LMG, Hermans J, Houbiers JGA, van den Broek PJ, Bouter H, Boer F, Harvey MS, Huysmans HA, Brand A. Beneficial Effects of Leukocyte Depletion of Transfused Blood on Postoperative Complications in Patients undergoing Cardiac Surgery. Circulation 1998:97:562-68.
12. The Bypass Angioplasty Revascularization Investigation (BARI) Investigators. Comparison of coronary bypass surgery with angioplasty in patients with multivessel disease. N Engl J Med 1996;335:217-25.
13. Postma MJ. Assessment of the Economic Impact of AIDS at National and Multinational Level (thesis). Zutphen: Koninklijke Wöhrmann bv 1998.
14. Rutten-van Mölken MPMH, van Busschbach JJ, Rutten FFH. From Costs to Effects: a guide for evaluationstudies in health care (Van kosten tot effecten: een handleiding voor evaluatiestudies in de gezondheidszorg: in Dutch). Maarssen: Elsevier Gezondheidszorg 2000.
15. Owens Owens DK. Interpretation of cost-effectiveness analyses. J Gen Intern Med 1998;13:716-17.

LEGAL AND REGULATORY ASPECTS OF BLOOD TRANSFUSION

M.L. Kavanagh[1]

Introduction

The use of blood and blood components has contributed hugely to advances made in medicine and surgery but, as has been discovered, their use is certainly not without risk. Contaminated blood and components can transmit disease and, as our knowledge increases, more risks can be identified.

An example of this is the theoretical risk of transmission of variant Creutzfeldt Jakob Disease (vCJD) by blood components or blood products. Each newly identified risk provokes a corresponding precautionary or remedial measure and, in the UK, the response to the vCJD problem has been to implement universal leukocyte depletion and to stop the collection from UK donors of plasma for fractionation.

In the light of the enormous benefits provided by blood transfusion services throughout the world but also bearing in mind the known unknown risks, it has been recognised that there is a need to take appropriate steps to ensure the supply of safe, high quality blood and blood components. Different approaches have been taken in various countries with many using a legal regulatory framework, while various guidance documents have also been published to assist in achieving the good of safety and supply in the blood transfusion chain.

Guidance and Regulation

There are many national and international organizations involved in the regulation of blood and blood components, including the World Health Organization (WHO), the Council of Europe, the European Commission, the Pharmaceutic Inspection Convention/Co-operation Scheme (PIC/S) and the competent authorities of individual countries and states.

In 1975, the World Health Assembly adopted resolution WHA28.72 on the utilization and supply of human blood and resulting from this, the 'Requirements for the Collection, Processing and Quality Control of Human Blood and Blood Products' [1] were published in 1978. These recommendations of the WHO Expert Committee have since been expanded and are regularly updated.

---

1. Medicines Control Agency, Department of Health, London, UK.

The Council of Europe currently numbers 41 member states and over the years has adopted a number of Recommendations covering various aspects of blood transfusion. In particular Recommendation No. R (95)15, adopted on 12 October 1995, covered the preparation use and quality assurance of blood components; guidelines were published as technical appendix to this Recommendation [2]. These guidelines contain a section on Good Manufacturing Practice (GMP) for blood components.

Medicinal products derived from human blood or human plasma (fractionated products) are covered by European legislation (Directive 89/381/EEC) and the collection of plasma for fractionation is subject to inspection and regulation by the component authorities of the member states. The Rules Governing Medicinal Product in the European Community apply to these products and particularly relevant is Volume IV, the 'Guide to Good Manufacturing Practice, for Medicinal Products' [3].

Annex 14 of the Guide specifically covers the manufacture of medicinal products derived from human blood or human plasma. The Committee for Proprietary Medicinal Products (CPMP) also publishes Notes for Guidance of particular relevance to blood products manufacture are guidelines on virus validation studies, plasma-derived medicinal products and plasma pool testing.

Although fractionated blood products are covered by European legislation, blood and blood components are excluded. However, there have been several initiatives taken by the Council of the European Union and the European Commission to develop a harmonised policy on the regulation of blood and its components. These have included Commission communications in May 1993 and December 1994, resolution of the European Parliament in July 1995 and April 1996 and a Council resolution in November 1996 which followed a colloquium on blood safety and self-sufficiency, held in Adare, Ireland in September 1996.

The Council Resolution of 12 November 1996 reiterated the statement that Community self-sufficiency must be based on the principle of voluntary, unpaid donors and requested that rapid progress be made in taking the work forward.

In the absence of European legislation covering blood and blood products, many member states apply their own national regulations, as do countries out of the European Union.

In the United Kingdom, blood transfusion services are regulated under the Medicines Act of 1968, which requires that these have a Manufacture's 'Specials' Licence. This is a licence for a manufacturer to produce medicinal products, which do not have a product licence (or marketing authorisation). There are specific conditions applied to holders of 'Specials' licences but the manufacturer must still operate to an acceptable level of GMP in terms of product quality and safety.

There are four blood transfusion services in the UK: the National Blood Services in England the Scottish National Blood Transfusion Service, the Welsh Blood Service and the Northern Ireland Blood Transfusion Service. Each of them holds a Manufacturer's 'Specials' Licence which names the various blood centres which constitute the services. The centres are subject to regular GMP inspections on a two-yearly cycle to ensure that they continue to operate in compliance with the principles and guidelines of GMP.

In addition to the EC Guide which offers guidance on the general principles of GMP, the blood transfusion services of the UK, in association with the National Institute for Biological Standards and Control (NIBSC) have produced 'Guidelines for the Blood Transfusion Services in the United Kingdom', which is a comprehensive guide to the standards expected in the production of blood components. The 'red book', as it is commonly known, is now in its fourth edition and is used by MCA inspectors during their inspections of blood centres.

Another document of relevance has been produced by PIC/S. Within the PIC/S, there is a group of inspectors known as the PIC/S Expert Circle on Blood and Blood Products. This group has produced a GMP Guide for blood centres. The final draft of this document was produced in May 2000 and is currently being circulated to interested parties for comment. When it is finally adopted by the PIC/S Committee of Officials, this guide will be used by inspectors in PIC/S member countries to aid their inspections of blood centres.

Although mainly the legal and regulatory framework for blood centres in the UK has been described, many member states in the European Union and other countries world-wide operate similar systems for regulating the operations of their blood transfusion services.

Future Developments

Although blood and blood components have been subject to regulation in the UK and elsewhere for many years, the same controls have not been applied to tissues, including stem cells. There is a general movement to change this situation and tissue regulation was one of the topics discussed at the year 2000 meeting in Finland of the PIC/S Expert Circle on Blood and Blood Products.

Again, European legislation on the control of tissue banking seems some time away and, in the meantime, several countries are taking measures at a national level to address the issue. In the UK, the Department of Health is introducing an accreditation scheme for tissue banks which will be effective from 1 April 2001 and which will apply to public sector organisations supplying tissues to the Health Services.

The scheme will be administered on behalf of the Department of Health by the Medicines Control Agency and the scope of the scheme includes cardiovascular tissue, musculoskeletal tissue, skin, ocular tissues, immature gametes, foetal tissues and haemapoietic progenitor cells.

In order to facilitate the introduction of the accreditation scheme, a Code of Practice for tissue banks has been produced. The final draft of this document has been circulated for comment and the final version will be issued at the end of the year. Tissue banks which apply for accreditation will be inspected by MCA inspectors to ensure their compliance with the Code of Practice.

The Code of Practice itself is, in effect, a GMP guide for tissue banks, which is intended to ensure that tissue banks within the accreditation scheme operate to standard which will maximise the safety and quality of tissues. Chapters in the Code cover Quality Systems, Process Control, Facilities, Personnel, Donor Selection, Packaging, Labelling, Transport and Documentation.

A matter of discussion within the drafting group of the Code of Practice and also at the PIC/S Expert Circle meeting has been the environmental requirements for the aseptic of processing of tissues, such as stem cells, which do not have terminal microbial inactivation. The consensus of both groups was that such processing should be performed in a Grade A environment with a Grade B Background, which will present quite a challenge to many tissue banks.

There is no doubt that legal regulation, both of blood transfusion services and tissue banking operations, will become more widespread and accepted in the years ahead.

References

1. WHO Expert Committee on Biological Standardisation, WHO Technical Report Series 840, 1994.
2. Guide to the Preparation, Use and Quality Assurance of Blood Components, Council of Europe Publishing, Strasbourg, France. 6th Edition, 2000.
3. Commission of the European Communities. The Rules Governing Medicinal Products in the European Community Vol IV Good Manufacturing Practice for Medicinal Products, Luxembourg: Office for Official Publications of the EC, 1992.
4. Guidelines for the Blood Transfusion Services in the United Kingdom, The Stationery Office, London: 4th Edition, 2000.
5. PIC/S GMP Guide for Blood Centres (Draft).

DISCUSSION

J. Harrison (London, UK): A comment about a very simple method to improve reducing bacterial contamination that nobody has mentioned so far: cleaning the donor arm properly. We have been looking at this in the United Kingdom. We have examined the method we currently use for cleaning the donor's are and discovered that 37% of donors' arms were not cleaned effectively. We have established that there is a much better method. To adopt this method would mean an increase of only 25 pence in the cost of the method and it takes one minute longer. I think this is a very cost-effective method of reducing bacterial contamination.

J.P. AuBuchon (Lebanon, NH, USA): I am aware of these studies. We recently changed the arm prep in our institution to match what is being used in the United Kingdom for just those reasons. When there is an obvious threat and when there is something simple that can be done and particular when that does not cost very much why not use it. Another technique that is being investigated is diversion of the first few millilitres of blood collected into a side pouch with the thought that any skin plug that may have been picked up by the ultimately large bore needle and any bacteria associated could be diverted into the pouch and prevented from contaminating the entire unit. Studies at the American Red Cross would indicate that would have a positive effect that would reduce the risk of bacterial contamination. That is something that obviously would require the assistance of the bag manufacturers.

L. Corash (Concorde, CA, USA): Regarding the formal economical analysis a comment and a couple of questions. This analysis has been done from the perspective per donation, when I think it really should be looked at from the perspective of the therapeutic treatment of the patient or transfusion episode. Almost no one receives a single blood product unless it is a single donor platelet product. Generally, in the course of treatment of the patient there are multiple therapeutic exposures. So, somebody getting platelets support for treatment of acute leukaemia may see 8-12 transfusion episodes during induction of chemotherapy. So, the analysis needs to be reconfigured from that point of view. The other thing, of course, is that when you look at the technical viral inactivation you really should think of pathogen inactivation. You really should think of a broader array of pathogens including bacterial. Also look at protozoae which are important in other parts of the world particular in Africa and in India. Also I think you really need to look at leukocyte inactivation and whether or not these types of technologies would in fact have an impact on leukocyte depletion technologies and change the way we approach these. Lastly, nobody is really thinking about the fact of the next viral contaminant that enters the donor population and what would be the cost impact of that. That does not figure into these analyses but if you go back and you look at the impact of HIV infections at least in San Francisco in 1981, you get a very different analysis. Obviously the effect on quality adjusted life here.

J.P. AuBuchon: So, when we have pathogen inactivation techniques available we will still be doing all of the testing we are been doing and then will inactivate on top of that, knowing the way that our system tends to approach things. I understand that you are calling about patients receiving multiple units and that certainly is true. The analysis is constructed on a pre-unit basis, because of the relatively low frequency of transmission. It is highly unlikely that someone would encounter two contaminated units during a transfusion episode, during a lifetime given the low risk for at least HIV and HCV. So, the numbers would come out about the same. You could, however, state it differently in terms of dollars expended per patient going through the transfusion process successfully without coming in contact with any pathogen. That is an interesting notation.

C.L. van der Poel (Amsterdam, NL): I think it is an interesting discussion. I learned today that the standard would be in the United States about 50,000 dollars per QALY where it would be 30,000 guilders[1] in the Netherlands per QALY. The real issue is what are you willing to pay. Where would you draw the line of cost-effectiveness for interventions in blood safety that would be appropriate in developing countries as well as in developed countries. But we would still have to discuss how much we are willing to pay for a QALY. I would say HCV-NAT is already cost-effective if you relate the question to Norway where the production of plasma had to be blocked including the 15,000 donors involved in that production. HIV adding on top of that is much cheaper than Dr. Postma said. Cost-effectiveness analysis I think is a nice tool, but we still have to figure out where we hammer the nail with that tool.

M. Postma (Groningen, NL): One of the problems with thresholds is that there are different thresholds for different types of healthcare. So, in general the threshold is laid lower for preventive medicine than for curative medicine, for example we know that in the Netherlands heart transplantation costs much more than 30,000 per QALY gained but of course it occurs. So, different thresholds for different types of medicine. Maybe also we are going to a threshold for transfusion safety which could be different. So, that is a complicating factor.

J.P. AuBuchon: There are surely societal and psychological factors involved in deciding whether or not to provide a particular intervention in the case of hae-

1. 1USD = ± 2.40 DFl (Dutch guilder).

mophilia. This would be a situation where the individuals effected by the treatment or lack of treatment are very clearly identifiable. They are effected in a very visible and a very mediate way. So, people have a rational reaction to that and say yes, we want to treat haemophilia even though it may not look to be cost-effective.

K. Sazama (Houston, TX, USA): I would like to follow up on Mr. Kavanagh and Dr. Emmanuel. I was very interested in the review of the regulatory and legal oversights in the UK. I just like to ask the question do you regularly discover that there is a minority of blood transfusion centres that are unable to meet the GMP requirements and if so what happens as a consequence of those discoveries?

The second question which is really to Dr. Emmanuel: What is the role, if any, for accreditation, particularly in those countries who are just now developing blood transfusion schemes. Is it part and parcel of the plan that there be some sort of an accreditation process when countries begin to try to achieve the goals under WHO.

M.L. Kavanagh (London, UK): In answer to the first part of your question, we do find occasionally that there are failures following the principles and guidelines of cGMP in blood centres. The actions that are available to us could be at its most severe to remove a blood centre from the manufacturer's license of the blood service in question. We never had to do that. What normally happens is we identify the problem to the blood centre and ask them how they are going to address it. Thankfully so far, they have always managed to rectify the situation before we needed to take regulatory action. But it is available when considered necessary and all the blood services could survive if one centre was actually removed from the licence should that ever happen. The standards have actually improved dramatically over the last few years. This is largely due to the services themselves as well as the government regulatory action.

J. C. Emmanuel (Geneva, CH): WHO is not a regulatory body; it is more like the Council of Europe with recommendations, guidelines. It can self-regulate; it has done so in vaccines for instance for the international vaccination requirements that has imposed upon itself. But it is very rare that it would do that. Therefore, accreditation is not really possible for WHO, because by implication that means WHO is responsible for the accredited partner. But, having said that, WHO obviously is working very closely together with other organisations like Council of Europe and the EC. But it also has its norms and standards when it comes to pharmaceutically derived medicinal products. In those cases there are recommendations made by the Expert Committee on Biological Standards. We have the standards and norms that we are responsible for on a global basis, that are adopted by other agencies. So, on the side of pharmaceutically derived medicinal products we have very strict guidelines. We do not regulate countries, but we do develop guidelines and now we are trying to get in training workshops for national regulatory authorities. One of the major problems one has is that the regulatory authorities are not trained. Therefore they cannot even regulate what they are supposed to do. Now, the question of regulating blood transfusion services is more difficult because as you heard we have not got any models to really follow on how can it be regulated like a pharmaceutical process or what is the alternative. But, again we are working on producing these standards and norms that we can ask them to have oversight if you like. But certainly if any of the products be moved into the pharmaceutical derived medicinal products they have to adhere to that. So, in short what we are doing is to guide countries, train national regulatory authorities and help them to meet those standards, which we will set for them.

C.Th. Smit Sibinga (Groningen, NL): Mr. Lotgerink,.it is quite obvious that the basis of what has been discussed so far in this discussion is with the public and their representation at governments, the parliaments, the politicians. They should be regarded as kind of customers but also suppliers. Probably your view on that relates to how the public looks at the blood supply system, the perspective, the corporate image so to speak. Could you give us some advice?

Th.E.P. Lotgerink (Groningen, NL): Regarding the public image of blood supply, it is influenced by, as I stated in my presentation, earlier situations that are not in control, not within the circle of influence of blood supply organisations nor in the circle of influence of governments. Why not try to stop the water running where it started. There might be a way in educating existing donors and try to make them understand make the public understand what the risks are. I fully agree with informing the public about the real risk of blood donation and blood supply, but the role of existing donors within that information circuit is perhaps somewhat underestimated. My point would be why not use ambassadors that you already have, inform them more appropriately of the real risk of blood donation and calculate the decreasing cost of risk management because of that. That is something that I missed in the risk management presentations. It would be interesting I think to study whether informing donors better about life style and things like that would decrease risk to a certain amount. It is just the idea that I have and that might work; it is not based on scientific survey.

J.C. Emmanuel: I think the point that you raised is really important. There is a publication going to come out in the World Health Bulletin on an innovative approach towards blood donors and educating the public called Pledge 25. It started amongst school children and they give blood from 16 years of age and they pledge to give 25 times, which means they are captive audience beyond the school going age. They have a peer group and they do educating amongst their own peer group. It was started in Zimbabwe and it is gone all over and very well developed in South Africa too. To give an example: in the general blood donation public by similar age the prevalence of HIV is 25% positive. That is what you would be addressing if you did not have public education. Amongst the Pledge 25 it is less than 0.7% in the first time donor and less than 0.02% in the regular donor. Even those who are not donors amongst that group of peers, they have educated them into safer sex and life styles; they are not finding HIV in that group to the same level, even when they do not donate. I think partly of what you are saying is an educational campaign with taking this on board and it is gone beyond the dynamics of just blood donation.

F. Fritzson (Uppsala, S): Dr. Emmanuel, the Council of Europe, WHO and European Commission recommend unpaid donors or non-remunerated donors. I think that there are other important safeties like exclusion criteria for donors, non-repeat donors and testing and testing methods. What I want to know is the definition of non-remunerated and remunerated donors, because the interpretation is really different from country to country.

Question two is, is it really evident based that the risk is much higher with the remunerated donors than non-remunerated donors?

J.C. Emmanuel: I am sure Dr. AuBuchon can answer much better on the prevalence amongst once paid donors and the non-paid donors. I think it would not take much imagination to know that if you started paying people in developing countries. I am talking about the 25% and remember there are no alternative testing sides. So, any donor questioning is completely irrelevant if you start paying somebody. Regarding the definition of volunteer non-remunerated donor – you are quite right, there has to be some kind of standard. I think that the ISBT in conjunction with the International Federation of Red Cross and Red Crescent Societies and WHO has come up with the simple definition that is: any form of payment or gifts that can be exchanged afor monetary gain could be considered remuneration. However, that is just a broad definition of payment. From the WHO perspective what we are saying is that it has to be voluntary and you cannot give any form of payment. We also discourage any thing that can be changed for monetary gains. So, that basically is anything that will stop somebody distorting the truth when you are doing a donor questionnaire. You are quite right, the repeat donor is the most valuable, but the questionnaire is very valuable and they have to understand it and answer honestly.

Now, if the payment or the reward system is greater than the understanding of altruism you may have a problem. I think the comment I made about the Pledge 25 shows that exactly: they do get a cap but that has not made them lie. You have got 25% HIV positivity amongst the donors if you paid in a situation like that; you would get 25% of the donors coming for to get paid. It has even been suggested once at WHO, that it is discrimination not to pay somebody and therefore you know one has to pay even the unemployed. Now the statistics I think speak for themselves and this has been an ongoing analysis of the current literature. But there is no question in developing countries and clearly the people in developed countries will speak for the dangers of paid donations.

F. Fritszon: Surely, all donors are voluntary, even if they are paid.

J.C. Emmanuel: That is true, but voluntary non-remunerated is what I am talking about. It is no question. Yes voluntary, even the army and the police can give voluntarily, even if they ordered this to the voluntary act. That is part of their drills. So, the question is not voluntary, it is always *voluntary non-remunerated.*

F. Fritszon: Just a comment. If you repay the costs that the donor has for the donation is that payment all right for remuneration or not?

J.P. AuBuchon: Are you speaking in terms of for example paying for the parking of the donor or paying for the direct expenses of the donor occurred in donating, would that be considered payment.

C.Th. Smit Sibinga: Cost made in reason as it is usually named. The legislation in the Netherlands for instance has such a phrase that where costs are made in reason by a donor who we have called specifically, they then should be reimbursed.

J.C. Emmanuel: I think that is what it is. Why would they bother to come to get paid just to get remuneration back for parking if they already were paid out? It is the incentive of the payment that makes them come, so therefore if it is ten times the cost maybe it is worth it. But whatever you are paying that makes them an untrue factor, giving you false information to the donor questionnaire.

Th.E.P. Lotgerink: Chairman, I like to add a little thing, because it might work the other way around when you start paying donors. If the value that the customer gets from achieving, using or processing a product or a service, if the customer value of giving blood is being a good citizen, whenever you start paying them you are reducing the customer value. So, you better think twice before you start doing that.

A.P.M. Los (Groningen, NL): Over the past years we have done a survey and asked donors what would you do if payment of blood would be the rule in the Netherlands. 25% of the donors responded they would stop donating blood voluntarily.

J-P. Allain (Cambridge, UK): Dr. Emmanuel, you have been mentioning the residual risk of blood transfusion with various viruses. My question is particularly addressed to hepatitis B which I think is a special case among the other, the three main viruses in the sense that in most developing countries the rate of infection is very high in particular in chronic infected individuals. But the risk is essentially seen as far as I can tell from the donor point of view. In fact, if you want to really estimate it, you have to look at the recipient point of view. I actually just finished a study in Ghana where the prevalence of HbsAg chronic infection is about 15%. But to my surprise I noticed that the prevalence of potential recipients – looking at the markers of hepatitis B, particularly anti-HBc and other markers – showed that by age 15 65% of the population had been in contact with hepatitis B virus and by age 40 100% of the population had been. This means that the risk of post-transfusion hepatitis B after age 40 is zero. So, I wonder whether this is something that is integrated into this estimation as far as WHO concerns.

J.C. Emmanuel: What you have done has been done before; At least 25 years ago it was mentioned that there was no need to be doing hepatitis B. This was a question of debate and the vulnerable in fact are the people, the children. Remember, in the developing countries the people who receive the most blood are women as a consequence of pregnancy, children and trauma victims. Estimated in the region about a quarter of a million women die as a consequence of haemorrhage or loss of blood every year. They are all very young women really in developing countries and they are at risk of receiving positive samples, so it is worth doing. We also think it is preventable, we are not sure if they all got immunity against it. You are right, we cannot argue that point, but hepatitis B is not an expensive test to do and when you look at what we are trying to promote, which is regular blood donation, they should be screened out in the first passage through. As they become regular donors there should not be any further risk of transmission. Now, it is only in an organised and well-run blood transfusion service that you have regular donor panels. There you can have strategies where you could test them every 3rd or 4th donation if you so wished. But in most of developing countries as you well know they are usually one-time donors and they do not repeat donation. The most expensive test is obviously the HCV test.

J-P Allain: I am not suggesting not to test for hepatitis B, I am just mentioning that eventually there are simple tests probably not meeting the standards of Western countries, where in fact the residual risk according to my calculation by just using a simple dipstick for HBsAg. In Ghana the residual risk in the overall population is one in 40,000, which is equal to what it is in Britain.

J.C. Emmanuel: Well, we have looked at that and that is exactly what we are working on with reference standard preparations with the US and lot of other workers in to giving standards for HIV, hepatitis B and hepatitis C to do exactly what you are saying; so I appreciate that.

J.P. Allain: It would be an interesting analysis to look at the cost or cost-effectiveness of providing universal hepatitis B vaccination for all children in an environment like that versus testing the blood supply for hepatitis B, where it had not been tested before.

C.Th. Smit Sibinga: For HCV as you know there is a rapid test, very simple test now basically available which we discussed last year at the symposium here, developed by Howard Field at the CDC[1]. The problem with HCV, however, is the variety of the types that are present in the world. So, the standard that you use to validate the test should be appropriate according to which part of the world you are in. That makes it more difficult in comparison to hepatitis B.

---

1. Fields HA, Khudyakov YE, Lopeneva E, Ulanova T, Talekar G, Ravash Y. Development of a new diagnostic method for the development of HCV antibodies: The rapid lateral flow test. In: Smit Sibinga CTh, Klein HG, eds. Molecular Biology in Blood Transfusion. Kluwer Academic Publ. Dordrecht, Boston, London, 2000:111-23.

J. Power (Cork, IRL): Mr Kavanagh coming back to tissue banking pretentious–ly as looked in the future, where are we going? It does very much seem as a 'déjà vue'. Tissue banking is really out where blood banking was five or six years ago and as you have mentioned we obviously had to enhance our practice greatly to meet the requirements around cGMP. That has come with understanding. I am just looking at the Code of Practice guidance document; it is a very comprehensive document, I think it is a very good document and it is coming in surprisingly on time. But there seem to be two schools working within the UK and I am just wondering how that is going to be managed; the tissue banks that are associated with the transfusion services and the tissue banks who are not. The understanding of the requirement for cGMP – the cost to put in proper cGMP structures and the need for it – I am just not seeing a reaction within the professions if we look at the orthopaedic surgeons, cardiovascular surgeons and others who have been the controllers of these non BTS typed tissue banks in the past. What is going to happen, are you going to shut these down or is there going to be an advanced and accelerated programme to try to get those structures in. It just seems that if you have two very different streams working to provide one type of service.

M. Kavanagh: The way the accreditation scheme is going to operate that is that there is going to be a statement put out by the Department of Health to the health service clinicians that they should only use tissues from banks which are accredited. It is a non-statutory scheme and the feeling is that a lot of the very small banks do not apply for the accreditation and therefore will just seize to be. The whole scheme has got a two years transitional period and we accept that it is bit like going back to the transfusion services as they were. We have to take a reasonably pragmatic approach, but the problems to view is that these important issues in these banks should operate to acceptable standards of cGMP, traceability and so on. So, they are determined that it should take place. It is difficult to even know how many tissue banks actually operate, because some of them are just a person with a freezer and some bones in it. So, we have not really got a handle on what the scale of the operation is; the best estimate is that there are about over 200. A good proportion of these will seize to operate once the scheme comes in. But yes, it is difficult, but it will be interesting both for the MCA and the tissue bankers.

C.Th. Smit Sibinga: A question to Mr. Los. I wonder what would you think be the customer values if you look at the essence of the presentation of Mr. Lotgerink and your community involvement. Could you name three?

A.P.M. Los: The donor customer value; well I think that the way donors are treated is one very important thing and it is also very important to measure the way donors perceive that they are treated. Another possibility is to educate the personnel with regard to the treatment of donors so that they know how donors will have to be treated.

C.Th. Smit Sibinga: Could the mechanism to create more feeling of ownership of the donors with respect to the blood supply be a possibility?

A.P.M. Los: I do not know whether or not this is a feeling of ownership, because when the donor is in the donor centre and is a regular donor and the donor is treated well, he feels at home; they have a certain bond or connection with the personnel. So, you can look at a donor as a customer and then you can apply all marketing principles for keeping them in your donor centre, of course. But, that some marketing techniques have some methodology and that you can use for improving the way donors are treated. When these marketing techniques are used for improving the way donors are treated, and I think I think that would be appropriate.

Th.E.P. Lotgerink: A very short comment. Customer value is a very difficult concept and it is used in various ways. Mostly it is used in the definition what the value of the customer to the organisation is. In blood supply organisations how many times does the person in question give blood. Another concept is the life-time value of a customer. What I was talking about was what does the customer get out of giving blood. What is the value that he receives for giving blood and what is in it for him. That has got something to do with pride, has something to do with good citizenship.

One of the things that I would argue would be recognition by peer groups, by environment of being a donor, and that has something to do with communication.

A.P.M. Los: I like to add that to the Pilliavin[1] and Oswald[2] reasons for donating blood. What Mr Lotgerink is saying are exactly the reasons that are found in surveys for the last 40 years. So, when we address to those reasons and also the self-respect of the donor; altruism in itself is good citizenship as you say. Those are not new findings, those are findings that have been forthcoming for the last forty years. So, you can have a look at the literature and then you have also the reasons and the possibilities for addressing the donor.

J.C. Emmanuel: Just a plea for 80% of the world: they have not got the confidence that they are going to a blood transfusion service where it is blood is regarded a national resource. They keep their blood because they go to the nearest hospital. If they have given their blood and they go to that hospital they are asked to donate again. Therefore, they see themselves as custodians of their own family and their friends and social circle. So, really I would say that the organisation and the management have to convey a sense of confidence that they are using the blood in the correct way and that is where we come from.

---

1. Piliavin JA, Callero PL. Giving blood. The development of an altruistic identity. John Hopkins University Press, Baltimrre, MD, USA, 1991.
2. Oswalt RM. A review of blood donor motivation and recruitment. Transfusion 1977; 17:123-35.

J.D. Cash (Amsterdam, NL): Well, two comments. One is I actually believe we need in the context of customer to separate quite clearly blood donors and what I call the real customers the clinicians, the patients, the hospitals, because both sets can make completely different demands. The way we actually are committed or whatever to respond is profoundly different. I like to see blood donors rather like Friesian cows; we are looking after them, we are cuddling them regularly, we are really looking after them, we are feeding them well, we give them a warm reception and so on. It is about human relationships, whereas I think increasingly it is the market place that in fact drives the other sort of customers and I think that is really very important.

The second thing I like to say is that I dream that eventually there will be doctors, scientists working together in the future, that will in fact deliver which they now to best practice. That is the best you can have. And that behind them or in front of them – it does not matter – are an informed group like the economics people who will say that is mashing, we will give you a feeling for value for money. Because, ultimately society has got to pay up and there is no sense in having people like econometrists unless there is not a third body that actually receives their information and makes decisions. And the notion of gyms well what we have got to do is try to educate the people that an extra test is four pence extra. That is pine in the sky and I would like to ask our Dutch colleagues is there a body in the Netherlands that is just waiting for your data that says well we have had a customer that is saying I demand leukocyte-depleted blood for instance and the national body can look at this and say no or yes based on parliamentary or societal reasons. I cannot imagine that ever existing in the USA as I know it, but I can imagine it in those countries that have opted for national blood transfusion services with national regulations.

H.J.C. de Wit (Amsterdam, NL): Part of the answers are given in the lecture by Dr. Emmanuel. The system that you asked for is different in different countries depending on laws, on tradition, on culture and what you can afford. For the Netherlands I can give a clear answer: yes, there is a body waiting for pharmaco-economic studies like presented here by Dr. Postma. Yes, we need evaluations of quality adjusted life years and cost for new safety measures to be taken in the field of blood transfusion but also in other fields of health care. That body is our government, because in the Netherlands with the law on blood transfusion, blood transfusion and other health care aspects too are regulated by the Ministry of Health. So, our discussion as a blood transfusion organisation is mainly with the Ministry of Health, who will reimburse all costs of blood and blood transfusion in hospitals. If they do not accept a new costly safety measure, hospitals will not be reimbursed. It is then very hard to introduce it and that is the situation at this moment for universal leukocyte depletion, where the discussions are going sky high.

II. TECHNICAL AND PHARMACEUTICAL DEVELOPMENTS

FREEZING AND VITRIFICATION OF RED CELLS, RECOLLECTIONS AND PREDICTIONS

H.T. Meryman[1]

The subject of red cell freezing has been reviewed repeatedly since the first report of glycerol cryoprotection by Audrey Smith in 1950 [1]. At least four books on the subject have been published [2-5] and the science, the technology and the applications have been so exhaustively documented that yet another review of red cell freezing seems largely redundant. What is still missing, however, are those obscure and statistically insignificant events that never found their way into print, often for good reason, and known only to a few of the rapidly diminishing ranks of octogenarians who were there at the creation. The goal of this review, therefore, is not only to summarize the topic as it is understood today but also to recall the human side of some of the milestones in the development of red cell freezing, many of them autobiographical.

The real pioneers of red cell freezing were Basil Luyet, Max Strumia, JJ Griffitts et al and Carl Walter and John Gibson, all of whom first reported their early experiences in the proceedings of a conference held by the Committee on Blood and Blood Derivatives of the (US) National Research Council in 1949. Luyet [6] had recovered intact red cells following ultra-rapid freezing and thawing, but the conditions were so demanding that only minute volumes could be frozen. Strumia [7] showed that red cells could be frozen at -3°C for at least 24hrs without hemolysis. Griffitts et al [8] reported that 16% human serum albumin plus saline or glucose enabled human red cells to be quick frozen at -60°C and thawed at +45°C with a "considerable proportion of cells surviving as measured by the degree of hemolysis." Three of these reports were unwittingly exploiting vitrification long before its potential role in red cell freezing was recognized.

During the 1950s, another approach with real clinical potential emerged: glycerol cryoprotection.

Cryoprotection by glycerol was discovered at the Mill Hill laboratories outside of London by Chris Polge, Audrey Smith and Allan Parkes [10]. Parkes, later to be Sir Allan, was the Director of the Laboratories. Chris Polge, whose interest was animal breeding, was looking into the possibility of freezing fowl sperm.

1. Cryopreservation and Transfusion Program, Naval Medical Research Center, Silver Spring, MD, USA.

Years later, Jim Lovelock, who spent several years at Mill Hill, told me the following account of the experiments.

A microscope with a freezing stage was designed so that the freezing process could be directly observed and photographed. Multiple spears of ice could be seen to shoot through the suspension of sperm cells until the image turned opaque. As the ice melted, only lifeless forms remained. The possibility that the sperm were actually being speared by the ice was considered. Sugars and other solutes were added in an attempt to change the way the ice grew but dead sperm were always the result. At one point, probably to the relief of the frustrated investigators, the experiments were temporarily suspended because of competing priorities.

Some time later, the project was revived where it had left off. The bottle containing the most recent mixture of sugars was retrieved from the fridge and some of its contents added to a sperm suspension on the cold stage. Ice moved across the field of view. The image turned opaque. The ice retreated. And there, amazingly, were the spermatozoa, wiggling away as though nothing had happened. The experiment was repeated again and again and it worked every time. Parkes was ecstatic and a few days later one of the titled ladies who was a laboratory sponsor was brought in to see the show. It was the breakthrough of the century!

By now the reagent in the bottle was almost gone and a new batch was made up. But it didn't work. The old stuff worked, the new stuff didn't. It was a crisis. Ultimately, an embarrassed technician confessed that, when he had gone to the fridge to get the original bottle, he found that the labels had fallen off of many of the bottles and he had put them back where he thought they belonged. So now no one knew what the magic elixir was.

Two floors down was a world-famous analytical chemist. Polge took the mystery bottle down to him. He explained the gravity of the situation; the potential for frozen storage of many living things that could revolutionize biology and medicine, endless horizons, fame and fortune for Mill Hill. "I understand," replied the chemist, "I hope I can tell you what's in it. Give me the bottle." Then, somehow, between hand and hand, the bottle slipped, fell onto a soapstone laboratory bench and shattered. There was a moment of silence. "Well," said the chemist, "I guess we'll never know. But I'll tell you one thing. Did you notice the odor when the drop fell on the hot plate? It's got glycerol in it."

Later, in his autobiography, Parkes described the discovery of glycerol [11]. It was a sanitized account compared to Lovelock's. Precisely where the truth lies I can't be sure, but I prefer Lovelock's version.

Shortly thereafter, in 1950, Audrey Smith reported a single experiment with human red cells, demonstrating recovery after freezing in 15% glycerol [12] and triggering a flurry of experiments by others. In 1951, Sloviter [13] repeated Audrey's experiments, also with a final concentration of 15% glycerol, frozen relatively rapidly using dry ice, thawed rapidly and deglycerolized by dialysis against a succession of four diminishing concentrations of glycerol in isotonic saline. Very shortly thereafter, Mollison and Sloviter [14] reported the first successful transfusion of frozen red cells, using 250ml of cells in 15% glycerol, deglycerolized by dialysis over a 24hr period. They reported a 70% recovery and in vivo survival of the remaining cells comparable to unfrozen controls. Clinically feasible red cell freezing could now be safely predicted.

In 1952, Mollison, Sloviter and Chaplin [15] reported good in vivo survival after storage at –79°C for 6 months although recovery was only about 50% since, as we now know, the glycerol concentration was too low for storage at that temperature. Lovelock [16], that same year, simplified deglycerolization by adding hypertonic sodium citrate to the thawed cells, anticipating our own 'break-through innovation' years later of hypertonic saline addition as the first step in deglycerolizing [17]. Careful rereading of the early literature can be sobering.

In 1953, Chaplin and Mollison [18] raised the final glycerol concentration to 40% and demonstrated good storage stability for over 3 months at a temperature as high as -20(°. True colligative freezing in which ice formation could not cause lethal cell dehydration at any temperature had at last been achieved. The final important advance took place that same year when Chaplin and Veall [19] deglycerolized red cells using a continuous-flow washing technique developed in 1950 by Buckley, Gibson, D'Hart and Tinch [20]. They rotated an Ehrlenmeyer flask about its long axis so that the blood stood against the walls of the flask. Wash solution was introduced at the periphery and collected from near the axis, an approach essentially identical to the eventual Haemonetics system. Nearly all of the important developments in red cell freezing techniques during the subsequent 5 decades were anticipated during those three early years.

However, understanding the mechanism of action of glycerol did not come easily. It was obvious that glycerol reduced the amount of ice formed on a purely colligative basis. Lovelock [21] proposed that red cells were denatured by salts that were concentrated by the freezing out of water. Reducing the amount of ice reduced the concentration to a tolerable level. Subsequent studies by Mazur [22] and by Meryman [23, 24] demonstrated that cell injury correlated not with salt concentration per se but with osmotic dehydration of the cells. Although the precise mechanism has yet to be elucidated, it is generally now agreed that, at an osmolality much above 1200 mosm, the resulting cell dehydration and cell volume reduction leads to membrane alterations, an influx of otherwise impermeant solutes, and ultimate hemolysis.

A colligative cryoprotectant must therefore meet two criteria. It must penetrate the cell otherwise it will itself cause dehydration, and it must be non-toxic at the multi-molar concentrations required. These are demanding criteria. Glycerol is remarkably non-toxic. A facilitated transport mechanism [25] is apparently responsible for its passage into red cells but it penetrates most other cells very slowly or not at all. Dimethyl sulfoxide (DMSO), first proposed as a cryoprotectant by Lovelock and Bishop [26], penetrates most cells very rapidly but becomes toxic at much over 1M. A number of other solutes have been tested as cryoprotectants, particularly sugars, glycols and alcohols. Those that do penetrate cells readily, such as methanol and ethanol, protect against freezing injury as predicted but rapidly reach toxic concentrations [24], generally at concentrations too low to be useful.

Vitrification

To some extent, the concentration of colligative cryoprotectants and therefore the toxicity of cryoprotectants like DMSO can be reduced by increasing the rate of freezing. Cells do not contain ice nuclei. In the absence of nuclei, pure water will super cool to -40°C. Since ice nuclei are present in the extracellular solution, ice always forms first outside the cells. As it grows, increasing the extracellular osmolality, water flows from inside the cells to contribute to the extracellular ice. If the rate of cooling is increased, less time is available for the movement of water and a low, stabilizing temperature may be reached before lethal cell dehydration has taken place.

For unfrozen, freezable water to be stable, it must have become a glass, i.e., be vitrified. This occurs when lowering the temperature has, for all practical purposes, increased the viscosity of the solution until the translational movement of water molecules effectively ceases at a point termed the glass transition temperature, Tg'. Tg' for pure water is somewhere around -160°C [27] but increasing the solute concentration, especially with solutes such as sugars and polymers that contribute to viscosity, can raise Tg' to very high temperatures. Seeds, for example, owe their stability to glass transition temperatures well above ambient [28]. Freezing platelets with 5% DMSO depends on the establishment of extracellular vitrification as does the 'low glycerol' red cell freezing method which will be discussed shortly. Both require rapid cooling and warming rates and low storage temperatures.

The ultimate application of this principle is found in the ultra-rapid freezing and thawing of cells which can, in extreme cases, be accomplished in the complete absence of cryoprotectant [6]. My own serendipitous introduction to both red cells and to cryobiology was via this route.

Cryopreservation of Red Cells by Vitrification

In 1948 I was an electron microscopist at the Naval Medical Research Institute in Bethesda, Maryland, struggling with the first electron microscope made in the US, the RCA EMB. O-rings had yet to be available and the EMB used flat rubber gaskets coated with grease. The EMB had a 90% down time because of vacuum leaks. Its high voltage tank sat on the top of the instrument and in the humid Washington summer, it would periodically arc over with an explosion heard throughout the institute. As a result, I acquired the only air-conditioned lab in the building.

At that time it was generally agreed that electron microscopy had no applications in biology since the specimens were hydrated and were incompatible with the high vacuum. Being young, naive, and therefore fearless, I built a liquid nitrogen-cooled stage for the EMB as well as a vacuum evaporation system where replicas could be made at liquid nitrogen temperature [29,30]. We took pictures of bacteria, bacterial viruses and a variety of ice surfaces. We even did freeze-fracturing of tissues a decade before Branton received but we had neither the resolution nor the insight to appreciate what we were seeing.

At that time, a well-known physiologist named Melvin Knisely was studying a remarkable phenomenon that he called 'sludged blood' in which red cells stuck together in clumps in certain diseased states such as pneumococcic pneumonia, CML and Plasmodium malaria [31]. With a slit lamp one could easily see the clumps flowing jerkily through the bulbar conjunctival vessels, sometimes momentarily blocking them. A colleague of Knisely's, E. H. Bloch, spent the summer of 1952 with us in order to look at them with the EM. One of the 'diseased states' is acute hangover (Knisely was a teetotaler on the basis of that observations) so we had no problem getting good blood samples at the Navy Base. Sure enough, in the EM, by both transmission and replication, the frozen red cells had fuzzy coats [32] whereas normal cells were crisp and clean. But it was almost a year before it dawned on me, oblivious to Luyet's earlier observations, that those red cells, frozen to liquid nitrogen temperature, were intact. We decided to try scaling up the procedure.

I had an elderly technician, Emanuel Kafig, whom I had pirated from an applied physics laboratory to help me set up the electron microscope. Manny had been a chicken farmer and a free-lance photographer in a prior life. He was without formal education but he was ingenious. He constantly tried impossible things without telling me, like heating a vacuum or thawing red cells in urine because it was a natural body fluid, but every so often he would announce out of the blue, "Doc, it worked!" and I would have to figure out what he had done. I also had my own lathe, mill and drill press right in my lab. Mr. Kafig and I built a motor-driven device (Figure 1) that sprayed blood onto the surface of liquid nitrogen where the little droplets would dance around on the surface for a moment until they sank to the bottom. When the frozen droplets were retrieved and sifted into warm saline, the recovery was good. Adding 7 gm% glucose resulted in 97% recovery. If the cells could survive after transfusion, we were on our way to Stockholm.

In vivo survival studies using ^{51}Cr were pretty new and I had some misgivings about being my own guinea pig but there were no other volunteers. To spray-freeze enough blood for the study, we built a liquid nitrogen tank out of a used 55 gallon oil drum insulated with cotton wool. We inserted a funnel-shaped insert at the bottom to collect the droplets as they froze and sank, ending up in a brass cup. The cup had a screen for a bottom and a little crank like a pepper grinder. When the time came for thawing, we could fish it out of the nitrogen and sift the frozen droplets into a dish of warm saline that was being agitated in a warm water bath.

Ray Schulman, later to be a distinguished hematologist at the NIH, was my neighbor at the Navy laboratory. He did the venipuncture as I lay on a laboratory bench. Mr. Kafig caught the blood in an open beaker containing anticoagulant and glucose (Figure 2). Then it was poured into the syringe that fitted into the spraying system. We all stood around the oil drum as the sprayer rotated, watching the droplets dancing on the surface of the liquid nitrogen, freezing and sinking. I looked across at my number two technician, Willy Platt. He had a cigarette in his mouth and ashes were sifting down into the drum along with my blood.

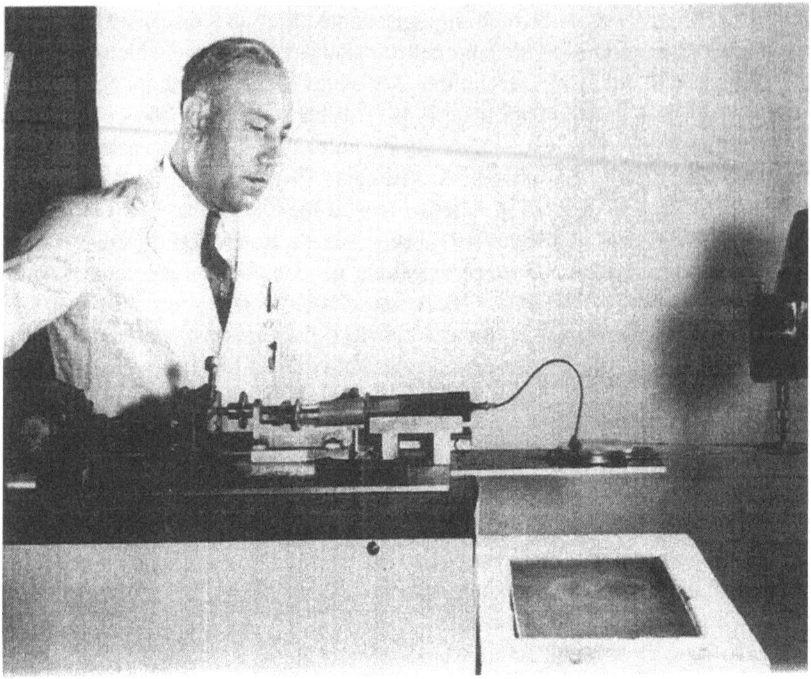

Figure 1. Emanuel Kafig operating the blood spraying device. Blood is pumped through the loop of tubing seen on the right by a motor-driven syringe. The vinyl tubing has been drawn to a point to create a thin stream of blood that freezes in 1-2mm droplets on the surface of liquid nitrogen in the pan as the sprayer is rotated by a motor and belt at the right of the sprayer from underneath the syringe.

In vivo survival studies using ^{51}Cr were pretty new and I had some misgivings about being my own guinea pig but there were no other volunteers. To spray-freeze enough blood for the study, we built a liquid nitrogen tank out of a used 55 gallon oil drum insulated with cotton wool. We inserted a funnel-shaped insert at the bottom to collect the droplets as they froze and sank, ending up in a brass cup. The cup had a screen for a bottom and a little crank like a pepper grinder. When the time came for thawing, we could fish it out of the nitrogen and sift the frozen droplets into a dish of warm saline that was being agitated in a warm water bath.

Ray Schulman, later to be a distinguished hematologist at the NIH, was my neighbor at the Navy laboratory. He did the venipuncture as I lay on a laboratory bench. Mr. Kafig caught the blood in an open beaker containing anticoagulant and glucose (Figure 2). Then it was poured into the syringe that fitted into the spraying system. We all stood around the oil drum as the sprayer rotated, watching the droplets dancing on the surface of the liquid nitrogen, freezing and sinking. I looked across at my number two technician, Willy Platt. He had a cigarette in his mouth and ashes were sifting down into the drum along with my blood I spent a restless night thinking about the radioactive chromium, the cigarette ashes and the frozen red cells that had never been transfused into anyone before. The next day we thawed the blood by sifting it into the open dish of warm saline. I got back on the laboratory bench while Ray hung up the bag of red stuff and put the needle in my arm. As the red stuff came down the tubing and disappeared into me, I had the sensation of heat around the needle, going up my arm, into my chest, and I felt I couldn't breath. "You damned fool," I thought, "you were going to be a hero and now you're going to die." "Ray," I croaked, "something's happening." Ray stopped the infusion and took my pulse as the sensation passed. The infusion continued and the 24-hr survival was normal [33].

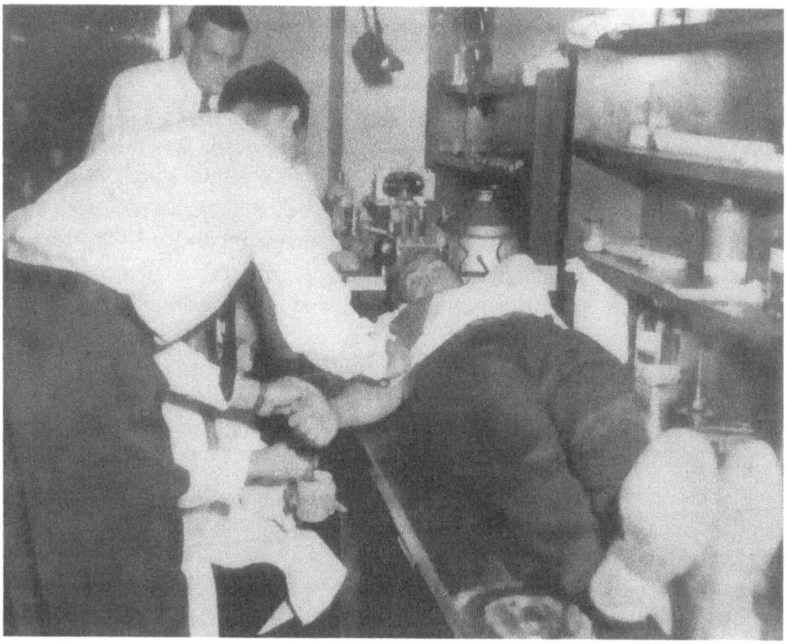

Figure 2. The author lies on a lab bench (behind the shoes). Ray Schulman administers the venipuncture. Manny Kafig catches the blood in a beaker while Willy Platt looks on.

The Office of Naval Research awarded the Linde Division of Union Carbide Corp. a multi-million dollar contract to develop the spray-freeze technique for clinical use. The Navy saw it as the answer to red cell storage, a '1-step' product that could simply be thawed and transfused. The Linde people built a fantastic device that sprayed blood from multiple needles onto a water-fall of liquid nitrogen. As a gadget it was an engineer's dream; as a potential clinical procedure it was a nightmare [34].

In our original experiments, we had achieved almost perfect recoveries when we added the polymer, polyvinylpyrrolidone (PVP), which had been used during the war by the Germans as a plasma substitute. The Linde group, which included Art Rinfret and Art Rowe, experimented with it, looking for some common denominator among cryoprotectants that could help explain the mechanism. Although understanding the mechanism remained decades away, they did confirm the fact previously observed by several other investigators [reviewed in 2,35] that the addition of polymers substantially reduced the required rate of freezing and thawing. This in turn enabled cells to be frozen in metal containers with a degree of asepsis unattainable with the waterfall [36]. A new class of cryoprotectants had been introduced; agents that remained extracellular, thereby avoiding the osmotic problems that made glycerol so difficult to introduce and remove. The only caveat immediately apparent was the requirement that the polymer be transfusable.

Max Strumia showed that sugars also permitted reduced cooling and thawing rates [37] but, unfortunately, concentrations high enough to be effective proved toxic in dog experiments [38]. An inclusive review of the reports of many investigators using a wide variety of cryoprotective agents was published in 1966 by Doebbler, Rinfret and Rowe [35].

Unfortunately, PVP, as well as the other polymers that were subsequently investigated by others, such as dextran by Strumia [39], serum albumin by Steinbuch and Quentin in France [40], and hydroxyethyl starch (HES) by Knorpp et al [41], all had the same Achilles Heel. Although recoveries after thawing as high as 97% could be reproducibly obtained with PVP [42], following transfusion, intravascular hemolysis of the order of 10 to 20 percent or more always occurred. In 1976, Allen et al [43] showed by electron microscopy that many cells frozen and thawed with HES had extensive membrane lesions although, remarkably, the cells had not lost their hemoglobin. It was not until 1975 that Bob Williams [44] in our laboratory unraveled the mystery, showing that the concentrated polymer raised the surface activity of the extracellular solution sufficiently above that of hemoglobin to create a stable interface so that hemoglobin remained within the boundaries of the cell despite major membrane disruption. With transfusion, this 'Band-Aid effect' was lost as the polymer was diluted, releasing hemoglobin from damaged cells.

The Allen and Weatherbee electron micrographs also showed very small, probably healable defects in red cells suspended in HES solution prior to freezing, suggesting that it is the polymer itself that is somehow responsible for the membrane damage and that the increase in polymer concentration during freezing serves to increase defect size beyond what might heal on thawing. The early studies of sludged blood by Bloch et al [32] also demonstrated the fuzzy coat on red cells suspended in PVP. The British Army maintained a research unit that for many years attempted to produce a clinically useful product, directed in succession by Colonels Witcher, Robson and Thomas. Despite extensive efforts by these and many other investigators, a way of preventing the membrane lesions and the subsequent intravascular hemolysis has yet to be found.

Although full units of red cells have been frozen in HES and transfused by both Sputtek [45] and Thomas et al [46] with acceptable 24-hr survival, the transfusion of multiple units results in hemoglobinuria. Furthermore, our own (unpublished) studies have shown that, after washing, the remaining cells are unstable during subsequent refrigerated storage, with hemolysis progressing rather rapidly. Plasma and Human Serum Albumin can delay this hemolysis but the percent hemolysis still rises above 1% within 2-3 days. It should be pointed out parenthetically, that attempts to freeze-dry red cells frozen with polymers will also have to deal with this form of freezing injury in addition to potential damage during drying and rehydration.

1-step freezing of red cells remains a tantalizing mirage. The development of new, automated red cell washing techniques has raised the possibility that a processing step fast enough and simple enough to preserve the essence of the 1-step method might help to salvage this potentially useful storage system, but the cause of and the prevention of the membrane lesions and the resulting post-thaw instability remain unresolved.

The Clinical Use of Frozen Red Cells

Red cells cryoprotected with glycerol are the only frozen red cells currently licensed. The principle obstacle to the widespread use of frozen red cells was and continues to be the deglycerolization process. In 1953, Chaplin and Veall [19] were obliged to performed 5-6 centrifugation steps over the course of as many hours in order to reduce the glycerol concentration to a transfusable level. The obstacle, of course, is cell swelling as the extracellular glycerol concentration is reduced below that present within the cells, so that deglycerolization becomes a tightrope walk between osmotic hemolysis and tedium.

Using their 'long traverse centrifuge', Chaplin and Veal were the first to introduce continuous flow washing. However, in 1954 a more sophisticated effort was reported by Tullis [47] in Boston, using the centrifugal device developed by A.D. Little for the automation of the Cohn plasma fractionation procedure. As later reported by Ketchel et al [48], the device was complex and the procedure time-consuming, taking 45-50 min to glycerolize and 90-120 min to deglycerolize, and served primarily to stimulate Latham to develop something better. The successor to the Cohn Fractionator was the Model 10, which mixed concentrated glycerol solution and isotonic saline according to a program etched on photographic film. The procedure still required nearly 90 minutes to deglycerolize. Part of the problem was the very slow initial sedimentation of the cells while they were still suspended in concentrated glycerol, an obstacle ultimately overcome by first adding hypertonic saline to shrink the cells as well as to partially dilute the glycerol [16,17].

Meanwhile, Huggins was utilizing the phenomenon of agglomeration for deglycerolization [49,50], having noticed how red cells clumped as red cells and glucose solution were simultaneously infused into a patient. Huggins was the first to produce a licensed product and his agglomeration apparatus was widely used. The Navy set up a frozen red cell station in Da Nang during the Vietnam War [51], demonstrating the potential for frozen red cells in combat. The agglomeration procedure suffered from relatively poor recovery because of cells that failed to form clumps and the cells were not stable during temperature rise from freezer malfunctions. However, it was Charlie Huggins who pioneered the clinical use of frozen cells, who convinced the blood banking and transfusion communities that frozen red cells were clinically effective and who prepared the stage for subsequent developments.

Another approach to simplifying deglycerolization was pursued more or less independently by Art Rowe [52], Jim Pert [53] and Herman Krijnen [54], all of whom reduced the glycerol concentration used to roughly half that 4M used by the Boston group and more comparable to Audrey Smith's original formula. Reducing the glycerol concentration sacrificed the stability of colligative freezing and required relatively rapid cooling in order to achieve vitrification. Rowe used large stainless steel canisters of thin cross section that were later replaced by a polyolefin plastic bag fabricated by Union Carbide Corp. Pert attempted to use plastic containers in metal frames but, at that time, only Teflon could withstand the low temperature and fabrication was a major problem. Krijnen developed a method using cylindrical metal containers based originally on the commercial spray can. All methods required rapid cooling and storage in liquid nitrogen to maintain the temperature below the glass transition temperature of the glycerol solution.

Linde, a manufacturer of liquid nitrogen as well as a pioneer in 1-step freezing, was active in the design of freezing storage and shipping apparatus. One of their counter-intuitive innovations worth recalling was the coating of the aluminum freezing containers with a thin layer of insulation. In practice, the metal container was dipped first in glycerol, then in PVP powder. The insulating layer thus created provided a sufficient temperature gradient so that boiling of the liquid nitrogen at the surface was minimized. Since the boiling nitrogen gas at an uncoated metal surface would produce far more insulation than that of a layer of PVP, the cooling rate was substantially increased. During thawing in a water bath, the insulating layer washed off to permit maximum heat transfer.

The requirement for liquid nitrogen storage was possibly a reason for the failure of the 'low glycerol' procedure to replace high glycerol in the United States. Freezers capable of temperatures below -80°C were unavailable at the time. Whereas the FDA permitted refreezing of high glycerol cells experiencing freezer failures of less than 24 hours duration, even a brief rise in the storage temperature of low glycerol cells results in total hemolysis. This method did simplify manual deglycerolizing by repeated centrifugation but, in practice, the same Haemonetics, IBM and Fenwal devices used for deglycerolizing the high glycerol product were generally used for the low glycerol so that major economies were not achieved.

Other attempts to deal with the obstacle of deglycerolizing were to use cryoprotectants such as DMSO that crossed the red cell membrane rapidly [55], thereby minimizing the osmotic effects that complicated the glycerol procedures. However, using concentrations high enough to provide colligative stability proved difficult.

The lion's share of the credit for the practical development of Audrey Smith's basic 'high glycerol' system goes to Allan 'Jack' Latham. Jack doggedly pursued his dream of frozen red cells beginning with the Cohn Fractionator in collaboration with Jim Tullis and the Protein Foundation, then the Model 10, followed by the stainless steel bowl and, ultimately, the disposable bowl. Very little of his work was published outside of committee reports. A substantial portion of his work was supported by the Navy and conducted at the Chelsea Naval Hospital in collaboration with Tullis, Surgenor, Haynes, Henderson,

Runck, Sproul, Valeri and others. The early engineering development was conducted by Arthur D. Little, Inc., in Cambridge where Jack was a Senior Engineer. Navy funding was then, as now, unreliable from year to year and much of the instrumentation came from Jack's beautifully equipped basement shop and funded from his own pocket. When development began to merge into production, A. D. Little spun Jack off into the 500 Company, (Jack told me that the name came from the number on their first check) and shortly thereafter Haemonetics was formed.

Those were the glory days of the stainless steel bowl. The addition of glycerol was conducted, and still is in many places, using the Burrell paint shaker, a brute force, low tech approach of great efficiency. But it was the Latham bowl that set the standard for elegance if not of practicality. It weighed 17 pounds, had to be disassembled, cleaned, reassembled, wrapped and autoclaved after every use. An adapter enabled it to be mounted in the PR-6 clinical centrifuge. And it worked.

At the Red Cross Blood Research Laboratory, to which I had moved in 1968 to optimize the deglycerolizing protocol [17], the Latham Bowl provided the crucial element required to create a clinically feasible system. It was time for FDA licensure.

We sent a letter to the FDA outlining our protocol and got our IND more or less by return mail. We made up some bag and tubing sets for our ^{51}Cr 24hr survival studies which we performed mainly on laboratory personnel. We provided the FDA with percent red cell recovery, osmolality as an surrogate measure of residual glycerol and our survival data. We cited storage data reported by Jim Tullis using the Cohn Fractionator to request a frozen storage shelf-life of 2 years. Period. Those were the good old days.

Three weeks seemed like an awfully long time to wait for a ruling from the FDA and we were getting impatient. Finally the call came from Lew Barker, then head of the Division of Blood Products. "Harry," he said, "I've got a little problem with your licensure request." "Oh?" I said, apprehensibly. "Yes, you want to freeze red cells at any time up to their 21-day expiration but you only gave us survival data on cells stored up to six days." Tibi Greenwalt and I chewed that one over. Another set of survival studies was not an attractive prospect. "Oh Hell," said Tibi, "Let's just go for the six days." And that's still the way it is 30 years later.

Boston was the first Red Cross Blood Center to try frozen cells. But they needed disposable bag and tubing sets. I bought a lot of tubing, bags and fittings from Fenwal and took them down to Goodwill Industries in Washington, D.C. along with some sample sets and bottles of cyclohexanone. They lined up a bunch of their handicapped workers at long tables and made 1000 sets for me, cheap. We had them sterilized by ethylene oxide and off they went, first to Allan Kliman and Irma Szymanski in Boston, then to Byron Myhre in Los Angeles. Ultimately there were 10 Red Cross Centers wrestling Latham Bowls into centrifuges. My long-time colleague, Marne Hornblower, also a talented watercolor

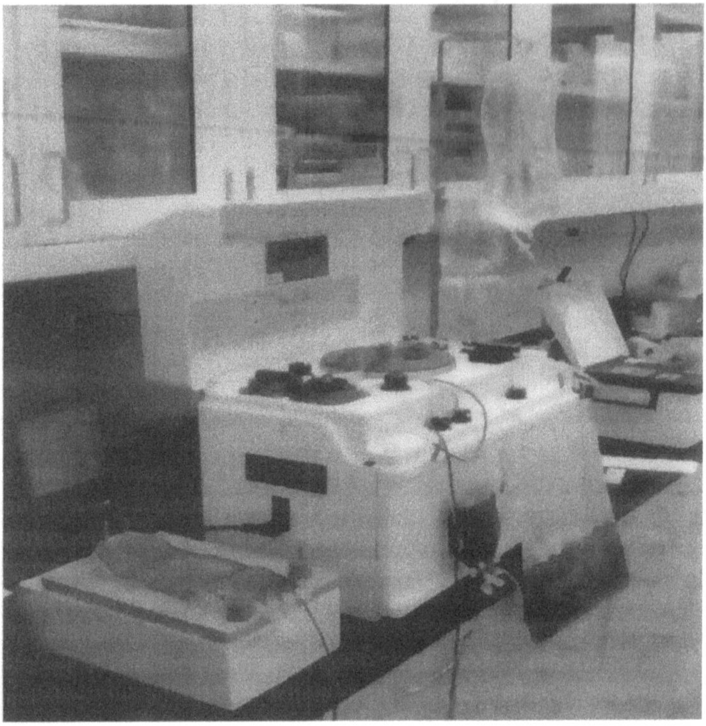

Figure 3. Haemonetics Model 215.

artist, made hand-painted color comparators for the Centers to use to estimate waste hemoglobin concentration.

The stainless bowl, like the Cohn Fractionator and the Model 10, was just a way station for Jack Latham. He was determined to make a disposable bowl. He first made one that was low and wide with rubber sides that fitted into a steel holder. When we checked it out, it washed cells with an efficiency equal to the theoretical maximum but it was clumsy to use. His ultimate goal was the polycarbonate bowl. The first designs didn't work too well. The angle and shape of the center post proved to be critical to efficiency and impossible to predict. Jack used to come down to Bethesda every couple of weeks with a new shape to test until he got it right and the Model 15 was born.

Frozen and deglycerolized red cells turned out to have some virtues other than prolonged storage. At the time, they provided the best leukocyte reduction available [56] and it was suspected, but never adequately proven, that they were less likely to transmit hepatitis B [58]. In their peak year, 1977, approximately 200,000 units of red cells were frozen in the US. Valeri introduced the concept of 'rejuvenating' outdating red cells with a brief incubation in a solution containing inosine, pyruvate, glucose and phosphate to restore ATP and 2,3 DPG and to improve survival [58]. Since the solution was not transfusable, the cells were washed, acquiring a 24-hr outdate, then frozen to provide additional storage time.

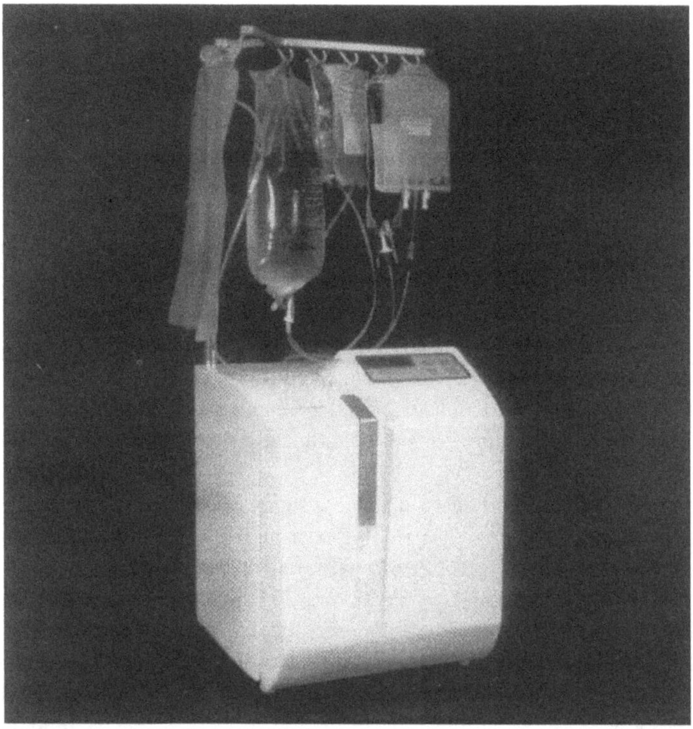

Figure 4. Mission Medical Model 1000.

Over the past 30 years, basic red cell freezing has changed little. The Haemonetics and the Cobe (originally developed by George Judson of IBM [59]) devices have remained pretty much the same since the late 1970s. The Fenwal Eleutramatic developed by Charlie Schlutz and David Bellamy [60] circumvented the rotating seal by use of the ingenious 'jump rope' which also enabled two units to be deglycerolized at the same time. That apparatus was quite effective but the complexity of the assembly and its higher cost were obstacles to widespread use. Valeri modified the Red Cross Protocol in several ways [61] for use by the Navy but still using the Haemonetics Model 15 and its successor, the 115.

A major shortcoming of frozen cells has always been the use of spikes to enter bags or bottles which, although aseptic, could not be considered sterile, or 'closed.' Lacking a closed system, a 24 hour outdate was imposed on the product because of the risk of microbial contamination. The 'sterile docking' device now available from Haemonetics and the use of 0.2(m bacterial filters for the introduction of solutions resolves this problem. The rotating seal required in both the Haemonetics and the Cobe machines, which was for years an obstacle to classifying the systems as closed, has now been approved as sterile, at least for the latest Haemonetics device, opening the door to extended refrigerated storage after deglycerolization.

At least 2 companies are now developing automated closed systems for processing frozen red cells. Haemonetics' Model 115 has metamorphosed into the Model 215 (Figure 3). Mission Medical, Inc., a new player from Fremont, CA, is using hollow fibre technology rather than centrifugation in its M-1000 (Figure 4), an approach that achieves deglycerolization in 30 min compared to 60 for the 215. In both systems, the red cells to be glycerolized are initially attached to the processing sets by sterile connection. Both devices maintain sterility during the introduction of glycerol and wash solutions through the inclusion of 0.2(m bacterial filters. Both systems can glycerolize and deglycerolize with the same apparatus. Both systems resuspend the washed cells in a licensed red cell storage solution. A fringe benefit of the hollow fibre system is its ability to deglycerolize sickle trait units using its standard protocol. Sickle cells pack in a centrifugal field unless special precautions are taken [62]. Neither system is as yet licensed for use and the ultimate post-thaw shelf-life has yet to be defined.

The sophistication of modern control systems is offering opportunities for automation and cost savings that did not exist in 1970. The ability to store red cells for weeks after deglycerolization will remove one of the major shortcomings.

Whether or not the 1-step freezing procedure using extracellular cryoprotectants can ever become competitive remains to be seen. Washing after thawing is a significant compromise, the loss of cells is not insignificant and the instability of the cells after washing seriously limits their usefulness. The development of a means for preventing the membrane lesions could breathe new hope into the method. The availability of mechanical freezers capable of maintaining -120°C or below can eliminate the need for liquid nitrogen storage, but the rapid and total hemolysis of the frozen cells during temperature rise is an unavoidable shortcoming of any freezing procedure that depends on vitrification.

Fifty years later, the progeny of Audrey Smith's glycerol procedure continue to be the dominant red cell freezing methods. Although the current procedures are still technically demanding and time-consuming, the imminent availability of closed systems with extended post-thaw storage and automation that can eliminate the need for skilled technicians will make frozen red cells more attractive for many special situations. In many countries the increasing shortage of safe donors and of adequate donor testing has created serious problems of blood supply, especially for small permanent military or civilian missions, problems that could be solved by maintaining stocks of easily mobilized frozen red cells. The increasing frequency of blood shortages has already led some blood banks to maintain a small emergency reserve of frozen red cells. The changing economics of blood collection and the critical problems faced in supplying safe transfusions may serve to re-establish frozen red cells as an important specialty blood component. Although cost remains an inevitable obstacle, reducing the need for skilled technicians and extending the post-thaw shelf life eliminates two of the serious deficiencies that have previously limited the use of this clinically effective product. And it was fun getting there.

References

1 Smith AU. Prevention of hemolysis during freezing and thawing of red blood cells. Lancet 1950;2:910-11.
2. Turner AR. Frozen blood. New York: Gordon and Breach, 1970.
3. Red cell freezing: A technical workshop. Washington, DC: American Association of Blood Banks, 1973.
4. Valeri CR. Blood banking and the use of frozen blood products. Cleveland: CRC Press, 1976.
5. Clinical and practical aspects of the use of frozen blood. Washington, DC: American Association of Blood Banks, 1977.
6. Luyet BJ. Effects of ultra-rapid and of slow freezing and thawing on mammalian erythrocytes. Biodynamica 1949;6:217-23.
7. Strumia M. Freezing of Whole Blood. In: The preservation of the formed elements and of the proteins of the blood. Washington, DC: American National Red Cross, 1949:160-66.
8. Griffitts JJ, Hornibrook JW, Downs JJ. Freezing and thawing red blood cells. In: The preservation of the formed elements and of the proteins of the blood. Washington, DC: American National Red Cross, 1949:167-68.
9. Walter CW, Gibson JG. Freezing of red blood cells. In: The preservation of the formed elements and of the proteins of the blood. Washington, DC: American National Red Cross, 1949:169.
10. Polge C, Smith AU, Parkes AS. Revival of spermatozoa after vitrification and dehydration at low temperatures. Nature 1949;164:666.
11. Parkes AS. Off-beat biologist. Cambridge: Galton Foundation, 1985:438-39.
12. Smith AU. Prevention of hemolysis during freezing and thawing of red blood cells. Lancet 1950;ii:910-11.
13. Sloviter HA. Recovery of human red blood cells after freezing. Lancet 1951;i:823-24.
14. Mollison PL and Sloviter HA. Successful transfusion of previously frozen human red blood cells. Lancet 1951;ii:862-84.
15. Mollison PL, Sloviter HA, Chaplin H. Survival of transfused red cells previously stored for long periods in the frozen state. Lancet 1952;ii:501-05.
16. Lovelock JE. Re-suspension in plasma of human red blood cells frozen in glycerol. Lancet 1952;i:1238-39.
17. Meryman HT, Hornblower M. A method for freezing and washing red blood cells using a high glycerol concentration. Transfusion 1972;12:145-55.
18. Chaplin H, Mollison PL. Improved storage of red cells at -20(. Lancet 1953;i:215-18.
19. Chaplin H, Veall N. Removal of glycerol from previously frozen red cells: a modified method. Lancet 1953;i:218-19.
20. Buckley E, Gibson JG, D'Hart MD, Tinch RJ. "Long Traverse Centrifuge" Proc. 2nd conf. on the separation of the formed elements of the blood. 1950. Boston, MA.
21. Lovelock JE. The mechanism of the protective action of glycerol against haemolysis by freezing and thawing. Biochem Biophys Acta 1953;11:28-36.
22. Mazur P. Causes of injury in frozen and thawed cells. Fed Proc 1965:24(2,pt.3): S175-82.
23. Meryman HT. The exceeding of a minimum tolerable cell volume in hypertonic suspension as a cause of freezing injury. In: Wolstenholme GEW, O'Conner M, eds. The frozen cell. London: J & A Churchill, 1970:51-64.
24. Meryman HT, Williams RJ, Douglas M StJ. Freezing injury from "solution effects" and its prevention by natural or artificial cryoprotection. Cryobiology 1977;14:287-302.
25. Hunter FR. Facilitated diffusion in pigeon erythrocytes. Amer. J. Physiol. 1970;218: 1765-72.

26. Lovelock JE, Bishop MWH. Prevention of freezing damage to living cells by dimethyl sulfoxide. Nature 1959;183:1394-95.
27. Dowell LG, Rinfret AP. Low temperature forms of ice as studied by X-ray diffraction. Nature 1960;188:1144-48.
28. Williams RJ, Bruni F, Leopold AC. Changes in the vitreous state of dry dormant seeds with germination. Cryobiology 1990;27:656.
29. Meryman HT. Replication of frozen liquids by electron microscopy. J Appl Physics 1950;21:68.
30. Meryman HT, Kafig E. The study of frozen specimens, ice crystals and ice crystal growth by electron microscopy. Research Report: Naval Medical Research Institute, Bethesda, MD. 1955;13:529-44.
31. Knisely MH, Elliot TS, Bloch EH. Sludged blood in traumatic shock. Arch Surg 1945;51:220.
32. Bloch EH, Powell A, Meryman HT, Warner L, Kafig E. A comparison of the surfaces of human erythrocytes from health and disease by in vivo light microscopy and in vitro electron microscopy. Angiology 1956;7:479-94.
33. Meryman HT, Kafig E. Rapid freezing and thawing of whole blood. Proc. Soc. Exp. Biol Med 1955;90:587-89.
34. Rinfret AP, Doebbler GF. Observations on the freezing and thawing of blood in droplet form. Biodynamica 1960;8:181-93.
35. Doebbler GF, Rowe AW, Rinfret AP. Freezing of mammalian blood. In: Meryman HT, ed. Cryobiology. New York: Academic Press,1966:407-50.
36. Rinfret AP. Some aspects of preservation of blood by rapid freeze-thaw procedures. Fed Proc 1963;22:94-101.
37. Strumia MM, Colwell LS, Strumia PV. The preservation of blood for transfusion. V. Post-transfusion survival of red cells modified with sugars, frozen, and stored in the frozen state. J Clin Med 1960;56:587-93.
38. Pert JH, Moore R, Schork,PK. Low temperature preservation of human erythrocytes. Bibl Haemat 1964; 23:674-82.
39. Strumia MM, Strumia PV. Recovery and survival of human red cells frozen with albumin, dextran, and lactose-albumin. Bibl Haemat 1962;19:61-8.
40. Steinbuch H, Questin M. Recherches sur la congelation du globule rouge en milieu macromoleculaire. Vox Sang 1958;3:123-42.
41. Knorpp CT, Merchant WR, Gikas PW, Spencer HH, Thompson NW. Hydroxyethyl starch: extracellular cryophylactic agent for erythrocytes.Science 1967;157:1312-13.
42. Bloom, ML, Witebski E, Rinfret AP, Doebbler GF, Cowley CW. Rapidly hard-frozen blood: evaluation of progress and clinical survival. Bibl Haemat 1965;23:642-45.
43. Allen Ed, Weaterbee L, Spencer HH, Lindenauer SM, Permoad PA. Large unit red cell cryopreservation with hydroxyethyl starch. Cryobiology 1976; 13:500-06.
44. Williams RJ. The surface activity of PVP and other polymers and their antihemolytic capacity. Cryobiology 1983;20:521-26.
45. Sputtek A, Körber Ch, Rau G. Cryopreservation of human erythrocytes with hydroxyethylated starches under variation of starch modification and concentration, electrolyte content, hematocrit, and cooling rate. Cryobiology 1990; 27:667-68.
46. Thomas MJG, Parry ES, Nash SG, Bell SH. A method for the cryopreservation of red blood cells using hydroxyethyl starch as a cryoprotectant. Transfus Sci 1995;17:385-96.
47. Tullis JL. Use of Cohn fractionator in connection with the preservation of red cells in glycerol. In: [Proceedings 9th] Conference of the plasma proteins and cellular elements of the blood. 1954;Cambridge, Mass., Protein Foundation:25-26.
48. Ketchel MM, Tullis JL, Tinch RJ, Driscol SG, Surgenor DM. Use of biomechanical equipment for the long-term preservation of erythrocytes. JAMA 1958;168:404-08.
49. Huggins CE. Preservation of blood by freezing with dimethyl sulfoxide and its removal by dilution and erythrocyte agglomeration. Vox Sang 1963;8;99-100.

50. Huggins CE. A system for the preservation of blood by freezing. Bibl Haemat 1965;23:662-66.
51. Moss GS, Valeri CR, Brodine CE. Clinical experience with the use of frozen blood in combat casualties. N Engl J Med 1968;278:747-52.
52. Rowe AW, Eyster E, Kellner A. Liquid nitrogen preservation of red blood cells for transfusion; a low glycerol-rapid freeze procedure. Cryobiology 1968;5:119-28.
53. Pert JH, Schork PK, Moore R. Low temperature preservation of human erythrocytes: biochemical and clinical aspects. Bibl Haemat 1964;19:47-53.
54. Krijnen HW, de Wit JJFrM, Kuivenhoven ACJ, Loos JA, Prins HK. Glycerol treated human red cells frozen with liquid nitrogen. Vox Sang 1964;9:559-72.
55. Huggins CE. Preservation of transfusions by freezing with dimethyl sulfoxide. Bibl Hemat 1964;19:69-74.
56. Meryman HT, Bross J, Lebovitz R. The preparation of leukocyte-poor red cells: a comparative study. Transfusion 1980;20:285-92.
57. Meryman HT, Yoshinari M, Tokunaga E, Roht L. The effects of red cell freezing and deglycerolizing or of saline washing on post-transfusion hepatitis (abs). Transfusion 1979;19:656
58. Valeri CR. Metabolic regeneration of depleted erythrocytes and their frozen storage. In: The human red cell in vitro. Greenwalt TJ and Jamieson GA, (eds). New York, Grune and Stratton, 1974:281-321.
59. IBM, the CPU that processed blood. Datamation 1973;19:110.
60. Schlutz CA, Bellamy D. Continuous flow cell washing system. Transfusion 1968;8: 299-303.
61. Valeri CR. Simplification of the methods for adding and removing glycerol during freeze-preservation of human red blood cells with the high or low glycerol methods: Biochemical modification prior to freezing. Transfusion 1975;15:195-218.
62. Meryman HT, Hornblower M. Freezing and deglycerolizing sickle-trait red blood cells. Transfusion 1976;16:627-32.

PLASMA FRACTIONATION

P.R. Foster[1]

Introduction

It was in May 1941 at The Walter Reed General Hospital in Washington that a young man with serious injuries became the first person to be treated with Human Albumin supplied from the laboratories of Edwin Cohn at Harvard University. By November 1941, 50 patients had been treated, but on 8th December every bottle available in Boston was flown to the US naval base at Pearl Harbour for the treatment of military casualties. This was administered to a number of severely burned patients, all of whom showed prompt and sustained clinical improvement. On 5th January 1942, after reviewing clinical data from 87 patients, the US National Research Council recommended that Human Albumin be adopted by the armed forces immediately and that output should be increased by transfer of the technology to a number of commercial manufacturers under the general direction of Dr Cohn [1,2].

It was Cohn's vision that the procedure used to prepare Albumin should also be capable of providing a wide range of potentially useful components from human plasma, all in a biophysical state and dose form suitable for clinical administration. This concept, that plasma could be sub-divided or 'fractionated' into individual components to provide a more effective and efficient utilisation of a valuable resource resulted in the wartime provision to the US armed forces of Normal Immunoglobulin for the prevention of measles as well as Human Albumin for the treatment of shock and Fibrin Foam/Thrombin for use as a haemostatic agent. Other products envisioned by Cohn included specific immunoglobulins such as antibodies to mumps, hepatitis and the Rhesus factor; immunoglobulin made suitable for intravenous administration and a range of coagulation factors for the treatment of haemophilia and other disorders of haemostasis [2].

It is a remarkable testament to the foresight, quality and scientific rigour of this work that the methods developed by Cohn and his co-workers not only formed the basis of the plasma fractionation industry that emerged after World

---

1. Scottish National Blood Transfusion Service, Protein Fractionation Centre, Edinburgh, UK.

Table 1. Current products of plasma fractionation.

Product	Clinical indications
Albumin	Volume replacement, albumin replacement
Plasma protein fraction	Volume replacement
IgG (broad spectrum)	IgG deficiencies, prevention of hepatitis A
IgG (specific)	Prevention of Rh(D), treatment of infections eg. Tetanus, hepatitis B, zoster, cytomegalovirus, rabies, pertussis
Factor VIII	Haemophilia A, factor VIII deficiencies
Factor IX	Haemophilia B
Factor IX complex	Anti-coagulant reversal, coagulation disorders
Factor VII	Factor VII deficiency
von Willebrand Factor	von Willebrand's disease
Anti-thrombin III	Antithrombin III deficiency, DIC
Alpha-1-antitrypsin	Alpha-1-antitrypsin deficiency
Fibrinogen	Fibrinogen deficiencies
Thrombin	Haemostasis
Fibrin sealant	Haemostasis
Factor XIII	Factor XIII deficiency
C1-inhibitor	Angioedema

Table 2. Quantity of human plasma fractionated worldwide 1984-1999 [3].

Year	Quantity of plasma (10^6 litres)		
	For profit	Not for profit	Total
1984	9.1	2.9	12.0
1987	10.7	4.2	14.9
1990	12.0	5.5	17.5
1993	14.5	6.3	20.8
1996	14.8	6.5	21.3
1999	18.4	7.7	26.1

Table 3. Distribution of plasma fractionation capacity 1999 [3].

Year	Fractionation capacity (10^6 litres plasma/year)		
	For profit	Not for profit	Total
Europe	7.7	5.2	12.9
North America	10.6	0.2	10.8
Asia	4.8	3.3	8.1
South America	0.1	0.5	0.6
M. East/Africa	0.3	0.5	0.8
Oceania	0.6	–	0.6
Total	24.1	9.7	33.9

War II, but remain the backbone of established practice 60 years later. Today, plasma fractionation is a heavily regulated sector of the pharmaceutical industry, producing a wide range of clinical products (Table 1). In 1999, 26 million litres of human plasma were processed world-wide [3] (Table 2), providing Albumin and Immunoglobulins in tonnage quantities as well as a variety of coagulation factor concentrates for the treatment of haemophilia and other disorders of haemostasis.

Despite these advances many challenges remain. Further advances in product quality should be attainable and new products are under investigation, together with new or improved process technologies. Although the threat of infection from major pathogens such as HIV and the viruses of hepatitis B and hepatitis C has been conquered, concerns remain over the potential for new diseases to be transmitted. Plasma products are expensive and with 70% of the world's fractionation capacity being located in Europe and the USA [3] (Table 3) life-saving products remain unavailable to much of the world's population. In the developed world, sophisticated technologies have been introduced to overcome risks of virus transmission and to provide highly purified products, but less complex methods of manufacture would be more affordable and easier to implement in developing countries. The knowledge base now exists to design processes for this purpose, without detriment to product quality; harnessing the expertise necessary may be the greater problem.

The Origin of Plasma Fractionation

Albumin

In the spring of 1940, in anticipation of the entry of the USA into World-war II, the Transfusion Committee of the National Research Council wondered if a substitute might be found for human plasma. Advice was sought from Edwin Cohn, who pointed out that serum albumin was responsible for 80% of the colloid osmotic pressure of plasma. Based on his already extensive knowledge of the solubility behaviour of proteins [4,5] Cohn immediately began to devise a method for the fractionation of plasma from which albumin and other potentially useful constituents could be obtained. In order to separate proteins according to their solubility behaviour it was necessary to control the solution pH, ionic strength, protein concentration and temperature in the presence of an additive which could reduce protein solubility. Two types of precipitation agent had already been well studied by Cohn, neutral salts such as ammonium sulphate and alcohols such as ethanol. To be suitable for clinical use the agent selected would have to be removed from the product which must also be free from products of bacterial contamination; dialysis, the only technology available for the removal of ammonium sulphate was prone to bacterial contamination, however, the volatile nature of ethanol allowed it to be readily removed by procedures which could be operated much more hygienically such as sublimation during freeze drying. Consequently, ethanol was selected as the precipitation agent, with operation at reduced temperatures to avoid protein denaturation. Basic schemes for the fractionation of plasma according to these principles were developed rapidly during 1940. Initially this work was done with bovine plasma as the military authorities were primarily interested in using bovine albumin in the belief that this would be tolerated in humans. To avoid antigenic reactions a high degree of purification was required, this was the first criteria that the fractionation method had to achieve, the second concerned the product dose form. Cohn proposed a crystalline preparation, but the Subcommittee on Blood Substitutes preferred a 25% solution [1]. This decision was to prove critical in that the solution would have to remain stable in the heat of North Africa and South East Asia. Therefore the fractionation process was designed to ensure the complete removal of heat sensitive constituents, an accelerated test of heat stability devised and research undertaken on further product stabilisation. From the outset Cohn was sceptical that an animal product would be tolerated by humans and he established a parallel programme of work to develop Human Albumin as an alternative [2]. Cohn's judgement proved to be correct when the bovine albumin project was terminated following an unacceptable number of adverse reactions in trials in prison volunteers, including one fatality [1].

Formulation and Pasteurisation of Human Albumin

In order to provide an isotonic solution, a concentration of 0.15M sodium chloride was originally specified and a mercurial preservative added to comply with the requirements of the National Institute of Health. Stability of the product was determined visually after heating for 12 hours at 50°C. Heat sensitive constituents were removed both by partitioning over multiple precipitation steps as well as by depth filtration procedures introduced to clarify the resultant solutions. Heating at 50°C proved a rigorous test of product quality, which proved difficult to meet consistently on the scale-up and transfer of the technology to commercial operation. It was observed that stability could be improved at increased concentrations of sodium chloride and this was therefore raised to 0.3M sodium chloride in March 1943. Subsequently, there were clinical concerns over both the high salt content and the presence of merthiolate in the product [6].

In order to accurately control the adjustment of pH during precipitation Cohn had devised a system of acetate buffers which required a re-precipitation step to remove residual acetate ions. In the course of experimental studies using an intermediate albumin fraction from which acetate had not been removed, Dr Murray Luck at Stanford University found that acetate gave a greater stability than chloride and, following a suggestion from John Edsall, he began a systematic study of longer-chain aliphatic acids which culminated in the discovery that enhanced stability to heat could be obtained in the presence of sodium caprylate and sodium acetyltryptophanate [7]. As well as allowing sodium chloride to be returned to an isotonic concentration, it was suggested by Dr George Scatchard of the Massachusetts Institute of Technology that the product could also be heated in the final container to inactivate bacterial contaminants eliminating the need for a mercurial preservative and with the possibility that the virus of serum hepatitis might also be destroyed [2,8]. The revised formulation, together with heat treatment at 60°C for 10 hours were introduced in 1945, with the recommendation by Cohn that studies be undertaken to determine the conditions required to destroy the agent of hepatitis [1]. Subsequently Gellis and co-workers, using plasma known to be infective, observed no transmission of hepatitis from albumin which had been heated at 60°C for 10 hours [9], findings which were later confirmed by Dr Roderick Murray in a series of extensive experiments using prison volunteers [10,11].

The view is widely held today that pasteurisation was developed by Cohn specifically to remove the risk of hepatitis transmission; for example, Douglas Starr in his epic history of blood [12] states:

"In the early 1940's, as Dr Edwin Cohn prepared albumin for the military, he refused to release the substance until his men could find a way to pasteurize the product, even during the wartime emergency."

As we have seen, Human Albumin issued between 1941 and 1945 was not subjected to pasteurisation. Nor was it concern over hepatitis that drove the research on formulation, but the imperative of making the solution stable for storage in hot climates and the avoidance of bacterial contamination, together with clinical concerns associated with a high salt content and the use of merthiolate as a bacteriostat. It was fortuitous that hepatitis viruses were inactivated under the conditions selected for heat treatment; findings which were confirmed [10] only after Cohn's death in October 1953.

Safety of Albumin

The impressive safety record of Human Albumin is usually ascribed to the fact that the product is pasteurised at 60°C for 10 hours. However, blood samples from Murray's study [10] were subsequently assayed for the presence of hepatitis B surface antigen (HbsAg) to determine more precisely the dates on which volunteers who had been given unheated material were infected. From the relationship between incubation time and virus titre [13] Hoofnagle and Barker were able to estimate that 5 to 6 logs of hepatitis B virus (HBV) had been removed by the manufacturing process prior to pasteurisation [14], implying that the safety of Human Albumin may be determined more by adventitious elimination of viruses over the fractionation process than by pasteurisation. Process steps which may play a role in this regard include partitioning of viruses over precipitation [15], adsorption of viruses to depth filters [16] and inactivation of viruses on freezing and thawing of ethanol precipitates [17]. These observations are still relevant today, especially where process changes to albumin or immunoglobulin products are envisaged, as new procedures must be shown to have a capacity for virus elimination comparable to that of a safe, established process in its entirety, not just the pasteurisation step.

Although Human Albumin is a long established product which is believed to be free from any risk of virus transmission, a number of issues remain to be resolved. The effectiveness of pasteurisation against some non-enveloped viruses is limited [18] and it is not ideal for product safety to be dependent on procedures which may be less robust than a well designed process for virus inactivation. Ultimately, the safety of a plasma product can only be established by extensive monitoring of recipients for evidence of infection. Although this type of surveillance is now commonplace for coagulation factors [19], it has not normally been undertaken with Human Albumin, leaving room for a degree of uncertainty over the true safety of this product.

Transfusion Transmitted Infections

Although problems of infectious disease transmission are being dealt with more fully by other presentations at this symposium, no review of plasma fractionation over the last century would be complete without some reference the tragedy of AIDS, the impact of which cannot be overstated. In her introduction to the Proceedings of the 1983 Congress of the World Federation of Hemophilia in Stockholm, Margareta Blombäck [20] captured the prevailing mood when she wrote:

"During the last two decades, new developments have assured a better general life for the hemophiliac patient. New concentrates are available which have made possible surgery for the disabled, treatment at home and prophylactic treatment. This has increased the life expectancy and quality of life of the hemophiliac, and increased the possibility to better accommodate to society in general. Still there are problems to be solved. The hemophiliacs in the countries with poor economies suffer greatly. Nor are there enough concentrates for all hemophiliacs due to lack of blood and to economic problems. The side effects of treatment with blood products such as liver damage through hepatitis and acquired immune deficiency syndrome, AIDS, are like dark clouds scattered in the sky."

We now know that as Dr. Blombäck penned these words, most haemophiliacs subsequently found to be infected with the human immunodeficiency virus (HIV) had already seroconverted to the virus [21,22] and that the haemophilia community world-wide was on the brink of being engulfed by this terrible disease. However, HIV was soon to be discovered, donor screening tests were developed and plasma products made safe by heat treatment, despite concerns that greater harm would result from exposing sensitive proteins to such conditions [23]. Today, some 20 years after the epidemic began in the USA, some 34 million people have been infected word-wide; the spread of the disease has not been halted, there is still no vaccine available, nor has a satisfactory cure being developed; by contrast, in one of the few successes in the fight against AIDS, blood products were made safe within months of HIV being discovered.

It is also estimated that 200 million people are infected with Hepatitis C world-wide. Although the virus responsible was discovered 10 years ago, a vaccine has still to be developed and no satisfactory treatment is available; by contrast, methods were developed to inactivate hepatitis C virus (HCV) in labile concentrates of coagulation factors even before the virus had been isolated.

Plasma Products

As Cohn had foreseen, once technology for plasma fractionation had been established, plasma products began to play an increasingly important role in modern medicine. Anti-D immunoglobulin was introduced for the prevention of haemolytic disease of the new-born and a range of hyperimmune immunoglobulins introduced for the prevention and treatment of specific infections such as hepatitis B, tetanus, rubella, varicella-zoster, cytomegalovirus and rabies [24]. Prekallikrein activator was discovered to be the cause of vasoactive reactions associated with albumin products [25] and also with adverse reactions which occurred when immunoglobulin prepared by ethanol fractionation was administered intravenously [26], a finding which was key to the development of immunoglobulins suitable for intravenous administration. Advances in ultrafiltration technology also enabled undesirable contaminants, such as aluminium [27] to be removed from albumin [28] and residual ethanol to be removed from albumin and immunoglobulin products with a lower degree of protein aggregation than after freeze drying.

The discovery that calcium is integral to the stability of factor VIII [29] and that the labile nature of factor VIII during manufacturing was primarily due to the use of citrate for anticoagulation [30], led to the determination of solution conditions that allowed factor VIII solutions to be processed much more extensively without substantial loss of yield [31, 32]. The ability to achieve stable formulations of factor VIII was important in the application of advanced dry heat treatment for the inactivation of HCV [33] as well as in the application of chromatographic methods for further purification. The concurrent development of chromatography media with high specificity or high capacity provided a means of removing toxic virucidial chemicals, resulting in coagulation factor concentrates being treated to inactivate pathogens, such as HIV, HBV and HCV and purified to a degree which had not previously been possible [34-36].

Future Product Developments

Although modern plasma products are generally well tolerated, there are a number of areas where further improvement would seem desirable. For example, the development of inhibitors to factor VIII is one of the most serious problems of haemophilia treatment and there is evidence that at least in some instances this may be product related [37]. Therefore there is a need to develop *in vitro* control tests for product selection and batch release and ideally to develop concentrates which are non-immunogenic, even when used by patients who may be especially susceptible to inhibitor formation. Factor IX concentrates have a risk of causing thrombogenic reactions [38] and although this problem has not been observed with highly purified products [39], the absence of validated *in vitro* control tests leaves the possibility that a thrombogenic batch might still be released. The pharmacokinetics of plasma products is also an area that deserves more attention. The half-life of manufactured products is invariably much shorter than that of the endogenous protein in a normal individual. If product half-life could be increased, patients would require fewer infusions, treatment would be less expensive and more product would be available.

For many years, the development of new products was inhibited by a risk of viruses being transmitted to patients in whom the benefit of treatment was unknown. The development of virus inactivation technologies which can be applied to new products has altered this situation and a number of potentially new products are now under evaluation. These include fibrinogen coated albumin spheres as a substitute for platelets [40]; fibronectin based products for wound healing [41] and tissue repair [42]; immunoglobulin M [43], immunoglobulin A [44] and mannose-binding-lectin [45] for the treatment of infections, apotransferrin for the reduction of iron overload [46], inter-alpha-trypsin inhibitor for the treatment of endotoxic shock [47] and ceruloplasmin for replacement therapy in deficiency states [48].

Process Technologies

The preparation of multiple biopharmaceutical products from a common feedstock requires a series of process functions to be performed in a highly integrated manner, with each process stage being carefully designed to meet predetermined objectives of quality, capacity and cost [49]. Protein separation is obtained by fractional precipitation and fractional extraction, with solid-liquid separation being achieved by centrifugation and depth filtration. Chromatographic methods may be employed for further purification or in some instances for adsorption of labile proteins directly from the plasma pool.

The intermediate products that result must be treated to inactivate viruses (Table 4) and then processed to remove toxic chemicals and undesirable solutes such as ethanol, salts and metal ions, as well as to obtain the product potency, concentration and dose form desired. Ultrafiltration, diafiltration and chromatography are now the predominant procedures used for this latter purpose, with suitable equipment becoming generally available over the last 10 to 15 years.

Table 4. Principal technologies for the inactivation of viruses in plasma products.

Product	Virus inactivation technology	Period
Albumin	Terminal pasteurisation, 60°C/10 hours	1945-
Coagulation factors	Pasteurisation, 60°C/10 hours	1979-
	Terminal (dry) heat, 60-68°C/24-72 hours	1983-1992
	Terminal (dry) heat, 80°C/72 hours	1985-
	Solvent/detergent treatment	1985-
Immunoglobulins (IV)	pH4 (+epsin) treatment	Early 1980's
	Solvent/detergent treatment	Mid 1990's
Immunoglobulins (IM)	pH4 treatment	Late 1990's
	Solvent/detergent treatment	Late 1990's

One key technology, not always appreciated, is membrane filtration for the removal of bacterial contaminants. The introduction of cartridge filters during the late-1970's was of enormous importance, providing a much greater capacity and rate of filtration than could be achieved with earlier disc or sheet systems. The subsequent development of synthetic membranes with low-protein-binding characteristics has enabled highly purified concentrates of coagulation factors to be filtered without the protection of protein additives such as albumin.

Following aseptic dispensing, coagulation factors and some immunoglobulin products are freeze dried to ensure that the product remains stable for it's designated shelf-life. Again there have been major advances in equipment design over the last 10 to 15 years, with the introduction of sterilisable driers, enhanced monitoring of process parameters and increased automation. Such advances made an important contribution to the quality of freeze drying that was required to support the application of terminal dry heat treatment for virus inactivation, as well as providing greater reliability and assurance of product safety. It is likely that further advances in product formulation will enable more products to be supplied as solutions, possibly reducing future requirements for freeze drying.

Future Developments in Process Technology

Changes in process technology usually represent a major and costly undertaking. In addition to being suitable for it's intended purpose, new equipment and procedures must be shown to be compatible with surrounding operations and consistent with subsequent downstream processes. Products which may be effected need to be assessed to demonstrate that no detriment has occurred as a result, with the possibility that clinical studies of product efficacy and safety may be required. Although opportunities for change may be restricted by such impediments a number of desirable improvements can be identified.

Industrial centrifuges used for the recovery of protein precipitates at low temperatures tend to have a small solids-holding capacity with respect to the volume of suspension to be processed. The fact that solids removal is a manual procedure adds to the difficulty, making the recovery of precipitates an arduous and hazardous task. In the absence of significant developments by centrifuge manufacturers, many fractionators have replaced centrifugation with depth filtration. Although depth filters have a much greater unit capacity, concerns remain over the need to use filter aid and the limited extent of automation and containment. Refrigerated centrifuges capable of discharging solids semi-continuously, under automatic control, are at an advanced stage of development, promising advances in yield and containment as well as in economy of operation.

Although chromatographic processes are used in the manufacture of many plasma products [50] a number of limitations have still to be resolved. The use of affinity ligands from biological sources introduces a theoretical risk of contamination from animal pathogens. In addition, some chromatographic media having limited tolerance to sanitization regimes necessary to prevent the possibility of adsorbed viruses being carried forward into a subsequent product batch. The difficulty of destroying agents of prion diseases, such as variant Creutzfeldt-Jakob disease (vCJD) will pose a considerable challenge in this regard. Ideally, chromatographic media should either be cheap enough to discard after each use or should be designed to withstand treatment capable of destroying the agent of vCJD, such as autoclaving in the presence 2M NaOH [51]. Some advance in this regard may be possible by utilising synthetic ligands obtained using new approaches to ligand discovery [52].

Although chromatography processes can be automated to perform a predetermined sequence of events, they are incapable of being controlled to correct deviations during processing as changes taking place within the packed bed cannot be monitored. This difficulty can be exacerbated by variations in packing and fluid flow that can occur within the bed. It may be possible to overcome limitations of this type by using ligands bound to membranes rather than to particles, with the prospect that affinity ultrafiltration could become a more robust and less expensive process operation than chromatography for protein purification [53].

Elimination of Viruses

The high degree of safety now enjoyed by plasma products has been achieved by the development of a number of virus inactivation technologies [54] (Table 4) as well as by the adventitious removal of viruses by procedures used for protein purification [15,55]. Despite these advances, concerns remain over the risk of transmission of new viruses [56] and known viruses which are not inactivated by solvent-detergent or low pH treatment and which are relatively resistant to heat treatment. Included in the latter category are the hepatitis A virus (HAV), the human B19 parvovirus and the bovine polyoma virus, a frequent contaminant of cell culture media [57]. In addition, the transmission of hepatitis B virus by a pasteurised factor IX concentrate [58] has led European regulatory authorities to offer the following advice [59]:

"It will be desirable in many cases to incorporate 2 distinct effective steps which complement each other in their mode of action such that any virus surviving the first step would be effectively inactivated or removed by the second."

Some manufacturers are now using two virus inactivation steps in the manufacture of coagulation factor concentrates, such as solvent-detergent treatment plus dry heat treatment at 80°C. It would seem to be a good practice for this principle to be applied to all plasma products.

There is considerable interest in using membrane filters to remove viruses which may not be destroyed by current virus inactivation procedures [60]. At the present time, filters of this type are expensive, they have a low capacity and cannot yet be applied to all plasma products. Their effectiveness in removing all virus particles of concern may be limited by a distribution in pore size which can be broad enough to allow some virus particles to pass through the membrane. Such 'leakage' of virus may be more likely to occur in routine large-scale operation than in small-scale equipment used for the measurement of virus removal, because the latter equipment usually operates with a greater degree of concentration polarisation at the membrane surface, a feature which acts as a secondary filter. It is for this reason that current nanofiltration technology should be regarded as providing a reduction in virus load, rather than absolute removal. To advance this technology further, less expensive membranes with a much more uniform pore size would be desirable.

Processes for the inactivation of viruses are preferred over those which function by virus removal, as the former type of technology is normally better defined in its mechanism of action and is therefore more capable of being operated and controlled with a high degree of assurance. New technologies, aimed specifically at inactivating non-enveloped viruses, are expected to emerge over the next few years; candidate technologies for this purpose include chemical treatments aimed at destroying nucleic acid [61] and continuous-flow UV-C irradiation [62].

Prion Diseases

It was in 1985 that evidence emerged that Creutzfeldt-Jakob disease (CJD) had been transmitted by human pituitary derived growth hormone [63]. Since then the possibility that CJD might also be transmissible by blood products has resulted in range of actions being taken by regulatory authorities and in numerous studies aimed at defining the risk of transmission by this route [64]. There is now a growing consensus that there is little or no risk of long established forms of CJD being transmitted by blood or blood products but this opinion does not extend to the disease of new variant CJD (vCJD) which emerged in the UK following the epidemic of bovine spongiform encephalopathy (BSE).

It is now accepted that BSE and vCJD are caused by the same prion agent. It has been estimated that over 100 000 people in the UK might develop the disease [65], but in the absence of a suitable diagnostic test, the incidence of pre-symptomatic vCJD is not known. This lack of knowledge concerning the epidemiology of vCJD, together with evidence of a higher concentration of abnormal prion protein in the tonsils of vCJD patients [66] caused the UK Government to conclude that there was a theoretical risk of vCJD being transmitted by blood products. Consequently, leukocyte depletion of all UK blood components was introduced and UK donor plasma was banned for use in the manufacture of fractionated products. Since then, preliminary findings have been reported that the BSE agent can be transmitted by whole blood transfusion between sheep [67], however, given the difficulty of these experiments and the very long incubation period of diseases of this type, it may be very many years before the true risk of transmission in humans is known.

Currently there are 82 confirmed cases of vCJD in the UK and only 3 cases outwith the UK. Nevertheless, given the export of animal feedstuffs, meat and livestock from the UK and the extent of international travel, it cannot be assumed that vCJD will be contained within the UK. The possibility that other agents of prion disease could enter the blood supply , such as the agent of Wasting Elk disease found in the USA [68], cannot be excluded.

In these circumstances, manufacturers of plasma products will have to address the possibility of there being at least a theoretical risk of vCJD being transmissible by plasma products regardless of the source of plasma. There is a pressing need for a diagnostic test suitable for screening blood donors. Although a number of groups are active in this field, difficulties in obtaining the sensitivity and accuracy necessary and the time required for validation of putative methods means that it may be some years before a suitable test is available [69]. There is evidence that prion agents can be removed by many of the processes used in plasma fractionation [70, 71], but further validation studies are required and new methods for eliminating prion agents from protein solutions may need to be developed. Ultimately the most difficult challenge will be to establish sufficient containment between batches to prevent infective material from one donor contaminating subsequent batches of product. To achieve this, all process equipment and materials should be designed to withstand severe sterilisation [51] or be sufficiently affordable to be replaced after each use.

Conclusions

The foundations of plasma fractionation were laid down by an exceptional body of scientists working under the pressure of a wartime emergency. New products were developed and the treatment of old diseases transformed. Set against this was the pervasive threat from transfusion transmitted infections, which culminated in the tragedy of haemophiliacs dying from AIDS and many thousands being infected with hepatitis C. Further scientific and technological advances have enabled today's plasma products to be manufactured without risk from HIV, HBV or HCV.

Although plasma fractionation is now an advanced sector of biopharmaceutical manufacturing industry, there are new problems to be solved. Non-enveloped viruses remain an issue and additional virus elimination technology is needed to provide increased assurance against emerging viruses. Action against the theoretical risk from vCJD seems inevitable.

The demand for plasma products continues to grow despite the impact of recombinant products and concerns over disease transmission. Meeting all of these demands, with products available for all world-wide, will present a substantial challenge to the fractionation community for many years to come.

Acknowledgements

The author would like to thank Dr Fred Rothstein for kindly providing me with information on the work of EJ Cohn and his co-workers. The author is grateful to Druscilla Rodger and to Kirsty Glass for their assistance in the preparation of this manuscript.

References

1. Coates JB, McFetridge EM. Blood programmes in World War II. Washington DC: Office of the Surgeon General, Department of the Army, 1964:325-57.
2. Cohn EJ. The history of plasma fractionation. In: Andrus EC, Bronk DW, Carden GA, et al., eds. Advances in military medicine, volume I. Boston: Little, Brown and Co., 1948:364-443.
3. Marketing Research Bureau. International directory of plasma fractionators 1999. Orange CT: Marketing Research Bureau, 2000.
4. Cohn EJ. The physical chemistry of proteins. Physiol Rev 1925;5:349-437.
5. Cohn EJ. The solubility of proteins. In: Cohn EJ, Edsall J, eds. Proteins, amino acids and peptides. New York: Reinhold, 1943:569-85.
6. Janeway CA. Human Serum Albumin: Historical review. in.Sgouris JT, René A, eds. Proceedings of the workshop on albumin. Washington: US Govt Printing Office, 1976: 3-21. (DHEW publication no. (NIH) 76-925).
7. Boyer PD, Lum FG, Ballou GA, Luck JM, Rice RG. The combination of fatty acids and related compounds with serum albumin. I. Stabilization against heat denaturation. J Biol Chem 1946;162:181-98.

8. Edsall JT. Stabilization of Serum Albumin to heat, and inactivation of the hepatitis virus. Vox Sang 1984; 46:338-40.
9. Gellis SS, Neefe J, Stokes J, Strong LE, Janeway CA, Scatchard G. Chemical, clinical and immunological studies on the products of human plasma fractionation. XXXVI. Inactivation of the virus of homologous serum hepatitis in solutions of normal serum albumin by means of heat. J Clin Inv 1948;27:239-44.
10. Murray R. Viral hepatitis. Bull N Y Acad Med 1955;31:341-58.
11. Pennell RB. The distribution of certain viruses in the fractionation of plasma. In: Hartman FW, LoGrippo GA, Mateer JG, Barron J, eds. Hepatitis frontiers. London: Churchill Ltd, 1957:297-310.
12. Starr D. Blood, an epic history of medicine and commerce. London: Little, Brown and Co. 1999:332.
13. Barker LF, Murray R. Relationship of virus dose to incubation time of clinical hepatitis and time of appearance of hepatitis associated antigen. Am J Med Sci 1971;263: 27-33.
14. Hoofnagle JH, Barker LF. Hepatitis B virus and albumin products. In : Sgouris JH, René A, eds. Proceedings of the workshop on albumin. Washington: Us Govt Printing Office, 1976:305-14. (DHEW publication no. (NIH) 76-925).
15. Foster PR, Cuthbertson B. Procedures for the prevention of virus transmission by blood products. In: Madhok R, Forbes CD, Evatt BL, eds. Blood, blood products and HIV, 2nd edition. London: Chapman and Hall, 1994:207-48.
16. Savage M, Hinskens W. Use of structured depth filters for virus removal. European patent application 1997: 0 798 003.
17. Morgenthaler JJ. Effect of ethanol on viruses. In: Morgenthaler JJ,ed. Virus inactivation in plasma products. Basel: Karger, 1989:109-21.
18. Ng PK, Dobkin MB. Pasteurisation of antihaemophilic factor and model virus inactivation studies. Thromb Res 1985;39:439-47.
19. Foster PR, Cuthbertson B, McIntosh RV, MacLeod AJ. Safer clotting factor concentrates. In: Forbes CD, Aledort L, Madhok R, eds. Hemophilia. London: Chapman and Hall, 1997:307-32.
20. Blombäck M, ed. New frontiers in hemophilia research: The World Federation of Hemophilia Congress Stockholm, 27 June- 1 July 1983. Scand J Haematol 1984:33 (Suppl 40).
21. Kroner BL, Rosenberg PS, Aledort LM, Alvord WG, Goedert JJ. HIV-1 infection incidence among persons with hemophilia in the United States and western Europe, 1978-1990. Multicenter Hemophilia Cohort Study. J Acquir Immune Defic Syndr 1994;7:279-86.
22. Darby SC, Ewart DW, Giangrande PL, Dolin PJ, Spooner RJ, Rizza CR. Mortality before and after HIV infection in the complete population of UK haemophiliacs. Nature 1995;377:79-82.
23. Bird AG, Codd AA, Collins A. Haemophilia and AIDS. Lancet 1985;i:162.
24. McCleland DBL, Yap PL. Clinical uses of immunoglobulins. Clinics in Haematol 1984;13:39-73.
25. Alving BM, Hojima Y, Pisano JJ, et al. Hypotension associated with prekallikrein activator (hageman factor fragments) in plasma protein fraction. N Engl J Med 1978; 299:66-70.
26. Alving BM, Tankersley DL, Mason BL, Rossi F, Aronson DL, Finlayson JS. Contact-activated factors: contaminants of immunoglobulin preparations with coagulant and vasoactive properties. J Lab Clin Med 1980;96:334-46.
27. Fell GS, Maharaj D. Trace metal contamination of albumin solutions used for plasma exchange. Lancet 1986;ii:467-68.
28. Welch AG, McBay WE, Angus KR. Improvement in the quality of albumin solutions (stable plasma protein solution) using ultrafiltration. Proceedings of the XXth Congress of the International Society of Blood Transfusion, London July 1988. Manchester: British Blood Transfusion Society, 1988:69.

29. Mikaelsson ME, Forsman N, Oswaldsson UM. Human factor VIII: a calcium-linked complex. Blood 1983:62:1006-15.
30. Foster PR, Dickson IH, McQuillan TA. Stability of factor VIII during the preparation of an intermediate-purity factor VIII concentrate. Br J Haematol 1983;53:343 (abstract).
31. Foster PR, Dickson IH, McQuillan TA, et al. Studies on the stability of VIII:C during the manufacture of a factor VIII concentrate for clinical use.. Vox Sang 1988;55:81-89.
32. McIntosh RV, Foster PR. The effects of solution formulation on the stability and surface interactions of Factor VIII during plasma fractionation. Transfus Sci 1990; 11:55-66.
33. McIntosh RV, Docherty N, Fleming D, Foster PR. A high-yield factor VIII concentrate suitable for advanced heat treatment. Thromb Haemost 1987;58:306 (abstract).
34. Schreiber AB. The preclinical characterisation of Monoclate factor VIII:C, antihemophilic factor (human). Semin Hematol 1988;25(suppl 1):27-32.
35. Griffith M. Ultrapure plasma factor VIII produced by anti-FVIIc immunoaffinity chromatography and solvent/detergent viral inactivation. Characterization of the Method M process and Hemofil M antihemophilic factor (human). Ann Hematol 1991;63:131-37.
36. Burnouf T, Burnouf-Radosevich M, Huart JJ, Goudemand M. A highly purified factor VIII:c concentrate prepared from cryoprecipitates by ion-exchange chromatography. Vox Sang 1991:60:8-15.
37. Raut S, Di Giambattista M, Bevan SA, Hubbard AR, Barrowcliffe TW, Laub R. Modification of factor VIII in therapeutic concentrates after virus inactivation by solvent-detergent and pasteurisation. Thromb Haemost 1988;80:624-31.
38. Lusher JM. Thrombogenicity associated with factor IX complex concentrates. Semin Hematol 1991;28(suppl 6):3-5.
39. Philippou H, Adami A, Lane DA, et al. High purity factor IX and prothrombin complex concentrate (PCC): pharmacokinetics and evidence that factor IXa is the thrombogenic trigger in PCC. Thromb Haemost 1996;76:23-28.
40. Levi M, Friederich PW, Middleton S, et al. Fibrinogen-coated albumin microcapsules reduce bleeding in severely thrombocytopenic rabbits. Nat Med 1999;5:107-11.
41. Ding M, Burstein N. Review: Fibronectin in corneal wound healing. J Ocular Pharmacology 1988:124:201-02.
42. Underwood S, Afoke A, Brown RA, MacLeod AJ, Dunnill P. The physical properties of a fibrillar fibronectin-fibrinogen material with potential use in tissue engineering. Bioprocess Eng 1999;20:239-48.
43. Jackson SK, Parton J, Barnes RA, Poynton CH, Fegan C. Effect of IgM-enriched intravenous immunoglobulin (Pentaglobin) on endotoxaemia and anti-endotoxin antibodies in bone marrow transplantation. Eur J Clin Invest 1993;23:540-45.
44. Johnson S, Sypura WD, Gerding DN, Ewing SL, Janoff EN. Selective neutralisation of a bacterial enterotoxin by serum immunoglobulin A in response to mucosal disease. Inf Immun 1995;63:3166-73.
45. Kilpatrick DC. Isolation of mannan binding lectin, serum amyloid P component and related factors from Cohn fraction III. Transfus Med 1997;7:289-94.
46. Fellman V, von Bonsdorff L, Parkkinen J. Exogenous apotransferrin and exhange transfusions in hereditary iron overload disease. Pediatrics 2000;105:398-401.
47. Jourdain M, Carrette O, Tournoys A, et al. Effects of inter-alpha-inhibitor in experimental endotoxic shock and disseminated intravascular coagulation. Am J Respir Crit Care Med 1997;156:1825-33.
48. Sasaki H, Yamatani K, Kato T, Kawanami T. Hereditary ceruloplasmin deficiency – a new type of diabetes mellitus. Intern Med 1996;35:596-97.
49. Foster PR. Blood plasma fractionation. In: Howe-Grant M, ed. Kirk-Othmer encyclopedia of chemical technology, 4th edition. New York: Wiley, 1994:990-1021.

50. Burnouf T. Chromatography in plasma fractionation: benefits and future trends. J Chromatogr B Biomed Appl 1995;664:3-15.
51. Taylor DM. Inactivation of prions by physical and chemical means. J Hosp Infect 1999;43(suppl): S69-76.
52. SprouleK, Morrill P, Pearson JC, et al. New strategy for the design of ligands for the purification of pharmaceutical proteins by affinity chromatography. J Chromatogr B Biomed Sci Appl 2000;740:17-33.
53. Galaev IY. New methods of protein purification. Affinity ultrafiltration. Biochemistry (Mosc) 1999;64:849-56.
54. Cuthbertson B, Reid KG, Foster PR. Viral contamination of human plasma and procedures for preventing virus transmission by plasma products. In: Harris JR, ed. Blood separation and plasma fractionation. New York: Wiley-Liss, 1991:385-435.
55. Burnouf T. Chromatographic removal of viruses from plasma derivatives. Dev Biol Stand 1993;81:199-209.
56. Allain JP. Emerging viruses in blood transfusion. Vox Sang 2000;78(suppl 2):243-48.
57. Schuurman R, van Steenis B, van Strien A, van der Noordaa J, Sol C. Frequent detection of bovine polyomavirus in commercial batches of calf serum by using the polymerase chain reaction. J Gen Virol 1991;72:2739-45.
58. Jantsch-Plunger V, Beck G, Maurer W. PCR detection of a low viral load in a prothrombin complex concentrate that transmitted hepatitis B virus. Vox Sang 1995;69: 352-54.
59. Committee for Proprietary Medicinal Products. Note for guidance on plasma derived medicinal products, CPMP/BWP/269/95, version 2. London : European Agency for the Evaluation of Medicinal Products, 1998.
60. Burnouf T. Value of virus filtration as a method for improving the safety of plasma products. Vox sang 1996;70:235-36.
61. Corash L. Inactivation of viruses, bacteria, protozoa, and leukocytes in platelet and red cell concentrates. Vox Sang 2000;78(suppl 2):205-10.
62. Rudge J, McLean C, MacDonald S, et al. Validation of a continuous flow device for UV-C virus inactivation process at production scale. Thromb Haemost 1999;82 (suppl):700.
63. Powell-Jackson J, Weller RO, Kennedy P, Preece MA, Whitcombe EM, Newsome-Davis J. Creutzfeldt-Jakob disease after administration of human growth hormone. Lancet 1985;ii:244-46.
64. Foster PR. Prions and blood products. Ann Med 2000;32:501-13.
65. Ghani AC, Ferguson NM, Donnelly C, Anderson RM. Predicted vCJD mortality in Great Britain. Nature 2000;406:583-84.
66. Hill AF, Butterworth RJ, Joiner S, et al. Investigation of variant Creutzfeldt-Jakob disease and other human prion disease with tonsil biopsy samples. Lancet 1999; 353:183-89.
67. Houston F, Foster JD, Chong A, Hunter N, Bostock CJ. Transmission of BSE by blood transfusion in sheep. Lancet 2000;356:999-1000.
68. Miller MW, Wild MA, Williams ES. Epidemiology of chronic wasting disease in captive Rocky Mountain elk. J Wildlife diseases 1998;34:532-36.
69. MacGregor I. Prion protein and developments in its detection. Transfus Med 2001: (in press).
70. Foster PR, Welch AG, Mclean C, et al. Studies on the removal of abnormal prion protein by processes used in the manufacture of human plasma products. Vox Sang 2000;78:86-95.
71. Lee DC, Stenland CJ, Hartwell RC, et al. Monitoring plasma process steps with a sensitive Western blot assay for the detection of prion protein. J Virol Methods 2000; 84:77-89.

VIRAL MARKER SCREENING: IS MORE TESTING SAFER?

J-P. Allain[1]

Introduction

Following the discovery of hepatitis B virus (HBV) in 1970, immunoelectrophoretic method and subsequently, enzyme immunoassays (EIA) were developed and applied to the screening of the blood supply. Hepatitis B surface antigen (HBsAg) is currently screened world wide in blood donations. Post-transfusion hepatitis declined by approximately 75% following the implementation of the test. With time and the development of new technologies including monoclonal antibodies for HBsAg capture, microtitre plates or more efficient solid phase such as microparticles, the sensitivity of the test increased by 1000 fold to now reach <0.1ng/ml.

The scenario briefly described here for HBsAg screening assay was later observed with antibody viral markers. Antibody to the human immunodeficiency virus type 1 (HIV-1) blood screening started in 1985. Both HIV-1 and HIV-2 antibodies were screened in 1986, finally, HIV-1 group O screening was added in 1995. As for HBsAg, sensitivity and specificity progressively improved between the first generation assays based on viral lysate as capture antigens to the second generation of EIAs based on recombinant proteins and peptides as sources of viral antigens. In the late 1980s, the improvement brought by third generation EIAs was related to a change in test format. Indirect detection of anti-HIV IgG by labelled anti-human IgG (called indirect EIA) used for first and second-generation assays was replaced by antigen 'sandwich' format. Taking advantage of the multivalence of captured antibodies, detection was obtained by directly labelled viral antigens. The test sensitivity improved by detecting the early rising IgM antibodies; concurrently, specificity was also improved.

When the clinical association between the human T lymphotropic virus type I (HTLV-I), an oncovirus within the family of human retroviruses, and adult T-cell leukaemia was established and the transmissibility of the agent by transfusion demonstrated, antibody screening assays were developed. It soon became apparent that these cultured viral antigen-based assays detected not only antibodies to HTLV-I but also to HTLV-II, another oncovirus, related to, but distinct from, HTLV-I. It was shown that when transmitted by transfusion, HTLV-I

1. Division of Transfusion Medicine. Department of Haematology, University of Cambridge, UK.

was apparently pathogenic only in immunocompromised recipients who may develop spastic paraparesis. Despite a low prevalence and disease penetrance, blood screening for antibodies to HTLV-I and HTLV-II was implemented in North America, Australia and some European countries. The high prevalence of HTLV-I infection in Japan justifies the screening.

The latest addition to blood screening by EIA followed the discovery of the hepatitis C virus (HCV) in 1989. Recombinant antigens were produced to detect specific antibodies. Here again, first, second and third generation EIAs appeared in close succession although changes mostly consisted of adding new capture antigens rather than modifying the indirect assay format [1]. Anti-HCV screening is implemented in all developed countries but the cost of the assay, the relatively mild pathogenicity, and low prevalence of HCV infection discouraged developing countries from implementing blood screening.

Surrogate Screening

ALT has been used as surrogate marker of non-A, non-B hepatitis prior to the discovery of HCV. Anti-HBc was shown to be associated with non-A, non-B hepatitis for epidemiological reasons. Both have been used as surrogate markers of viral hepatitis. Although clinical data indicated that since the implementation of anti-HCV screening, both ALT and anti-HBc became redundant, both tests continued to be performed on every blood donations collected in countries where they were implemented. With no demonstrable benefit, surrogate marker screening significantly complicates the testing process and increases the risk of errors.

At the same time, data was presented indicating that the addition of new screening assays was in itself increasing considerably the risk of errors related to the test themselves or to electronic information transmission (IT) or by manual transcription of results when appropriate IT was not available. Across developed countries, three to five viral markers (including HIV p24 antigen) detected by EIA and, in some, two surrogate markers are performed on every blood donation. While manual or partially automated method can still be used with acceptable level of performance with three screening assays, full automation and automatic transmission of results to release blood components becomes a necessity when four to seven assays are performed.

Blood Screening and Prevalence of Infection

At the present time, screening assays to insure the safety of the blood supply have been developed to cover the needs of high resource, generally low prevalence, areas of the world. Exception to this general rule is the high prevalence of HBV and HTLV-I infection in Japan. Assays are in general automated, using expensive and often delicate equipment, making the cost of assays high, despite the large sample throughput. The average cost is 1 USD/test. Because of the low prevalence of viral infection in Western blood donors, the critical element in the screening process is specificity. Unspecific reactions are the primary cause of blood waste. Except in the context of early detection of infection during the window period, sensitivity was not considered the priority in blood screening. The time required to perform assays was not a major issue since they were applied to post-donation blood samples.

The current assays are inappropriate to meet the needs of most of the world. The prevalence of HBV (all countries), HIV (SubSaharan Africa, Thailand), and HCV (in specific geographical pockets) ranges between 1 and 20%. The cumulated percentage of deferred blood donations according to Western criteria ranges between 5 and 25%. In this epidemiological context, screening assays should be rapid (less than 15 min), with high sensitivity (specificity tending to be high when prevalence is high), and performed without instrument (lack or frequent interruption of power). A dipstick able to simultaneously detect HBsAg, anti-HIV and anti-HCV would be the optimal system but is yet to be developed. At present, high performance separate dipsticks are commercially available for HBsAg and anti-HIV but distributed at a cost unaffordable by most developing countries. Rapid tests can be applied pre-donation, eliminating up to a quarter of the cost of blood collection and testing as well as blood waste [2]. The pre-donation approach might create some problems with HIV diagnosis because of its social stigmata, but not with hepatitis virus marker screening.

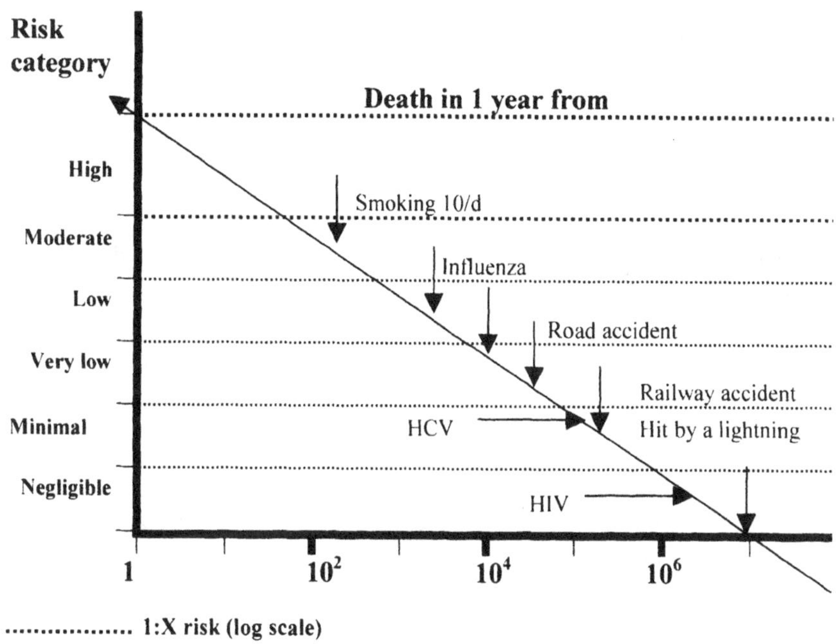

Figure 1. Relative risk of post-transfusion HIV and HCV infection compared to accepted risks in the UK.

The Residual Risk of Post-Transfusion Viral Transmission

At the present time, as a result of highly efficient EIAs, the residual risk of viral transmission by transfusion in Western countries is extremely small. It has been qualified as negligible for HIV (<1 per million transfusions), and minimal for HCV and HBV (ranging between 1:50,000 and 1:200,000 in England) (Figure 1).

The residual risk is similar in the USA although anti-HBc screening implemented in North America, but not in the UK, has an impact on post-transfusion hepatitis B [3]. In the absence of antibody screening, the risk of developing an HTLV-I or HTLV-II related clinical condition is in the order of 1:10 million. Yet, the risk is not zero and technologies theoretically permitting to eliminate this residual risk are available.

The residual risk is believed to be related to the background prevalence of an infection in the population. This assumes that incident infections (the only one with window period) occur within the age range of blood donors in correlation with the prevalence. It is also dependent on the proportion of susceptible recipients. In Asia or Africa, most HBV infections occur at birth or during the first years of life, accounting for the high prevalence of chronic carriers (5-20%). A relatively low proportion of the non-infected population is in contact with HBV through sexual or other contacts in blood donors ranging in age between 16 and 60. On the recipient side, approximately 60% of children have been in contact with the virus and, by age 40, virtually 100% of the population of West Africa, for instance, carry markers of HBV infection and is considered not susceptible to HBV infection. In that context, after EIA HBsAg screening, the residual risk of HBV infection by transfusion is approximately 1:40,000, not significantly different from the risk in Western countries. However, for each susceptible patient the risk of transfusion infection remains quite high.

The prevalence of HIV and HCV in Ghana is approximately 2% in blood donors [4]. The residual risk of posttransfusion transmission of each of the two viruses is 1:1500. In high-risk blood donors of KwaZulu Natal, South Africa the prevalence of HIV infection is 4% and the residual risk 1:700, despite HIV-1 p24 antigen screening. The prevalence of HIV in recipients being considered similar or higher than in the general population, approximately 80% of them are susceptible.

Genomic Screening: A New Step in Blood Safety

The current approach in reducing the residual risk of viral infection by transfusion is to add genomic screening by amplification methods to the serological screening. It is important to explore the potential benefits and limitations of this approach in high and low resource areas.

Since the late 70s, methods for the detection of specific nucleic acid targets from infectious agents have been developed but it is only in 1985 that nucleic acid amplification by polymerase chain reaction (PCR) was developed and applied to the detection of HIV sequences [5]. Since then, an extraordinary explosion of methods of amplification and their application to all fields of biology occurred. Despite its multiple steps, the relatively long assay time necessary to perform PCR, the problems of false positive reactions by cross-contamination and the high cost, nucleic acid amplification methods (NAT) have reached the field of transfusion and blood screening. In that context, automation, high throughput, affordable cost, and high specificity were paramount to the implementation of the new methods. Most of these requirements have been met (except low cost) and in 1999, HCV RNA screening became mandatory in developed countries [6]. In some, HIV RNA screening is implemented and HBV DNA will soon follow.

The impetus to apply NAT to blood screening did not originate from the need for extra safety. It essentially came in the aftermath of the HIV crisis in blood banking, and was driven by political considerations and, to some extent, commercial issues.

While the residual risk of transfusion was asymptotically tending towards zero in high resource countries, such was not the case in low resource/high prevalence areas covering most of the planet. The uncomfortable situation in which the cost of NAT testing can be afforded by populations who do not need it but cannot be afforded in areas where it would be effective is now reached. Calculations of the cost effectiveness of NAT for HCV and HIV infections done in the USA, France, Germany and Japan indicate a cost of several million dollars for each life year saved by NAT when it would be a few hundreds in many low resource areas.

The Residual Risk of Blood Borne Viruses in Transfusion

Irrespective of geography, the residual risk of post-transfusion viral infection has essentially four possible origins with widely different probability of occurring: pre-seroconversion window-period, donor immunosilence (infected but no serologic marker detectable), infection with a distant variant, and testing errors [7].

NATs are primarily intended for the detection of the infectious period of viraemia that precedes the development of antibodies during the initial phase of infection (window period). The potential efficacy of such screening depends on the prevalence of the infection in the population for first time donors, the incidence of infection in repeat donors, and the duration of the window period (Table 1).

Table 1. Relative impact of various factors in viral residual risk after transfusion in the USA; adapted from M. Busch.

	Window period (days)	Variants	Immunosilence	Testing errors
		(number of cases/10M donations)		
HIV	15	<0.6	<0.1	0.4
HCV	80	<1	0-20	11
HBV	63-150	<1	<1	1-3

Recent data concerning the viral kinetics during the pre-seroconversion window period have introduced various requirements in the level of performance to be met by NAT. Assay performance should enable the detection of most infected blood components that contain sufficient virus to establish an infection. Considerable data has been accumulated by the REDS group in the USA about the likelihood of closing the window period by NAT [7]. Such estimation is dependent on the sensitivity of the assays and the time separating the infection and the infectivity of the blood products. This interval is called the 'eclipse period' during which a virus is undetectable in the blood stream as it circulate at very low concentration or replicates at low level in tissue sanctuaries. The next window period of 'infectivity' extends between the end of the 'eclipse period' and the first positive enzyme immunoassay (p24 antigen for HIV, IgG antibodies for HCV, and HBsAg for HBV). This period of infectivity is estimated to be 6-10 days for HIV, 41-57 days for HCV and 30-45 days for HBV. Another important parameter is the time period during which a virus starts being shed in the blood stream and the time it becomes detectable by the genomic amplification assays. This period is directly related to the doubling time of viral replication, which is 0.3, 1 and 4 days for HCV, HIV and HBV respectively. The short doubling time of HCV and HIV suggest that the blind interval between the eclipse and infectious periods not covered by NAT may be as short as one day. Such a conclusion has been partially supported by ex-perimental data obtained in chimpanzees infected by HIV [8] in which demonstrable infectivity coincided with detectable HIV RNA by RT-PCR. Similar experiments are in progress for the other two viruses. There seems to be some degree of correlation between the viral doubling time and the level of viraemia achieved during the window period, prior to its modulation by the host immune system. The HCV window period level of viraemia ranges between 10^5 to 10^7 copies/ml, 10^2 to 10^7 for HIV, and 10^2 to 10^4 for HBV. This data has clear implications for the ability of NAT to close the window period, particularly when samples are diluted in plasma pools.

Immunosilence defined as the presence of persistent viral infection in the absence of detectable antibody marker has been described in HCV-infected blood donors [9]. Similar cases have been described in HIV infection in Africa [10] and may be considerably more frequent than initially thought. HBsAg-negative infectious blood can be found when virus is produced at a level below the sensitivity threshold of HBsAg assays. This situation corresponds to isolated anti-HBc donations that are positive by surrogate screening [11]. Recent data indicates that HBV DNA amplification might not be sensitive enough to insure identification of such cases [12].

The next potential cause of failure of detection by the current EIAs is patients infected by a variant virus too distant from the prototype virus(es) used to prepare antigens in the screening assays. This was described for HIV group O and, more recently group N [13]. Considering the wide phylogenetic distance between HIV-1 and HIV-2 and the presence of multiple simian immunodeficiency viruses potentially transmissible to humans, it is likely that other distant variants of HIV-1 and HIV-2 are still to be discovered. The relatively high frequency of blood donors with circulating HBV DNA in the absence of other markers of HBV infection suggests that not all such individuals are in the window period, but some may be infected with HBV variants. Therefore, designing NATs with primers targeted to sequences in highly conserved regions of the viral genome may help to identify variants that escape detection by EIA. However, given the low incidence of these events and the almost complete lack of relevant data, it is difficult to predict the number of additional infectious units that will be identified by a particular NAT-based test until it is implemented and surveyed on a large scale over time.

Table 2. Prevalence of viral markers in low resource countries of Africa.

Country	Prevalence in blood donors (%)			Total
	HBsAg	anti-HCV	anti-HIV	
Ghana replacement*	15	2.5	2.5	20
Malawi replacement	8	1	11.0	20
Botswana volunteer	5	1	10	16
South Africa volunteer**	4	0.5	4.5	9
Rwanda volunteer	2.9	3.5-15	1.5	8-19***

* Replacement of volunteer blood donors; ** high risk blood donors; *** anti-HCV prevalence varies considerably according to discreet geographical areas.

The last cause of viral infection missed by serological screening is testing errors: untested sample, test failure, recording failure, mislabelling, etc.

The impact of test failure has been evaluated and, as shown in Table 2, ranks second in frequency behind the window period.

Is NAT going to solve blood safety issues? Is antibody without detectable virus potentially infectious?

Clearly, NAT has a considerably higher potential for sensitivity than EIAs but even that has limitations. As it appears that HBV, HIV and HCV have very low threshold of infectivity, there are situations where a blood component is infectious but the viral genome is undetectable with the current NATs.

The pre-seroconversion level of HBV viraemia remains below 10^4 copies/ml and this level of viraemia could be difficult to detect, particularly in pools of plasmas.

Clinical post-transfusion hepatitis B is often traced back to a blood donation positive for anti-HBc, but without HBsAg or anti-HBs. These cases correspond to long-term chronic carriers whose level of HBsAg is below the threshold of sensitivity of the screening assays. Some individuals no HBV DNA can be detected by sensitive genomic amplification but were infectious by transfusion [12] but the relatively large volume of blood component transfused contains enough viral particles to be infectious. Recent data from this laboratory indicated that only 86% of HBsAg containing plasmas also contained detectable HBV DNA. Several hypotheses may explain that situation. Viral proteins may be synthesised from a mRNA from a small number of replicating hidden viral particles. There might be an unbalance between viral genome production and viral capsid protein related to abortive viral particles [14]. The capsid building blocks are produced and assembled but do not contain the viral genome. Parts of the HBV genome can be integrated into target cell genomes and produce HBsAg protein but not the complete range of viral proteins. This mechanism has been shown in patients with hepatocellular carcinoma. Although no clear clinical evidence of infectivity of such blood donation has been provided, they should be considered infectious.

Approximately 6% of random anti-HIV positive individuals have a viral load <500 copies/ml and 0.3% <20 copies [15]. Approximately 4% of HIV infected long term survivors have a viral load <20 copies/ml. This sub-population is more likely to present as blood donors.

In a small percentage of cases, patients recover from HCV infection. Detectable levels of antibodies to the N- and C-terminus of the hypervariable region are produced as well as antibodies able to block the attachment of the E2 envelop protein to target cells [16] which are probably critical in the viral neutralisation and elimination. Under these circumstances, antibodies to viral proteins are present but no virus and, presumably, no infectivity remains. However, short of clinical or experimental data, one can argue that, although at a concentration below detectability, the volume of the material transfused may contain virus above the threshold of infectivity. Some animal data may provide useful information to answer this question.

This data indicates that while NAT has the potential to provide a real improvement in blood safety, it cannot be used as only method of blood screening. Scientific evidence as well as the inherent prudence of regulatory bodies indicates that both serological and NAT blood screening will persist for the foreseeable future. As a result, the complication of blood screening operation will massively increase although serological and NAT screening are methods requiring totally separated equipment and facilities. However the shear number of tests and the number of parameters to be integrated prior to the release of blood is likely to increase the risk of testing errors and IT problems.

One can anticipate that some tests will be withdrawn, particularly surrogate tests that have been shown essentially redundant since the implementation of anti-HCV screening and even more so since the implementation of HCV NAT. A significant amount of data is currently collected indicating the complete overlap of HIV RNA and p24 antigen serological screening. This assay should no longer be used when HIV RNA screening is implemented.

Conclusion

In the near future, blood screening for safety is going to increase in number of tests by the duplication for each target virus of serological and genomic screening. To overcome the considerable operational burden involved, complete automation in complex, expensive, machine able to perform multiple assays simultaneously will be necessary. In parallel, the cost of blood will continue to increase, not only because of blood screening but also of the implementation of other safety measures such as universal leukocyte depletion and photochemical viral (and bacterial) inactivation. The cost efficiency of each extra unit of blood discarded compared to the EIA only era will become totally out of proportion and reason in the context of public health in developed countries. The political considerations will supersede sound evidence-based medicine and decision making for the foreseeable future.

The longer-term future can be quite different with the rapid development of new, miniaturised, multitarget, array testing on microchips. This approach can be adapted to both protein and nucleic acid testing with the major difference from the current approach that each potential donor can be individually screened for multiple target very quickly. This new era of pre-donation screening follows an approach similar to the currently developed scheme of serological screening in high prevalence areas [2]. Only donors passing a range of tests will be allowed to donate.

At the other end of the spectrum, one might imagine the addition to any blood of a compound that would simultaneously inactivate undesirable elements, being viruses, bacterias, or cellular nucleic acids. Although seductive by its simplicity, this approach may be put to difficult test when the bio-burden is high. Multiple layers of safety might then be needed to achieve the ultimate goal of zero risk for blood transfusion.

References

1. Allain JP. The status of hepatitis C virus screening. Transfusion Medicine Reviews 1998;12:46-55.
2. Adarkwa M, Sarkodie F. Larbi RA, et al. HBsAg and anti-HIV pre-donation screening in volunteer and replacement blood donors in Kumasi, Ghana. 26th Congress of the International Society of Blood Transfusion, Vienna. 2000; abstract 352.
3. Schreiber GB, Busch MP, Kleinman SH, Korelitz JJ. The risk of transfusion-transmitted viral infections. N Engl J Med 1996:334:1685-90.
4. Sarkodie F. Adarkwa M. Bedu-Addo G, Opare-Sem O, Acheampong JW, Allain JP. Screening for viral markers by EIA in volunteer and replacement donors in Kumasi, Ghana. 26th Congress of the International Society of Blood Transfusion, Vienna, 2000; abstract 351.
5. Lee H, Morse S, Olsvik Ø. Nucleic Acid Amplification Technologies: Application to Disease Diagnosis. Natick, MA: Eaton, 1997.
6. Muller-Breitkreutz K, Baylis SA, Allain JP. Nucleic acid amplification tests for the detection of blood-borne viruses. Vox Sang 1999;76:194-200.
7. Busch MP. Residual risks of viral transmission by transfusions and projected yields of additional screening tests. Trans Clin Biol 1996;3:7-11.
8. Murthy KK, Henrard DR, Eischberg JW, Busch MP, Alter HJ. Redefining the HIV infectious window in the chimpanzee model. Evidence to suggest that viral nucleic acid screening can prevent blood-borne transmission. Transfusion 1999:39:688-93.
9. Sugitani M, Inchauspe G, Shindo M, Prince A. Sensitivity of serological assays to identify blood donors with hepatitis C viraemia. Lancet 1992:339:1018-19.
10. Candotti D, Adu-Sarkodie Y, Davies F, et al. AIDS in an HIV-seronegative Ghanaian woman with intersubtype A/G recombinant HIV-1 infection. J Med Virol 2000;62: 1-8.
11. Iizuka H, Ohmura K, Ishijima A, et al. Correlation between anti-HBc titres and HBV DNA in blood units without detectable HBsAg. Vox Sang 1992;63:107-11.
12. Allain JP, Hewitt PE, Tedder RS, Williamson LM. Evidence that anti-HBc but not HBV DNA testing may prevent some HBV transmission by transfusion. Brit J Haematol 1999;107:186-95.
13. Simon F, Mauclere P. Roques P. et al. Identification of a new human immunodeficiency virus type 1 distinct from the group M and O. Nat Med 1998; 4:1032-37.
14. Sakamoto Y. Yamada G. Mizuno M. et al. Full and empty particles of hepatitis B virus in hepatocytes from patients with HbsAg-positive chronic active hepatitis. Lab Invest 1983;48:678-82.
15. Candotti C. Costagliola D. Joberty C. Bonduelle O. Rouzioux C. Autran B. the French ALT study group. Agut H. Status of long term asymptomatic HIV-1 infection correlates with viral load but not with virus replication properties and cell tropism. J Med Virol 1999;58:256-64.

16. Ishii K, Rosa D, Watanabe Y, et al. High titers of antibodies inhibiting the binding of envelope to human cells correlate with natural resolution of chronic hepatitis C. Hepatology 1998;28:1117-20.

INACTIVATION OF VIRUSES, BACTERIA, PROTOZOA, AND LEUKOCYTES IN LABILE BLOOD COMPONENTS BY USING NUCLEIC ACID TARGETED METHODS

L.M. Corash[1]

Introduction

Substantial increments in the safety of blood transfusion have been achieved through continued improvements in donor testing, yet residual concern about the safety of blood components persists. To further reduce the risk of transfusion-associated infection, additional measures, such as nucleic acid testing for selected pathogens, are being introduced. Transfusion of cellular components has been implicated in transmission of viral, bacterial, and protozoan infections [1]. While it is commonly recognized that hepatitis B virus (HBV), hepatitis C virus (HCV), cytomegalovirus (CMV), and the retroviruses, such as human immunodeficiency virus (HIV) and the human lymphotrophic viruses (HTLV) can be transmitted through cellular components, other pathogens are emerging as potentially significant transfusion-associated infectious agents. For example, transmission of protozoan infections due to trypanosomes [2-4] and babesia have been reported [5]. In addition to viral and protozoal infectious agents, bacterial contamination of platelet and red cell concentrates continues to be reported [6, 7], and may be an under reported transfusion complication [8]. More importantly, new infectious agents may periodically enter the donor population before they can be definitively identified and tested for to maintain consistent safety of the blood supply. The paradigm for this possibility is the HIV pandemic, which erupted in 1979. During the past decade a number of methods to inactivate infectious pathogens have been developed and have entered the advanced clinical trial phase.

Currently, prevention of transfusion-associated viral disease depends upon pre-donation evaluation of potential donors followed by serologic testing for infectious pathogens including: human immunodeficiency virus (HIV-1 and HIV-2), human T-cell lymphotrophic viruses (HTLV-I), hepatitis B virus (HBV), and hepatitis C virus (HCV). Cytomegalovirus (CMV) screening is generally performed after blood collection, when CMV sero-negative products are required. In addition to these agents, blood is tested for the syphilis pathogen (Treponema pallidum). Testing is not routinely done for parvovirus B19, hepatitis A virus (HAV), hepatitis G virus (HGV), hepatitis E virus (HEV), bacteria

1. Cerus Corporation and Department of Laboratory Medicine, University of California, San Francisco, CA, USA.

or protozoa. Although continuing improvements in testing have greatly reduced the transmission of viral disease by blood components, viruses may still contaminate the blood supply because diagnostic tests may be insensitive during the 'window period' before seroconversion of an infected donor. Even direct tests for a virus, such as the hepatitis B surface antigen (HBsAg) test, have a sensitivity threshold which allows contaminated components to escape detection. Recently, a case of HCV transfusion-associated transmission was documented despite nucleic acid testing of the donor [9]. Current estimates of the frequency of viral transmission due to transfusion of blood components, on a per donor basis, are 1 in 100,000 for HCV, 1 in 63,000 for HBV, and 1 in 680,000 for HIV [10] . The aggregate risk of receiving a blood component contaminated with one of the viruses for which sensitive tests are in place has been estimated to be 1 in 34,000 blood donors [11]. A recent US government report estimated that the average transfusion episode results in exposure to five donors [12]. Thus, per transfusion episode, the risk of receiving a component contaminated with virus may be as high as 1 in 6,800.

Bacterial contamination of platelet concentrates is a persistent problem due to room temperature (20°C-24°C) storage for up to five days prior to use. In addition, episodes of bacterial contamination of red cell concentrates continue to be reported [13]. Bacterial contamination may come directly from the donor or from an external source. A small number of contaminating bacteria can replicate to >107 per mL after five days of storage. A wide variety of bacteria have been cultured from patients with transfusion-transmitted septicemia [6, 14]. Although the number of reported cases of serious transfusion-transmitted sepsis is small, there are no routine laboratory tests to detect bacterial contamination of platelet units. Estimates of the frequency of bacterial contamination range up to 0.4% per platelet concentrate [15]. A 1991 survey by Morrow and co-workers identified bacterial contamination culminating in a septic response from 6 of 10,219 transfusions of pooled random donor platelets, a frequency of approximately 1 in 1,700 [14]. A prospective study of 3,584 platelet transfusions in 161 bone marrow transplant patients demonstrated the risk of symptomatic bacteremia as 1 per 16 patients, 1 per 350 transfusions, and 1 per 2,100 platelet units [16]. These frequencies are significant considering that over 8 million units of platelet concentrates are transfused annually in the United States alone [17]. The logistics and costs of continued expansion of testing processes, for example nucleic acid testing, have been questioned [10]. A recent report of the frequency of blood donations detected by nucleic acid methods but undetected by standard tests suggests that the yield of potentially infectious units will be in the range of 0.2 to 1.4 per 106 for HIV and HCV/HBV respectively [18]. Testing remains a reactive strategy to insure blood component safety, since new pathogens may enter the donor population before adequate tests can be implemented. Moreover, the sensitivity of all testing methods is limited inherently by the volume of blood that can be analyzed. A complementary approach to improving the safety of blood component transfusion is inactivation of infectious pathogens in blood components by using a process that treats the entire blood component. For example, treatment of plasma fractions with the solvent detergent process has demonstrated the benefits of this approach [19]. A robust inactivation technology that is compatible with current blood component processing procedures offers the potential for improving transfusion safety beyond that achievable by testing. Moreover, a nucleic acid targeted technology capable of inactivating residual leukocytes may confer additional benefits due to inhibition of cytokine synthesis, lymphocyte proliferation, and antigen presentation. Donor leukocytes are associated with a variety of adverse immune events ranging in severity from febrile transfusion reactions to allo-immunization and graft versus host disease [20, 21]. Although a number of measures have been implemented to reduce the likelihood of these adverse immune reactions, a robust nucleic acid targeted pathogen inactivation process offers the potential to inactivate all leukocytes, as well as infectious pathogens. Over the past decade a number of laboratories have reported efforts to apply pathogen inactivation technology to platelet and red cell concentrates. These efforts have now focused on several methods, three of which are in clinical trials (Table 1).

Table 1. Clinical trials of methods for inactivation of pathogens: platelet and red cell concentrates

Component	System	Trial phase
Buffy coat platelets	S-59	Phase 3
Single donor platelets	S-59	Phase 3
Red cells	S-303	Phase 1c
Red cells	PEN-110	Phase 1a

Potential Systems for Inactivation of Pathogens in Platelet Concentrates

Considerable effort has been devoted to investigations to develop methods for pathogen inactivation in platelet concentrates (Table 2, Table 3). The potential processes can be divided into two basic groups: psoralens and photodynamic methods. Recently, preliminary data have been reported using riboflavin as a nucleic acid associated photosensitizer to inactivate infectious pathogens [22]. The psoralen mediated processes generally utilize nucleic acid specific adduct formation while the photodynamic processes tend to utilize the production of active oxygen species as the primary effector mechanism for pathogen inactivation. The photodynamic methods generally do not provide sufficient pathogen inactivation and are associated with unacceptable levels of platelet injury [23]. The psoralen methods have been more extensively investigated and more progress has been made with psoralens than other systems.

Early investigations with psoralen mediated pathogen inactivation were conducted with 8-methoxypsoralen (8-MOP) based on the history of prior human use to treat psoriasis and cutaneous T cell lymphoma [24, 25]. These initial studies by Lin and co-workers established the principle of psoralen mediated pathogen inactivation, but 8-MOP photochemical treatment was not a sufficiently rapid process for treatment of platelet concentrates in clinical use [26, 27].

Table 2. Psoralen methods used to inactivate infectious pathogens and leukocytes in platelet concentrates

Photoreactive agent	Target	Reference
8-MOP	fd, R17, FeLV, E. Coli;,S. Aureus	[27]
8-MOP	MCMV, FeRTV	[45]
8-MOP	HIV	[46]
8-MOP	DHBV	[47]
8-MOP	12 pathogenic bacteria	[48]
AMT	VSV	[28]
AMT	HIV	[29,49]
AMT	VSV, Sindbis	[50]
PSR-Br	Bacteriophage	[51,52]
S-59	Pathogenic bacteria	[32]
S-59	Leukocytes	[33]
S-59	HIV, DHBV, BVDV, CMV, Bacteria	[32]

fd - bacteriophage, R17 - bacteriophage, MCMV - murine cytomegalovirus, FeRTV - feline rhinotracheitis virus, HIV -human immunodeficiency virus, HSV - herpes simplex virus, CMV - cytomegalovirus, VSV - vesicular stomatitis virus, FeLV - feline leukemia virus, Sinbis - Sindbis virus, 8-MOP - 8-methoxypsoralen, AMT - aminomethyltrimethylpsoralen, PSR-Br - brominated psoralens.v

Table 3. Photodynamic methods used to inactivate infectious pathogens in platelet concentrates

Photoreactive agent	Target	Reference
UVB	Poliovirus	[53]
Merocyanine 540	VSV	[54]
Merocyanine 540	HSV, MS2, F6	[28]
Methylene bleu	unspecified	[55]
Phtalocyanines	VSV	[56]
Riboflavin*	HIV-1, BVDV, PRV, PPV, HSV, Vaccinia	[22]

VSV - vesicular stomatitis virus, MS2 - bacteriophage, F6 - bacteriophage, HSV - herpes simplex virus, HIV - human immunodeficiency virus, PPV - porcine parvovirus, PRV - pseudorabies virus, BVDV - bovine viral diarrhea virus, and UVB - ulraviolet B light (280-320 nm).

* Nucleic acid targeted.

Several laboratories have investigated the use of AMT, a synthetic psoralen with enhanced nucleic acid binding efficiency [28,29]. While AMT has increased nucleic acid binding affinity compared to 8-MOP, it exhibits mutagenicity in the absence of light, and thus has an unfavorable toxicology profile. Several classes of new psoralens have been synthesized which offer potential advantages over AMT and 8-MOP. The halogenated psoralens do not appear to be sufficiently effective for viral inactivation and in preliminary studies demonstrate adverse effects on platelet viability [30, 31]. A new class of amino psoralens has been synthesized and shown to be highly effective for inactivation of pathogenic viruses, bacteria, and leukocytes in platelet concentrates [32, 33]. Recently, Lin and co-workers reported that human platelet concentrates (300 mL) contaminated with high titers of HCV (10 4.5) and HBV (10 5.5) treated with the S-59 process did not transmit hepatitis after transfusion into naive chimpanzees. Other studies demonstrated these novel psoralens inactivate high levels of T cells, inhibit leukocyte cytokine synthesis during platelet storage, and inhibit nucleic acid amplification [33]. More importantly, treatment of T cells with the S-59 process prevented transfusion-associated graft versus host disease in both immune competent and immune compromised murine transplant models [33].

Table 4. Methods used to inactivate infectious pathogens in red cell concentrates.

Reactive agent	Target	Reference
Dihematoporphyrin	HIV, HSV, CMV, SIV, T.cruzi	[57
Benzoporhyrin A	VSV, FeLV	[58]
Merocyanine 540	Friend LV	[59]
Merocyanine 540	HSV-1	[60]
Merocyanine 540	P. falciparum	[61]
Methylene blue	VSV	[62]
Methylene blue	VSV, Φ6, Sindbis, M13	[63]
Phthalocyanines	VSV	[64]
Phthalocyanines	VSV, Sindbis	[56]
PSR-Br	Φ6	[65]
Hypericin	HIV	[66]
DMMB	VSV, PRV, BVDV, Φ6, R17,EMC	[38]
Inactine	Porcine parvovirus, BVDV, HIV-1, VSV	[39]
S-303	HIV, DHBV, BVDV, Bacteria	[42]

One of these novel psoralens, S-59, has entered human clinical trials [34]. Phase 1 and 2 studies using S-59 treated, five day-old platelets transfused in healthy subjects have shown adequate viability. In these studies, photochemically treated platelets were well tolerated during and after transfusion of full doses (300 mL, 3.0×10^{11} platelets). The therapeutic efficacy of S-59 platelets was examined in a pilot study of profoundly thrombocytopenic patients. This clinical trial was designed to evaluate the hemostatic efficacy of S-59 treated platelet concentrates. In this study of eighteen patients, transfusion of S-59 treated platelet concentrates resulted in shortening of markedly prolonged cutaneous bleeding times, adequate platelet count increments, and acceptable intervals to the next platelet transfusion [35]. The S-59 platelet concentrates were well tolerated.

Two randomized, controlled, blinded, clinical trials to determine the therapeutic efficacy of multiple transfusions of S-59 treated platelet concentrates have been undertaken. A European trial using pooled random donor platelets prepared by the buffy coat method has been completed. This trial enrolled 103 thrombocytopenic patients with a broad spectrum of hematologic malignancies who required up to eight weeks of platelet transfusion support. Patients were randomized to transfusion with either S-59 treated or standard platelet concentrates. Buffy-coat platelet concentrates were pooled, leukocyte depleted, treated with S-59 and stored for up to 5 days before transfusion. Photochemical treatment was used in place of gamma irradiation for prevention of graft versus host disease in the experimental treatment group. The primary endpoint of this trial was the platelet count increment 1 to 2 hours after transfusion. Secondary endpoints included the platelet count increment 24 hours after transfusion, clinical hemostasis, refractoriness to transfusion, the inter-transfusion interval, and the frequency of acute transfusion reactions. All patients were followed for adverse events for four weeks after the last study platelet transfusion, and were eligible for a second cycle of transfusion to the assigned treatment product if additional platelet support was required while the study was open.

A larger study enrolling 600 patients is underway in the United States. In this study, thrombocytopenic patients are randomized to receive up to four weeks of platelet transfusion support with either S-59 platelets or standard single donor platelets. The primary endpoint in the U.S. trial is the proportion of patients with grade 2 bleeding during the period of platelet support. The selection of this endpoint required a larger patient group to achieve adequate statistical power. The secondary endpoints include the proportion of patients with high grade bleeding, platelet count increments, and the same spectrum of endpoints as in the European study. This study is expected to complete enrollment early in 2001.

Potential Systems for Inactivation of Pathogens in Red Cell Concentrates

A number of laboratories have investigated the application of pathogen inactivation to red cell concentrates (Table 4). Red cells present a difficult environment for pathogen inactivation due to the absorption spectrum of hemoglobin and the viscosity of packed red cells. Photodynamic mediated damage may be further increased during prolonged red cell storage. Significant defects of the photodynamic systems have included incomplete inactivation of pathogens, damage to red cells resulting in hemolysis and potassium leakage, increased binding of immunoglobulins, long treatment times, and the necessity to work at a reduced hematocrit or in a thin layer configuration to facilitate light activation. Cellular damage, due to active oxygen species, can be ameliorated by use of scavengers or quenchers [36, 37]. Wagner et al have described the use of a new phenothiazine compound, dimethylmethylene blue (DMMB), which exhibits an improved inactivation spectrum compared to methylene blue and demonstrates less hemolysis and immunoglobulin binding during storage after treatment [38].

To date, most efforts have relied on photodynamic methods, but more recently several groups have developed nucleic acid targeted processes. The latter approach offers the potential to minimize non-specific damage to red cell and plasma proteins. Inactine, a stable mono-alkylator compound, was reported to inactivate a series of model viruses in red cell suspensions [39]. This compound is nucleic acid targeted and does not require light for activation. A second study was conducted to evaluate the effect of inactine on red cell viability [40]. Baboon red cells were treated with the inactine compound PEN 110 and stored for 28 days. Following storage, the red cells were radiolabeled with ^{51}Cr and transfused. Post transfusion recovery and life span of the inactine treated cells were comparable to that of untreated red cells. A phase 1 clinical trial was initiated recently. This study will enroll 16 healthy subjects in a randomized cross over design to evaluate the effect of inactine treatment on red cell viability after 28 days of storage.

Cook and Wollowitz have developed a class of compounds known as anchor linker effectors (ALE) or frangible anchor linker effectors (FRALE) [41]. These compounds are activated by a pH shift after addition to packed red cells suspended in residual plasma and red cell additive solutions. FRALES are nucleic acid targeted and form covalent adducts with DNA and RNA. The FRALE compounds rapidly degrade to an inactive, negatively charged species (S-300) after reaction thus preventing further binding to DNA and RNA. To provide the highest safety margins for this process, the negatively charged breakdown molecule is reduced to very low levels using a compound absorption device (CAD). The lead compound, S-303 (100 ug/mL), upon addition to packed red cells (60% hematocrit) inactivated high titers of cell-free and cell-associated HIV, DHBV, VSV, HSV, BVDV, and both gram negative and gram positive bacteria. Using a murine transfusion model, S-303 treated red cells exhibited post transfusion recovery and life span comparable to untreated red cells [41]. In a second series of studies, dog red cells treated with S-303 exhibited post transfusion recovery comparable to untreated red cells [42]. Dogs transfused multiple times with allogeneic treated S-303 red cells failed to develop antibodies to S-303 treated autologous red cells, but some dogs did develop allo-antibodies to untreated donor cells indicating an intact allo-immune response not directed against S-303 treated red cells. Other dogs transfused with S-303 treated red cells (10 mL/kg) twelve times over a one month period had no evidence of clinical or histopathologic toxicity. In addition, replacement of 80% of the blood volume of dogs with S-303 treated red cells using treatment concentrations up to 500 ug/mL resulted in no toxicity.

Two Phase 1 clinical trials using S-303 treated red cells have been completed in healthy subjects. In the first study, 42 healthy subjects donated whole blood that was prepared as packed red cells and treated with either standard methods or S-303 and stored for 35 days at 4°C [43]. After 35 days of storage, the subjects were transfused with an aliquot of radiolabeled red cells to measure the recovery 24 hours after transfusion. S-303 red cells were tolerated and demonstrated post transfusion recovery greater than 75%. In the seocnd study, 28 subjects from the first study were re-enrolled and donated a unit of whole blood that was prepared as packed red cells and treated with S-303 [44]. The treated red cells were placed in storage and on days 7, 14, and 21 after donation, subjects were transfused with 15 mL of S-303 treated red cells. On day 35 after donation, the subjects were transfused with 15 mL of ^{51}Cr labeled red cells. Before each transfusion during the 35-day storage period, serum samples were obtained and assayed for detection of antibodies directed against S-303 red cells. The average post transfusion recovery was comparable to that of the first study for both control and S-303 treated red cells [44]. No detectable antibody against S-303 treated red cells was observed after four or five transfusions. The next study in this program will measure the tolerability of full unit transfusions in healthy subjects using the commercial components of the system.

Conclusions

Considerable progress has been made in the development of technology to inactivate infectious pathogens in platelet and red cell concentrates. These technologies have now entered the clinical trial phase, and the platelet system is now in the latter part of Phase 3. These inactivation systems have the potential to markedly change the way in which blood components are prepared.

References

1. Dodd RY. Will blood products be free of infectious agents? In: Nance SJ, ed. Transfusion Medicine In The 1990's. Arlington,VA: American Association of Blood Banks, 1990:223-51.
2. Schmunis GA. Trypanosoma cruzi, the etiologic agent of Chagas' disease: status in the blood supply in endemic and nonendemic countries. Transfusion 1991;31:547-57.
3. Grant IH, Gold JMW, Wittner M, et al. Transfusion-associated acute Chagas disease acquired in the United States. Ann Intern Med 1989;111: 849-51.
4. Nickerson P, Orr P, Schroeder ML, Sekla L, Johnston JB. Transfusion-associated Trypanosoma cruzi infection in a non-endemic area. Ann Intern Med 1989;111:851-53.
5. Mintz ED, Anderson JF, Cable RG, Hadler JL. Transfusion-transmitted babesiosis: a case report from a new endemic area. Transfusion 1991;31:365-68.
6. Goldman M, Blajchman MA. Blood product-associated bacterial sepsis. Transfus Med Rev 1991;5:73-83.
7. Blajchman MA, Ali AM. Bacteria in the blood supply: an overlooked issue in transfusion medicine. In: Nance SJ, ed. Blood Safety: Current Challenges. Bethesda, MD: American Association of Blood Banks, 1992: 213-28.
8. Sazama K. Reports of 355 transfusion-associated deaths: 1976 through 1985. Transfusion 1990;30:583-90.
9. Schuttler GC, Caspari C, Jursch CA, WR WRW, Gerlich WH, Schaefer S. Hepatitis C virus transmission by a blood donation negative in nucleic acid amplification tests for viral RNA. Lancet 2000;355:41-42.
10. AuBuchon JP, Birkmeyer JD, Busch MP. Safety of the blood supply in the United States: opportunities and controversies. Ann Intern Med 1997;127:905-09.
11. Schreiber GB, Busch MP, Kleinman SH, Korelitz JJ. The risk of transfusion- transmitted viral infections. N Engl J Med 1996;334:1685-90.
12. Chan K. Blood Supply: FDA Oversight and Remaining Issues of Safety. In: U.S. General Accounting Office, 1997.
13. Roth VR, Arduino MJ, Nobiletti J, et al. Transfusion-related sepsis due to Serratia liquefaciens in the United States. Transfusion 2000;40:931-35.

14. Morrow JF, Braine HG, Kickler TS, Ness PM, Dick JD, Fuller AK. Septic reactions to platelet transfusions: a persistent problem. JAMA 1991;266:555-58.
15. Blajchman MA, Ali A, Lyn P, Bardossy L, Richardson H. Bacterial surveillance of platelet concentrates: quantitation of bacterial load. Transfusion 1997;37(Suppl):74s.
16. Chiu EKW, Yuen KY, Lie AKW, et al. A prospective study of symptomatic bacteremia following platelet transfusion and of its management. Transfusion 1994;34: 950-54.
17. Wallace EL, Churchill WH, Surgenor DM. Collection and transfusion of blood components in the United States, 1992. Transfusion 1992;35:802-12.
18. Seifried E, Roth WK. First statistical survey of HCV, HBV, HIV-1 NAT screening of blood donors in the Red Cross Blood Service Centers in Germany. Vox Sang 2000; 78(Suppl 1):80.
19. Horowitz B, Wiebe ME, Lippin A, Stryker MH. Inactivation of viruses in labile blood derivatives I. Disruption of lipid-enveloped viruses by tri(n-butyl)phosphate detergent combinations. Transfusion 1985;25:516-22.
20. Heddle NM, Kalma L, Singer J, et al. The role of plasma from platelet concentrates in transfusion reactions. New Engl J Med 1994;331:625-28.
21. Ohto H, Anderson KC. Survey of transfusion-associated graft-versus-host disease in immunocompetent recipients. Transfus Med Rev 1996;10:31-43.
22. Goodrich RP. The use of riboflavin for the inactivation of pathogens in blood products. Vox Sang 2000;78(Suppl 2):211-15.
23. Corash L. Photochemical decontamination of cellular blood components. Anaesth Pharmacol Rev 1995;3:138-49.
24. Edelson R, Berger C, Gasparro F, et al. Treatment of cutaneous T-cell lymphoma by extracorporeal photochemotherapy. N Engl J Med 1987;316:297-303.
25. McEvoy MT, Stern RS. Psoralens and related compounds in the treatment of psoriasis. Pharmac Ther 1987;34:75-97.
26. Alter HJ, Morel PA, Dorman BP, et al. Photochemical decontamination of blood components containing hepatitis B and non-A, non-B virus. Lancet 1988;ii:1446-50.
27. Lin L, Wiesehahn GP, Morel PA, Corash L. Use of 8-methoxypsoralen and long wavelength ultraviolet radiation for decontamination of platelet concentrates. Blood 1989;74:517-25.
28. Dodd RY, Moroff G, Wagner S, et al. Inactivation of viruses in platelet suspensions that retain their in vitro characteristics: comparison of psoralen-ultraviolet A and merocyanine 540-visible light methods. Transfusion 1991;31:483-90.
29. Margolis-Nunno H, Bardossy L, Robinson R, Ben-Hur E, Horowitz B, Blajchman MA. Psoralen-mediated photochemical decontamination of platelet concentrates: inactivation of cell-free and cell-associated forms of human immunodeficiency virus and assessment of platelet function in vivo. Transfusion 1997;37:889-95.
30. Goodrich RP, Yerram NR, Tay GB, et al. Selective inactivation of viruses in the presence of human platelets: UV sensitization with psoralen derivatives. Proc Natl Acad Sci U S A 1994;91(12):5552-56.
31. Goodrich RP, Yerram NR, Crandall SL, Sowemimo-Coker SO. In vivo survival of platelets subjected to virus inactivation protocols using psoralen and coumarin photosensitizers. Blood 1995;86 (Suppl 1):354a.
32. Lin L, Cook DN, Wiesehahn GP, et al. Photochemical inactivation of viruses and bacteria in platelet concentrates by use of a novel psoralen and long-wavelength ultraviolet light. Transfusion 1997;37:423-35.
33. Grass JA, Hei DJ, Metchette K, et al. Inactivation of leukocytes in platelet concentrates by psoralen plus UVA. Blood 1998;91:2180-88.
34. Corash L, Behrman B, Rheinschmidt M, et al. Post-transfusion viability and tolerability of photochemically treated platelet concentrates (PC). Blood 1997;90(Suppl 1):267a.

35. Slichter SJ, Corash L, Grabowski M, et al. Viability and hemostatic function of photochemically treated (PCT) platelets in thrombocytopenic patients. Blood 1999; 94(Suppl 1):376a.
36. Rywkin S, Ben-Hur E, Reid ME, Oyen R, Ralph H, Horowitz B. Selective protection against IgG binding to red cells treated with phthalocyanines and red light for virus inactivation. Transfusion 1995;35:414-20.
37. Ben-Hur E, Rywkin S, Rosenthal I, Geacintov NE, Horowitz B. Virus inactivation in red cell concentrates by photosensitization with phthalcyanines: protection of red cells but not of vesicular stomatitis virus with a water-soluble analogue of vitamin E. Transfusion 1995;35:401-06.
38. Wagner SJ, Skirpchenko A, Robinette D, Mallory DA, Cincotta L. Preservation of red cell properties after virucidal phototreatment with dimethylmethylene blue. Transfusion 1998;38:729-37.
39. Zhang QX, Edson C, Budowsky E, Purmal A. Inactine – a method for viral inactivation in red blood cell concentrate. Transfusion 1998;38(Suppl 1):75S.
40. Edson CM, Purmal A, Brown F, Valeri CR, Budowsky E, Chapman JR. Viral inactivation of red blood cell concentrates by Inactine: mechanism of action and lack of effect on red cell physiology. Transfusion 1999;39(Suppl 1):108s.
41. Cook D, Stassinopoulos A, Merritt J, et al. Inactivation of pathogens in packed red blood cell (PRBC) concentrates using S-303. Blood 1997;90(Suppl 1):409a.
42. Cook D, Stassinopoulos A, Wollowitz S, et al. In vivo analysis of packed red blood cells treated with S-303 to inactivate pathogens. Blood 1998;92(Suppl 1):503a.
43. Greenwalt TJ, Hambleton J, Wages D, et al. Viability of red blood cells treated with a novel pathogen inactivation system. Transfusion 1999;39 (Suppl 1):109s.
44. Hambleton J, Greenwalt T, Viele M, et al. Post transfusion recovery after multiple exposures to red blood cell concentrates (RBCS) treated with a novel pathogen inactivation (P.I.) process. Blood 1999;94(Suppl 1):376a.
45. Londe H, Damonte P, Corash L, Lin L. Inactivation of human cytomegalovirus with psoralen and UVA in human platelet concentrates. Blood 1995;86 (Suppl 1):544a.
46. Lin L, Londe H, Hanson CV, et al. Photochemical inactivation of cell-associated human immunodeficiency virus in platelet concentrates. Blood 1993;82:292-97.
47. Eble BE, Corash L. Photochemical inactivation of duck hepatitis B virus in human platelet concentrates: a model of surrogate human hepatitis B virus infectivity. Transfusion 1996;36:406-18.
48. Lin L, Londe H, Janda M, Hanson CV, Corash L. Photochemical inactivation of pathogenic bacteria in human platelet concentrates. Blood 1994;83:2698-706.
49. Benade LE, Shumaker J, Xu Y, Dodd R. Inactivation of free and cell-associated HIV in platelet suspensions by aminomethyltrimethyl (AMT) psoralen and ultraviolet light. Transfusion 1992;32(Suppl 1):33S.
50. Margolis-Nunno M, Williams B, Rywkin S, Horowitz B. Photochemical virus sterilization in platelet concentrates with psoralen derivatives. Thromb Haemostas 1991; 65:1162(abstract).
51. Rai S, Kasturi C, Grayzar J, et al. Dramatic improvements in viral inactivation with brominated psoralens, napthalenes and anthracenes. Photochem Photobiol 1993;58 (1):59-65.
52. Yerram N, Forster P, Goodrich T, et al. Comparison of virucidal properties of brominated psoralen with 8-methoxy psoralen (8-MOP) and aminomethyl trimethyl psoralen (AMT) in platelet concentrates. Blood 1993;82 (Suppl 1):402a.
53. Prodouz KN, Fratantoni JC, Boone EJ, Bonner RF. Use of laser-UV for inactivation of virus in blood products. Blood 1987;70:589-92.
54. Prodouz KN, Lytle CD, Keville EA, Budacz AP, Vargo S, Fratantoni JC. Inhibition by albumin of merocyanine 540-mediated photosensitization of platelets and viruses. Transfusion 1991;31:415-22.
55. Klein-Struckmeier A, Mohr H. Virus inactivation by methylene blue/light in thrombocyte concentrates. Vox Sang 1994;67 (Suppl 2):36.

56. Horowitz B, Rywkin S. Margolis-Nunno H, et al. Inactivation of viruses in red cell and platelet concentrates with aluminum phthalocyanine (AlPc) sulfonates. Blood Cells 1992;18:141-50.
57. Matthews JL, Sogandres-Bernal F, Judy M, et al. Inactivation of viruses with photoactive compounds. Blood Cells 1992;18:75-89.
58. North J, Neyndorff H, King D, Levy JG. Viral inactivation in blood and red cell concentrates with benzoporphyrin derivative. Blood Cells 1992;18:129-40.
59. Sieber F, Krueger GJ, O'Brien JM, Schober SL, Sensenbrenner LL, Sharkis SJ. Inactivation of friend erythroleukemia virus and friend virus-transformed cells by merocyanine 540-mediated photosensitization. Blood 1989;73:345-50.
60. O'Brien JM, Gaffney DK, Wang TP, Sieber F. Merocyanine 540-sensitized photoinactivation of enveloped viruses in blood products: site and mechanism of phototoxicity. Blood 1992;80:277-85.
61. Smith OM, Dolan SA, Dvorak JA, Wellems TE, Sieber F. Merocyanine 540-sensitized photoinactivation of human erythrocytes parasitized by Plasmodium falciparum. Blood 1992:80:21-24.
62. Wagner SJ, Storry JR, Mallory DA, Stromberg RR, Benade LE, Friedman LI. Red cell alterations associated with virucidal methylene blue phototreatment. Transfusion 1993;33:30-36.
63. Wagner SJ, Abe H, Benade L. Differential sensitivity to methylene blue (MB) photosensitization. Photochem Photobiol 1993;57(Suppl):67S.
64. Horowitz B, Williams B, Rywkin S, et al. Inactivation of viruses in blood with aluminum phthalocyanine derivatives. Transfusion 1991;31:102-08.
65. Yerram N, Platz MS, Forster P, Goodrich T, Goodrich R. Selective viral inactivation in RBC, platelets, and plasma using a novel psoralen derivative plus ultraviolet A (UVA) light. Transfusion 1993;33 (Suppl 1):50S.
66. Lavie G, Mazur Y, Lavie D, et al. Hypericin as an inactivator of infectious viruses in blood components. Transfusion 1995;35:392-400.

ALTERNATIVES TO HUMAN BLOOD RESOURCES

P. M. Ness[1]

Introduction

The discovery of the acquired immune deficiency syndrome (AIDS) in the 1980's and its rapid evolution as a major concern for physicians and their patients has lead to many questions about the safety of the blood supply. The attention placed upon AIDS has resulted in new discoveries and technologies to reduce the risk of other transfusion complications such as hepatitis, bacterial contamination, and transfusion-associated graft versus host disease (TA-GvHD). Concerns about blood safety have focused much attention on alternative blood transfusion strategies such as autologous blood, viral inactivation, and artificial blood substitutes. In particular, there has been major interest in the development of alternatives to human blood resources such as blood substitutes. This paper will review the current status of human blood substitutes with particular emphasis upon red cell substitutes. The progress in the development of red cell substitutes will demonstrate that there will be some losses of functionality compared to human red cells, but some product characteristics may result in new therapeutic applications for these products.

Blood Preparation and Collection

Most of the blood collected for transfusion in the United States is collected at community blood centers; about half of these centers are maintained by the American Red Cross while the others are run by other non-profit community agencies. The remainder of blood collections are performed at hospitals. Plasma derivatives are provided by commercial vendors using paid plasma donors while the Red Cross provides plasma components from volunteer donations.

Blood collections and red cell usage declined in the mid 1980's. The AIDS epidemic made it easier to convince clinicians to use clinically appropriate indications for homologous blood, and autologous blood collections rose substantially. In 1997, approximately twelve million volunteer collections occurred in

---

1. Transfusion Medicine Div, Dept Pathology, Johns Hopkins Medical Institutions and Greater Chesapeake and Potomac Region, American Red Cross Blood Services, Baltimore, MD, USA. Dr. Ness is a consultant for Northfield Laboratories, Evanston, IL, USA.

the United States [1]. At the current time, collections and red cell usage are rising again, most likely as a result of more cancer and cardiovascular procedures being performed in our aging population.

Although current blood supplies are usually adequate to avoid unnecessary loss of life from unexpected hemorrhage, supply shortages are common at Christmas and during the summer months. In addition, group O red cells which can be used for any recipient is often in short supply despite the fact that group O is the most common ABO type. Chemical efforts to enzymatically remove the sugars which define ABO specificity, converting group A or B blood to group O, are in commercial development and could be important to alleviate blood shortages and avoid the rare ABO hemolytic transfusion reaction which still occur [2].

Red cell substitutes potentially could play an important role in supplying oxygen carrying capacity to patients where blood is not routinely available (military or civilian trauma sites). Even in developed countries, hospitals at long distances from blood centers may have minimal inventories of blood to facilitate major trauma stabilization or resuscitation. In addition, some patients with rare blood types or autoantibody problems may not have compatible blood available for immediate transfusion needs, such that a red cell substitute could provide critical temporary life support. A final consideration is the availability of blood substitutes for patients who refuse transfusions such as Jehovah's Witnesses. The availability of a perfluorocarbon solution or hemoglobin based oxygen carriers (HBOC) could be important for their therapy; many Witnesses will accept blood substitutes as a matter of conscience, even though their religious beliefs would not permit the transfusion of intact donor red cells.

Transfusion Alternatives

The only positive benefit of the AIDS epidemic and its associated publicity has been the increased utilization of alternatives to blood transfusion. In 1988, the National Institutes of Health held a consensus conference on 'Perioperative Red Cell Transfusion' [3]. The conference suggested that there was no evidence to support the widespread practice of using a hemoglobin concentration of less than 10 grams/dL as a transfusion indicator; 7 g/dL was suggested as a more reasonable alternative. Based upon this recommendation, most authorities advise physicians to forego transfusions unless the patient has symptomatic anemia or the hemoglobin concentration is below 7 g/dL. The conference also presented reaffirming data that mild to moderate anemia does not contribute to perioperative morbidity or delayed wound healing.

Based upon the increased perception of the infectious risks of transfusions, reduction of homologous blood transfusions was recommended and the increased utilization of alternatives to transfusion such as autologous blood was advocated.

Despite reassuring data from studies such as the Retrovirus Epidemiology Donor Study (REDS) [4], pressure to seek alternatives to transfusions has increased. This theme was given strong governmental support by the NIH Consensus Conference in 1988 which helped stimulate our current medical practices of reducing the transfusion trigger to levels based upon physiologic principles, minimizing donor blood exposure, and encouraging alternatives to blood transfusions (Table 1).

Table 1. Transfusion alternatives.

Perioperative autologous blood donation
Perioperative hemodilution
Blood salvage
Pharmacologic therapies
Apheresis to reduce donor exposure
Viral inactivation
Blood substitutes

Development of Blood Substitutes

Some believe that absolute transfusion safety will not be realized until blood substitutes can be infused. Current blood substitutes are oxygen carriers with a short intravascular lifespan and in only limited ways substitute for all of blood's functions [5]. Their toxicities are becoming better understood and formulations of hemoglobin-based oxygen carriers (HBOC)[6] and perfluorocarbons are undergoing clinical trials in trauma and elective surgery with minimal adverse effects [7].

The desirable characteristics of a red cell substitute have only partially been achieved [5]. One requirement of a blood substitute would be to replace all cellular functions; current formulations provide oxygen delivery and some blood volume expansion, but other blood or red cell functions are lacking. Although the destruction rate of transfused red cells is similar to the one per cent per day destruction rate of the recipient's own red cells, current red cell substitutes survive in the circulation only 12-24 hours. The goals of removal of antigenicity so that no compatibility testing is required and the elimination of disease transmission seem to be achievable with current blood substitutes under development. On the other hand, the desired result of no or minimal clinical toxicity has been difficult to reach and toxicity issues remain a major barrier to licensure for clinical use. A final goal of easy preparation and long shelf-life has been achieved, with the possibilities of prolonged room temperature storage featured in products under clinical investigation.

HBOC can be produced from outdated human blood, animal blood, or by recombinant technology. Most of the products under development are chemically modified by a number of steps to reduce their potential toxicity. The hemoglobin tetramer is cross-linked or polymerized to increase its intravascular survival and minimize the renal toxicity which occurs when the tetramer dissociates into dimers. Polymerization also permits infusion of a solution with a greater concentration of hemoglobin with oncotic properties similar to blood. It appears that vasoconstriction, one of the major toxicities of HBOC, can be reduced by polymerization or coupling to a large macromolecule such as polyethylene glycol. Vasoconstriction is lessened when the extravasation of the HBOC is reduced so that nitric oxide is not bound in the endothelial cell [8]. Some formulations of HBOC using a cross-linked hemoglobin tetramer led to many adverse consequences secondary to vasoconstriction [9]. A second mechanism whereby HBOC may produce vasoconstriction involves the autoregulation of capillary blood flow by oxygen [10]. In addition, some HBOC are chemically modified to enhance oxygen delivery with chemicals such as pyridoxal phosphate [11].

HBOC have a number of potential advantages. The shelf life would be much greater than the 42 day period for which red cells can be stored, room temperature storage would be permitted, the solutions would not have blood group antigens, and HBOC can be treated to achieve viral inactivation. On the other hand, they have a very short intravascular survival of only 12-24 hours compared to the 50 day half-life of the red cell, and their infusion can interfere with a number of laboratory tests in the chemistry laboratory [12].

Perfluorocarbon emulsions, in which large quantities of oxygen can be dissolved, have advantages in ease of production and absence of viral risks. However, their potential clinical use is limited by the toxicity of some of the emulsifying agents in the preparations, activation of the complement system, thrombocytopenia that may occur from uptake of the perfluorocarbon in the reticuloendothelial system, and the fact that current perfluorocarbon formulations would deliver enough oxygen only in patients breathing very high oxygen concentrations [5, 7].

Clinical Studies of HBOC

Although red cell substitutes have not been approved by the FDA, several HBOC are in phase III clinical trials. The two clinical applications that seem most likely to be approved are for patients with acute trauma where several blood volumes of HBOC have been infused without complications and in acute normovolemic hemodilution (ANH) protocols where the HBOC permits lowering of the patient's red cells for reinfusion after surgery.

Some of the clinical trials underway have demonstrated that HBOC could have major benefits in the treatment of hemorrhagic shock. Gould et al performed a randomized trial of polymerized human hemoglobin as a blood substitute in acute trauma or emergency surgery [13]. Patients were randomized to receive red cells or up to six units (300 g) of PolyHeme as their initial blood replacement. Patients receiving PolyHeme received a mean of 4.4 units which resulted in a plasma hemoglobin level of 3.9 g/dL or approximately 40% of their circulating hemoglobin. No serious or unexpected adverse events were noted.

Further investigations with PolyHeme have shown no major consequences with infusions of up to twenty units. In many of the studied patients, the red cell hemoglobin level has fallen to below 3 g/dL, a level often associated with mortality. With the adjunctive support provided by the HBOC and compensating levels of plasma hemoglobin, the likelihood of mortality was lessened substantially, even in patients with major trauma.

Another application of HBOC was demonstrated in a recent case report where a patient with life-threatening autoimmune hemolytic anemia (AHA) was sustained by infusions of a polymerized bovine hemoglobin [14]. This patient had encountered severe reactions to red cells and the dramatic fall in hematocrit necessitated this intervention. In addition to patients for whom compatible blood can not be obtained because of the interference of potent autoantibodies, there are occasional patients who present with allo-immunization to red cell antigens that delay the availability of compatible blood. The life-saving potential of HBOC in these situations is substantial, although efficacy may be difficult to prove since these cases are infrequent and controlled trials would be difficult to perform.

Many studies of HBOC or perfluorocarbons have explored the utility of these materials in elective surgery. Since HBOC or perfluorocarbons have short in vivo survival, their use will be limited to supportive functions until transfused red cells or the patient's own red cells can sustain life. Many of the studies to date have used relatively small infusions of HBOC or perfluorocarbons with the study endpoint being the reduction or elimination of allogeneic transfusions. In one published report, a polymerized bovine hemoglobin solution was infused in doses of up to 150 grams over a 96 hour period to patients undergoing aortic surgery [15]. With this protocol, 27% of patients receiving the HBOC avoided allogeneic blood while 100% of the controls required at least one unit of red cells. The current safety of allogeneic blood and the likely high costs of HBOC suggest that the use of HBOC as described is unlikely to have major impact on transfusion practice.

A more exciting possibility is the use of blood substitutes in conjunction with extreme acute normovolemic hemodilution, offering the potential to perform bloodless surgery for vascular and orthopedic procedures that typically use large volumes of allogeneic blood [16]. The concept of hemodilution is that during a limited period of anticipated blood loss a patient's blood can be partially replaced with an expendable substitute (typically colloid and crystalloid), after which the patient's own blood is returned. A more complete realization of this concept may now be on the horizon with the use of HBOC. These substances retain the advantageous low viscosity of diluted blood while providing increased oxygen carrying capacity. Extreme hemodilution with a blood substitute may become feasible regardless of cardiac or pulmonary status. Since candidate blood substitutes have a short in vivo survival, blood bank procedures could be modified to permit storage of autologous blood collected in the operating room for transfusion over several postoperative days as the substitute level decays and anemia develops. The dilution of coagulation factors would presumably be limiting, although the autologous plasma and platelets collected could offset some of the deficit [17]. We are currently performing a study in aortic aneurysm surgery where more than 40 participants have been hemodiluted with a target of six units of autologous blood to be collected using a polymerized human hemoglobin substitute in doses up to 300 grams of hemoglobin (the equivalent of six units of red cells).

Conclusions

Although the fears of patients and their physicians of the adverse consequences of allogeneic blood transfusions have lessened, the development of artificial oxygen carriers as an alternative to human blood resources is proceeding and the availability of HBOC and/or perfluorocarbons can be anticipated in the next few years. The major utility of these agents is expected to be for trauma and elective surgery cases with emphasis upon their use as an adjunct to hemodilution protocols. It is not unlikely, however, that these agents will be used for other medical purposes, taking advantages of their low viscosity and ability to circulate around obstructive lesions. Table 2 provides a list of potential clinical applications their potential utility in diverse situations [18]. Because of this wide variety of potential clinical applications, there is a medical imperative to develop red cell substitutes, even if blood were always available in adequate supply and had no known adverse effects.

Table 2. Potential clinical applications for red cell substitutes.

Trauma
Elective surgery (hemodilution)
Alloimmune or autoimmune hemolysis
Ischemic disease
Extracorporeal circulation
Sickle cell anemia
Organ perfusion
Tumor therapy
Cardioplegia

Adapted from reference 18

References

1. Sullivan MT, Wallace EL, Umana WO, Schreiber GB. Trends in the collection and transfusion of blood in the United States, 1987-1997. Transfusion 1999;39:1S.
2. Lenny LL, Hurst R, Zhu A, Goldstein J, Goldbraith RA. Multiple-unit and second transfusions of red cells enzymatically converted from group B to group O: report on the end of phase I trials. Transfusion 1995;35:899-902.
3. Consensus conference. Perioperative red blood cell transfusion.JAMA 1988;260: 2700-03.
4. Schreiber GB, Busch MP, Kleinman SH, Korelitz JJ, for the Retrovirus Epidemiology Donor Study. The risk of transfusion-transmitted viral infections. N Engl J Med 1996;334:1685-90.
5. Klein HG. The prospects for red-cell substitutes. N Engl J Med 2000;342:1666-68.
6. Gould SA, Moss GS. Clinical development of human polymerized hemoglobin as a blood substitute. World J Surg 1996;20:200-07.
7. Kaufman R. Clinical development of perfluorocarbon-based red cell substitutes. In Winslow R, Vandegriff K, Intaglietta M eds): Blood Substitutes: Physiologic Basis of Efficacy. New York: Birkhauser; 1995.

8. Keipert PE, Gonzales A, Gomez CL, MacDonald VW, Hess JR, Winslow RM. Acute changes in systemic blood pressure and urine output of conscious rats following exchange transfusion with diaspirin-crosslinked hemoglobin solution. Transfusion 1993; 33:701-08.
9. Sloan EP, Koenigsberg M, Gens D, et al. Diaspirin cross-linked hemoglobin (DCLHb) in the treatment of severe traumatic hemorrhagic shock: a randomized controlled efficacy trial. JAMA 1999;282:1857-64.
10. Winslow RM, Gonzales A, Gonzales ML, et al. Vascular resistance and the efficacy of red cell substitutes in a rat hemorrhage mode. J Appl Physiol 1998;85:993-1003.
11. Seghal LR, Rosen AL, Noud G, et al. Large volume preparation of pyridoxylated hemoglobin with high in vivo P50. J Surg Res 1981;30:14-20.
12. Ma Z, Monk TG, Goodnough LT, et al. Effect of hemoglobin and Perflubron-based oxygen carriers on common clinical laboratory tests. Clin Chem 1997;43:1732-37.
13. Gould SA, Moore EE, Hoyt DB, et al. The first randomized trial of human polymerized hemoglobin as a blood substitute in acute trauma and emergent surgery. J Am Coll Surg 1998;187:113-22.
14. Mullon J, Giacoppe G, Clagett C, McCune D, Dillard T. Transfusions of polymerized bovine hemoglobin in a patient with severe autoimmune hemolytic anemia. N Engl J Med 2000;342:1638-43.
15. LaMuraglia GM, O'Hara PJ, Baker WH, et al. The reduction of the allogenic transfusion requirement in aortic surgery with a hemoglobin-based solution. J Vasc Surg 2000;31:299-308.
16. Rottman G, Ness PM. Acute normovolemic hemodilution is a legitimate alternative to allogeneic blood transfusion. Transfusion 1998;38:477-80.
17. Triulzi DJ, Gilmor GD, Ness PM, et al. Efficacy of autologous fresh whole blood or platelet-rich plasma in adult cardiac surgery. Transfusion 1995;35:627-34.
18. Winslow RM. Red cell substitutes. In: Hoffman R, Benz EJ, Shattil SJ, et al, eds. Hematology: basic principles and practice, 3rd edition. Philadelphia: Churchill Livingstone, 2000:2343-48.

DISCUSSION

A. Brand (Leiden, NL): Dr. Meryman, is the damage random or is it particularly the elder population of red cells that is damaged - the freezing damage and the deglycerolisation damage?

H.T. Meryman (Bethesda, MD, USA): It is random, if you freeze and get 5% haemolysis and take the remaining cells and freeze them again you get another 5% haemolysis. So, it is some kind of a random process; maybe related to the proximity to the surface of the container, who knows. It is not a particular cohort of the cells.

C.L. van der Poel (Amsterdam, NL): Mr. Chairman, I think this really needs some further clarification, because the problem in the idea of Dr. Brand was if you would take young red cells you could focus on younger populations more towards reticulocytes. Would that be useful to have less damage?

H.T. Meryman: It does. Yes, indeed the younger populations do appear to be a little more resistant to injury. However, the injuries are still random by the test that I just mentioned, but the younger populations do appear to be a little bit sturdier. But the process of producing younger populations is so complex that it is not worth the effort just to pick up a few percent more of surviving cells. With the glycerol system it is so good already if properly done that there is not much point to it. We routinely get a total recovery at the end of the process of 95-97% and I might add that the secret to this kind of success is in the glycerolising and not the deglycerolising. This is something that struck investigators for years because they know haemolysis after they add the glycerol. They get a lot after they take it out so they say ‘gosh we get problems taking it out’. But in fact the injury was done during the addition of glycerol as a result of the hypertonic stress that the cells were put through. They would leak during the hypertonic stress, but not sufficient to cause haemolysis.

W.G. van Aken (Amsterdam, NL): Thank you very much. Dr. Foster, do you have data on the removal of TSE's from plasma during fractionation. You did not address that specifically; is it for a specific reason that you left it out?

P.R. Foster (Edinburgh, UK): I let it out just in the interest of time. In my manuscript I will give the references and people can look at the data. I will discuss that in more detail if you like.

K. Morris (Belfast, UK): Dr. Foster, do immunoglobulin preparations in general meet the requirement for two complementary viral activation steps, which are validated? I am really thinking about the pepsin pH step which manufacturers would use as well as solvent detergent.

P.R. Foster: Sure, manufacturers are making changes, not only starting intervening with the normal immunoglobins, the various intramuscular as well as the intravenous products. I cannot give you exactly which manufacturers have actually got two steps and which have not, but certainly the position most manufacturers are moving towards is for example getting combinations of solvent detergent and low pH treatment opposed to what was most common. We are introducing a new irradiation protocol.

The status of the low pH technique is that it is comparable to solvent detergent and its effectiveness in vast inactivation.

K. Morris: Therefore does it beat the EU directive July 1998[1] which talks about validated for viral inactivation and complementary in their modes of action. What I caught was were there complementary or different ways to describe processes and the second aspect was that it had to be validated, presumably through remodelling and spiking experiments.

P.R. Foster: That is correct.

K. Morris: Is that a yes or no for low pH pepsin. About intravenous immunoglobulin, you described the viral inactivation steps and they were low pH pepsin and there were the two viral inactivation steps in use for intravenous immunoglobulin.

P.R. Foster: Those steps to my knowledge have been well validated in terms of inactivating viruses which are markers and models for hepatitis C and HIV and a range of enveloped viruses. Now that solvent detergent treatment nor low pH treatment are effective against non- enveloped viruses, that is an area that still requires to be developed as it does with coagulation factors.

W.G. van Aken (Amsterdam, NL): Dr. Corash, in your final remarks of a very interesting presentation on new virus inactivation methods you mentioned that there would also be a certain economic benefit to this technology. I think we live in a country here where we are not only interested from the governmental side in evidence based medicine, but also in cost benefit and in cost effectiveness. So, it is very urgent for us to know what we may expect from this new

1. EU Directive 1998.

technology if the results of the clinical trials prove indeed what you have shown us. Would you briefly address what you think in terms of costs, extra dollars.

L. Corash (Concorde, CA, USA): I think the economic benefits to the platelet system could be the following. First of all because there is an added solution that is used you replace 65% of the plasma. So, you get more volunteer donor plasma, which is available for collecting. Secondly, because you have effective viral inactivation for CMV, all of your units would really be put into CMV-negative inventory. So, CMV serological testing would go away.

I think in addition, the effective inactivation of leukocytes means one can eliminate gamma-irradiation and avoid the problem of having two inventories of gamma-radiated and non-gamma-irradiated blood for immuno-incompetent patients. Another benefit is that leukocyte reduction is obviously being used right now for CMV. Some people do rely on it, other people still feel that it is not a complete technology. Then obviously for reduction of allo-immunisation and for prevention of certain types of febrile transfusion reactions. The TRAP trial demonstrated certainly that ultraviolet B, which is not as effective for inactivating leukocytes, prevented allo-immunisation.

So, I think the possibility arises, using this technology, to really re-examine the way in which we look at leukocyte depletion. So, each of these provides a potential area for an economic benefit.

W.G. van Aken: Can you already inform us about what sort of cost we should expect in dollars?

L. Corash: This technology has not gone through the final records for its process yet; it has not been put into a final commercial configuration, so I really cannot tell you what the cost would be. But I think it would be a cost which is very competitive with some of the cost expanded on testing and leukocyte depletion today; it will be very much in that range. So, I think it is an affordable technology.

W.G. van Aken: Thank you very much. Dr. Allain, you mentioned in your presentation also this technology and you addressed notably what the impact could be in countries with a high prevalence, which do not have all the resources. What do you think of this information.

J-P. Allain (Cambridge, UK): Well, I tell you Dr. Corash and I have discussed that on several occasions. The basic problem in developing countries is that the kind of product that is used is basically whole blood. I understand that the products Dr. Corash has discussed were either platelets or red cell concentrates.

The question I have actually is, if there was this kind of technology available to whole blood instead of components would that not be obviously of extreme importance for developing countries. So, what is the status on this kind of approaches in whole blood.

L. Corash: We are actually now doing some work with the military looking at modifying these compounds to whole blood. Obviously the biology of red cells, plasma protein solutions and human platelets is quite different and I do not know whether or not we will be able to accomplish this. I think though that if you look at a situation where at least you could make packed red cells and plasma, which I think requires a minimum of technology that one could practice and have two of your most important components. I mean forget about platelets for the time being in developing nations. If you just could have safe red cells and good plasma, you would be very far along.

J.C. Emmanuel (Geneva, CH): In this sort of spirit of cheerful disagreement I like to take up something that Dr. Allain said. He knows well that I am going to ask the question of pre-donation testing. My own experience outside WHO is that it is something really dangerous to do. Most developing countries, in fact all of them that I know of do not have alternative testing sites and therefore you can actually attract the very people you are trying to avoid.

The second point is that what we found in my previous existent country as well is that when hepatitis was around and syphilis, there was no real stigma involved in notifying people or having bleeds in factories or schools. The minute HIV came, and this is a question of perception when you talk about high prevalence, I mean in my perception if the prevalence in the donor population is 2% that is pretty good. To you that is astoundingly bad. High prevalence to me is 20% or 15% and that sure is a question of degree. But as soon as you have any kind of prevalence like 2-3% and the HIV interventions start taking place outside blood transfusion service, everybody you notify is assumed to be HIV with or without hepatitis B. They do not really believe what you are telling them. So in a factory the stigma and discrimination can mean people lose jobs and so on. Thus, the counselling becomes extremely difficult and the follow-up.

What I am asking you now is if you have done this and you found it works for hepatitis B, because in your setting HIV was lower, what kind of psycho-social study did you do. I mean was it just a question and answer or was it a really in depth; what was the impact if you went to a school or a factory and told people they had hepatitis B. Did the others really believe this? Because, from WHO perspective we had to have a generic on a global basis and what you are talking about is a very specific area.

J-P. Allain : First of all, we have already discussed these various approaches and we agreed to a slight disagree. But I think both approaches need to be looked at.

As far as the prevalence is concerned as I showed, and I think there is more data that needs to be collected, is that there is a clear relationship between prevalence and residual risk related to window period and that the difference is very quickly apparent. So, if you have 0.1%, if you go to 1% or 2% then the risk of pressure conversion units comes into 1:500, 1:1000, which makes the risk quite considerable. So, this relationship of correlation between residual risk and prevalence is very important and to me 1% is high.

The third question about the way you can approach from a social point of view pre-donation testing. What we did in Ghana for hepatitis B, because at the time that was all we had available, was particularly to go into schools, assemble the students and tell them what we are going to do. That we were going to do a test and the test would be to look for hepatitis B chronic infection and if they were positive then we did not want to collect their blood, because it was dangerous for the recipients. But in addition we could do something for them, which is to ask them to come to the hospital, be counselled and have ALT testing. And actually doing that we I think we served an important public health purpose, which is to find out who had liver disease, and tried to do something about it. So, I think it allows pre-donation testing in my experience in developing countries allows to do donor care, which otherwise most of the time you cannot do, because you cannot trust the donors.

I mentioned HIV and I agree with you that the immediate response is when something is wrong it is HIV. As you mentioned of the fact that Ghana and a couple of countries nearby have a very relatively low prevalence of HIV makes this quite less acute, but there is obviously a problem to that, which in thinking with a group of people from Ghana we thought to be able to solve in telling people we are screening for a number of viruses and if one test is positive then you come to the hospital for counselling. It is then that we can tell them which virus it is which by the way allows us to confirm and then do the counselling in an environment of confidentiality. So, I think it is possible to do.

C.Th. Smit Sibinga *(Groningen, NL):* Dr. Allain, what would you think would be the policy for providing standard reference material to the various parts in the world specifically for HCV testing, because there are various types of the HCV and its very prevalence in the world. For instance the type III in Egypt and the type VI in Vietnam and so forth. There need to be different standards as a reference, whether you use dipstick or lateral flow or ELISA. What would be a policy appropriate to these countries.

J-P. Allain: Well, it is actually difficult because of the epidemiology of HCV. As has been published recently the epidemiology in Egypt is related to essentially those of common transmission. You may have pockets of very high prevalences and 20 km away in another village where the practices of injections and so on are different you can have very low prevalence. So, it is very difficult to decide on a global policy for HCV. But there are problems with the testing and the performance of what I have seen as rapid test. It is considerably worse than HIV or HBsAg in part, because the general level of antibodies is lower. So, it is more difficult to test and you have lower specificity and sensitivity. I think it is premature to decide on rules as to the use of anti-HCV.

C.Th. Smit Sibinga (Groningen, NL): You did not have the time to go into the bacterial testing. I am aware of an upcoming rapid test for bacterial contamination screening based on DNA. Could you give some more information on this.

J-P. Allain: Yes, there are some new ways of testing for bacterial DNA using either hybridisation technique or other. The problem in my view with this is that you have to establish to a threshold, because if you look in particular without amplification techniques to any blood unit, you are going to find bacterial material. So, the question is where is it dangerous and where to put the threshold which can depend on the concentration of bacteria, also may vary from bacteria to bacteria. But probably most importantly these thresholds vary tremendously depending on the recipient. So, if you have an immunocompetent recipient the level of bacteria that they can afford without any problem is very high, but if you are an immunocompromised recipient then it can become a big problem. So the rules are different to set.

C.Th. Smit Sibinga: Dr. Meryman, you focused on the red cells. But the vitrification technology was also explored in an attempt to cryopreserve complete organs like kidneys. So, how far has that come?

H.T. Meryman: It is going about as far as the funding would permit it to. We were achieving a really very good rate of survival of rabbit kidneys re-implanted in the original donor after being vitrified. There is tubular damage, but those kidneys would support life in those rabbits. The project was terminated as a result of lack of interest by the funding agency. I think that it is possible, that this could be picked up and could be done. I do not look at that as an impossible goal.

C.Th. Smit Sibinga: So, you see a future for that.

H.T. Meryman: Yes, I think so. The attitude that we ran into the funding agent was who needs it. We got more recipients of organs than we have organs, and who wants to preserve them. That was the attitude that was taken.

D.B.L. McClelland (Edinburgh, Scotland): Dr. Allain, you quoted some contribution of procedural error to the failure to detect and you put a pretty low figure on that. But if you look at some of the data for example the data published where you find a majority of failure to detect in laboratories in some parts of the world. I think you are being very optimistic about the rate of technical failure and I just like to link that for discussion with your other point that NAT adds a lot more complication. Equally adds viral inactivation procedure a lot more complication to component processing. So, I think at least in the developing country context we do have to be very aware of the ability to operate complex systems in terms of just quality management.

J-P. Allain: Well, I think you are perfectly right; clearly the complication particularly now with EIAs on one side, NAT on the other. If you have any problem in your IT system then you can be really dead in the waters. So, it is a real very serious problem of the extraordinary level of sophistication we have in electronics, but if something goes wrong it can be very wrong and I think that is something to keep in mind.

K. Sazama (Houston, TX, USA): My question really is provoked by Dr. Corash's presentation, maybe very simplistic and I apologise to the audience if it is that way; but it is compelling to me to consider if one could isolate one solvent from the psychosocial environment in the regular environments in which we live. Your data suggest to me that we can just actually go into viral inactivation or to organism or DNA inactivation and eliminate all of the testing and all the donor screening. So, rely solely upon what is in the bag having been processed in a manner that makes it safe from living materials in it. If one could envision that, then it seems like the rest of the discussion is almost not necessary. Meaning more and more tests with more and more complexity and all of the complications we have dealt with because of the donor impact of the results of testing could vanish. Help me with this pine in the sky image that I have. What are the potentials for having a viral inactivation or living material inactivation, so that become the products that we transfuse and eliminate obviously we can all agree that we will never eliminate all the rest that has gone into it. But if we could start with just what you have in hand, why not have envision a world where we just treat what is in the bag and administer it; meaning we could not neglect all of the costs of all of the rest of the activities that we go wrong and simply start with what is in the bag and make it safe and transfuse it.

L. Corash: Well, I think it is possible to entertain that. Obviously when you develop products like this and you do laboratory studies for pathogen inactivation, you do clinical trials. But non of the clinical trials are organised around looking at pathogen inactivation because in the current state of blood component testing you have to have clinical trials with literally hundreds of thousands of people in it. So, I think you need to gain experience with this technology how in the real world before you can entertain re-assorting the test mix or even getting rid of the test. But if you look for example at the ELISA based serological tests, they are reasonably inexpensive and they are quite effective. When looking at p24 antigen testing in the United States and nucleic acid testing we are talking about picking up relatively few cases. I think there is an argument to me to use this technology in place of nucleic acid testing for example with inexpensive serological testing. When you go in the developing world then I think it becomes more rational to ask about using this technology as the only technology. And I think that it is a technology which is simple enough I mean the platelet technology obviously requires platelets and plasma require an illumination device. So you need electric power and you have a machine that delivers that has got a microprocessor. It is a relatively simple machine, but it is nonetheless a machine. The red cell system really is just add, shake and incubate overtime. It does not require much except a refrigerator to put the red cells in, which you should have anyway. So, that one is pretty approachable. I think in developing countries you might start with this technology and not adapt testing; so I think it is possible.

B.G. Solheim (Oslo, N): Dr. Corash, you mentioned the very high efficiency on viruses, but there were differences and I am sure there are some viruses where these methods are significantly less efficient against which you know of.

L. Corash: Yes, we for example hepatitis A virus in the psoralen methodology because for platelets and also for plasma actually the time of illumination is very critical and we cannot inactivate high titres of hepatitis A virus. The protein captured is extremely tight, but hand palms do not get in. If you incubate for a long period of time you can inactivate these viruses. So, there are some limitations, I do not think any system is a 100%. I think there is an advantage that these are not pooled products. If you are making pools for platelets it is very small pools. The other differences we saw with Gram positive and Gram negative bacteria. Most of these are largely small experimental differences or a matter of the titres that you can get for these. I do not think they are that different.

B.G. Solheim: With respect to the cost efficiency of the psoralen method for platelets, I missed one argument and that was the removal of bacteria. That should offer the prolongation of shelf life to seven days.

L. Corash: Yes, absolutely, that is a good point. There is that potential to change the inventory and obviously there are other benefits to be gained. You could look at this being sort of economic benefits. I mean if the number of febrile transfusion reactions goes down, because you have complete inhibition of cytokine synthesis for example. Post-transfusion fever in a patient has an economic cost to it, it means medication, it means cultures, it means increased observation times. So sure, there are benefits like that.

B.G. Solheim: The cytokine release, do you have good data that that is really blocked?

L. Corash: Yes, it is 100% inhibited.

B.G. Solheim: FRASE compounds for whole blood, what is the possibility? Because that would have been very interesting for developing countries.

L. Corash: We are trying to develop some new compounds. The military is very interested in being able to have an inactivation system where you can literary draw a unit of whole blood from a healthy soldier, add a compound to it, shake it up and give it somebody who needs blood. We are not there yet, but I think it is a type of chemistry, which has potential to get us to that point.

B.G. Solheim: Dr. Ness, you mentioned intra-operative haemoglobin in the aortic surgery study of over 8 grams per dl. What was the erythrocyte haemoglobin?

P.M. Ness (Baltimore, MD, USA): Well, we measured haemoglobin levels so that in most of the patient's haemoglobin was totally red cell. If they got haemoglobin it was a combination of whatever residual red cell they had plus the haemoglobin infused.

A. Brand (Leiden, NL): Dr. Corash, indeed photodynamic inactivation is becoming very near and I want to have your opinion on three aspects that you discussed. First, do you need for the psoralens to use platelet reconstitution solutions. We do not consider in the Netherlands platelet preservation solutions, so it should at least be equal compared to plasma.

Second, if you say the immune suppressive or non-immunising effect of photodynamic treatment can be at least, as proven by the TRAP study[1], equal to other approaches like leukocyte depletion you have to consider that if the leukocytes are still present and you manipulate them by photodynamic treatment, the absence of immunisation is of course by another mechanism than simply removing the leukocytes.

Third, you mentioned a study in which your are evaluating inactivated plasma for CTTP patients. You mentioned a study size of 30 and I wondered what will be your end-point because we tried to find out what is the best plasma solution for TTP and ended up with 250 patients in the studies.

L. Corash: Yes, first of all the platelet additive solution. The system is put together with a platelet additive solution for two reasons. First of all because you do increase inactivation efficiency by deluting plasma protein particularly for bacteria. You gain a lot of robustness by doing that. In the United States today we do not use platelet additive solutions at all, so the system will change if this technology is adopted. You are already using platelet additive solutions for some of your products. So I think it should be an easier change, but you gain efficiency. In addition, the platelet additive solution has a substrate acetate which is a better substrate for platelet storage for metabolism and control of pH. Particularly if you have adequate oxygen and maintain respiration. So that is an advantage that you get I think especially if you want to go to 7 days of storage.

Your second question regarding allo-immunisation. We know that psoralens inhibit for example presentation of antigens on the surface of leukocytes and activation antigen expression more effectively so than ultraviolet B illumination. There is data looking at psoralens in mouse transfusion studies showing inhibition of allo-immunisation in mismatched animal models. So, we are very optimistic about that as being effective.

Your last point TTP. The primary end point in our trial is proportion of patients in remission at day 30. So, these patients are randomised to plasma exchange for up to 30 days. If they are not in remission at 30 days they can be extended for another 30 days, but the primary end point is the proportion of patients in remission at day 30. Based upon remission rates in the United States, that we see with plasma exchange, which are somewhere around 70-75%. We basically develop a protocol with the FDA that would enrol 30 patients. As you probably know this is a sporadic disease and it is hard to accumulate a large number of patients. This is not a high powered study, but it has enough power to allow us to compare the remission rates.

---

1. The Trial to Reduce Alloimmunization to Platelets Study Group. Leukocyte reduction and ultraviolet-B irradation of platelets to prevent alloimmunization and refractoriness to platelet transfusion. N Engl J Med 1997:337:1861-69.

A. Brand: It sounds to me like a registration number and not like a clinical effectiveness number.

L. Corash: There is no doubt that one could gain more data and have a better study by doing several hundred patients, no question about that. But that would be a very difficult study to undertake. Particularly, when you want to limit exposure to any other type of plasma. We are also very selective in the types of patients that we take. We do not take patients who have bone marrow transplant related TTP, because that is a therapy that does not really respond very well to plasma exchange.

J.R. Aluoch (Nairobi, Kenya): Dr. Ness, regarding the use of substitutes particularly in the management of patients with sickle cell anaemia, it would be beautiful to be able to give them something that does not contain sickle haemoglobin. But about the high cost issue one gets wondering to what extend can this be reduced in future. Most of the effected sickle cell patients live in economically disadvantaged areas.

The second question is what about ß thalassaemia of thalassaemics and to what extent do these substitutes be useful in reducing the rate of haemochromatosis.

P.M. Ness: I do not know of any data in thalassaemia and even in sickle cell anaemia. What I was referring to because the short half-life of these materials I am not sure that they have any real meaningful use for chronic therapy. The situation I was referring to is a situation at least in the US we get into an elective surgery, where we often get patients who come to us, who are going to have elective major surgery and there is a concern that they could have chest syndrome after the surgery because of anaesthesia problems and post-operative complications. The therapy for many of these patients is to do an exchange transfusion. We do an exchange transfusion often with a limited blood supply, because they are already allo-immmunised by the time they get to surgery they have received if they are adult or even a large trial 5 or 6 units of blood. They then start having a delayed haemolytic reaction often, because we missed an antibody or they made another. My thought is that if we had these oxygen carriers rather than doing the exchange transfusion for an acute event or even for a chest syndrome, one could give an infusion of the material, raise the haemoglobin level, not raise the blood viscosity. And since it has a short half-life and since the operative period is relatively short, the short half-life problem which would effect the chronic use of these materials would not be a problem for this specific indication. So, I think there are limited ways at least for sickle cell patients in the way we transfuse them now in the United States at least; in developed countries this may be a very meaningful therapy.

J.R. Aluoch: So, in other words it would not be of use for example to consider using them in children with sickle cell anaemia or where stroke is about to shocked them.

P.M. Ness: I do not think it is a problem for those who we give transfusion therapy because of prevention of the next stroke to develop. Unless we can do something to do a major increase of the in vivo survival I do not think they will be that useful.

III. QUALITY PRINCIPLES AND RISK MANAGEMENT

QUALITY SYSTEMS AND MANAGEMENT: 2000 WHERE HAVE WE BEEN AND WHERE ARE WE GOING?

K. Sazama[1]

Introduction

Functioning quality systems are the expected norm of practice in blood centers and transfusion services in the United States (U.S.) in the year 2000 [1]. Beginning in the mid-1980's when the Joint Commission on Accreditation of Healthcare Organizations [JCAHO] refocused its vision to the quality of patient care, not just on the processes of providing services [2], quality initiatives have been introduced in all aspects of healthcare. Both governmental and private organizations have endorsed the language of quality and incorporated the assessment of quality activities and outcomes into their accrediting decisions. Along the way, the importance of having qualified personnel who are knowledgeable and committed to the principles of quality has been recognized.

To assist organizations in their quest for quality, terminology has become standardized to facilitate accurate and consistent communication (Table 1), and routine practices are evolving in a uniform manner, as evidenced in part by the increased frequency of positive accreditation and registration decisions. The value of integrating quality (doing the right thing right) into routine processes cannot be overemphasized in a world of instantaneous communication and information exchange, as evidenced by the competitive market edge enjoyed by the highest quality producers, those that have achieved the six sigma goal of excellence.

However, a review of the events of the 20th century that have led to the current state of practice reminds us that quality is neither a new concept nor a completed act – it is a quest that demands constant attention. Beginning in mid-century, the foundations for modern quality concepts were laid, especially in the U.S. where professional societies initiated peer review processes and quality control (QC) measures into routine practice, including requirements for voluntary accreditation. These concepts expanded about every 15 to 20 years, scaling the quality hierarchy by building from QC to quality assurance (QA), then to the current quality systems level. (Figure 1) Even certain U.S. governmental agencies (e.g., the Food and Drug Administration [FDA] and the Health Care

---

1. Department Laboratory Medicine, The University of Texas M.D. Anderson Cancer Center, Houston, Tx, USA.

Financing Administration (HCFA) have endorsed QA and a quality systems approach to transfusion medicine as a requirement for certification (which, in turn, is required for U.S. government financial support).

Future efforts to improve quality will require integrating the remaining levels of quality, namely, quality management (QM) and total quality management (TQM), into routine practice.

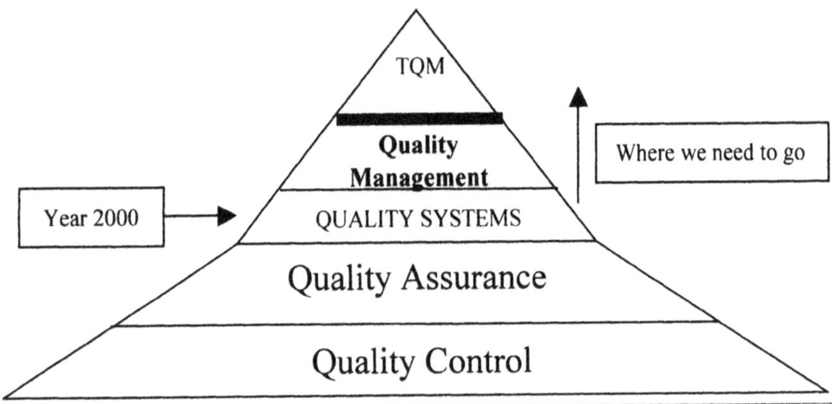

Total Quality Management(TQM) = Long term success through *customer satisfaction*
Quality Management (QM) = Adds *economic aspects* to activities listed below
Quality System = Comprehensive and coordinated efforts to *meet quality objectives*
Quality Assurance (QA) = *Planned/systematic activities* to provide confidence in quality
Quality Control (QC) = *Operational techniques* to fulfill requirements for quality

Figure 1. The quality hierarchy.

Historical Evolution of Quality Emphasis

In the past 100 years, transfusion medicine has emerged as a distinct medical practice and therapeutic entity. It has matured from a battlefield anomaly into an integral clinical modality for numerous acute and chronic disease conditions. Implicit in this maturation is an underlying commitment to quality of both product and practice. Some of the important milestones of the 20th century are shown in Figure 2, demonstrating that nearly the entire science of immunohaematology has been written in the past 100 years. The science of immunohaematology originated with Landsteiner's discovery of the A and B red blood cell antigens and progressed through development of the modern molecular methods now used to identify and define virtually all known red blood cell antigens, whether integral or adsorbed, as well as many platelet and leukocyte antigens. The immunology and biochemistry, as well as the cell-to-cell interactions and communications, of the immune system have been discovered and defined. Quality emphasis originated with the quality of the scientific method that produced verifiable information upon which this discipline has relied.

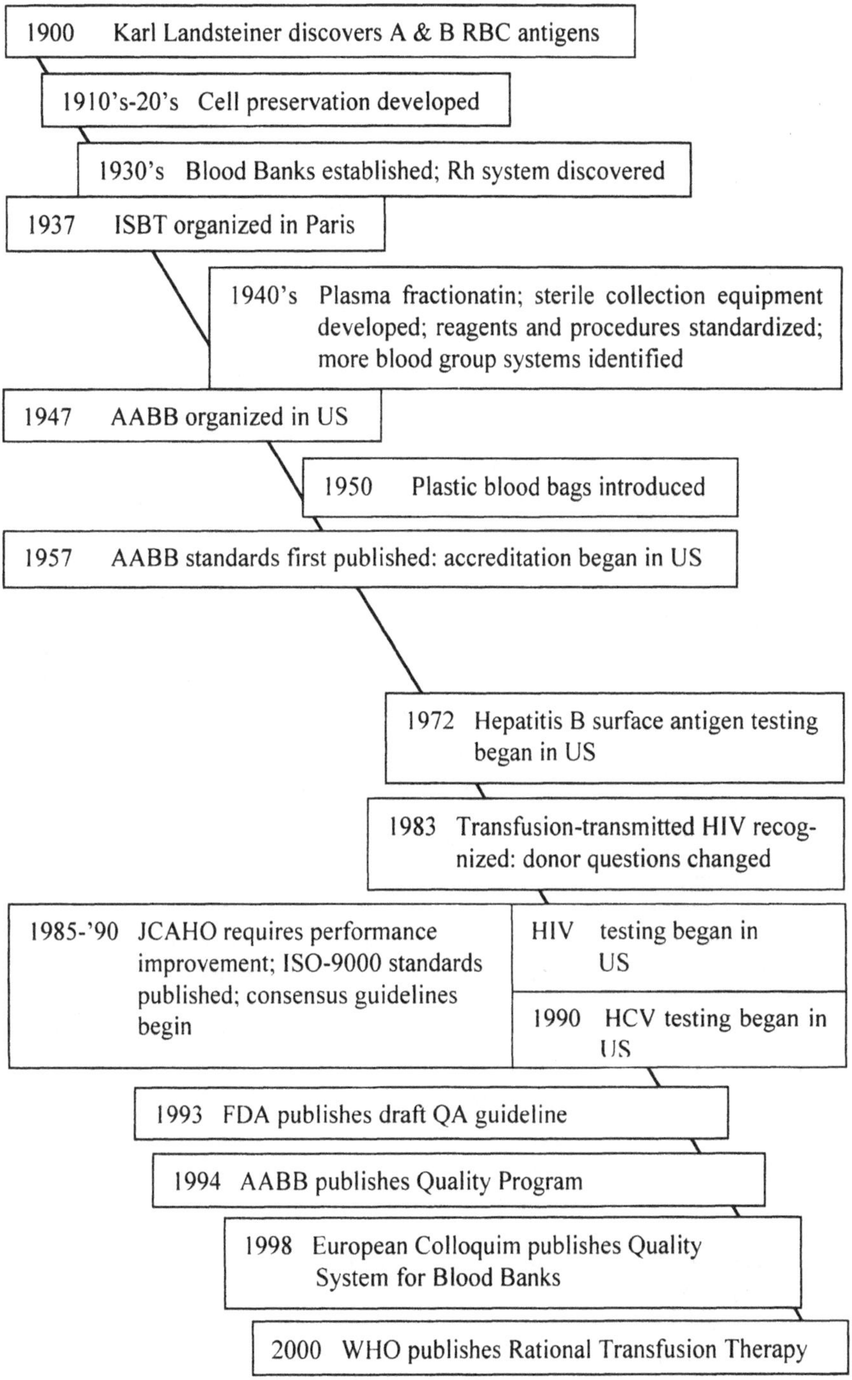

Figure 2. Selected quality milestones in blood banking and transfusion medicine in the twentieth century.

Other scientific breakthroughs included solving the problems of blood storage and cell viability (making possible the creation of 'blood banks' in the 1930's) and discovering a process to fractionate plasma and store it in more user-friendly packaging. The urgent need for plasma to support battlefield injuries during World War II gave impetus to broader application of transfusion therapies. By 1945, the separation and fractionation of plasma from whole blood was routinely performed, making plasma readily available in the military arena. With the end of hostilities, the civilian world reaped the benefits of this technology.

After the end of WWII, blood became readily available for civilian use, causing a predictable upsurge in blood utilization. This upsurge was supported by innovations such as the plastic storage bag and integral tubing, along with improved processing methods, permitting component preparation. All of these activities were dependent upon use of quality methods in development and manufacturing, most notably statistical process control. By the early 1970's, the U.S. FDA assumed an oversight responsibility for all aspects of blood collection and transfusion, publishing extensive regulations focused on standardization and quality control of blood for transfusion and for further manufacturing.

However, for professionals in blood banking, along with developing the capacity to safely store blood which made it readily available for transfusion, came the increasing awareness of the dangers of transfusion. From the earliest reports of transfusion practice in the early 1900's, problems with bacterial contamination, ABO incompatibility and infectious disease transmission (originally syphilis and hepatitis B) were recognized as significant hazards. Quality improvement measures (not named as such at the time) such as the introduction of 1) sterile equipment and routine use of aseptic collection techniques (which resulted in a significant reduction in the problem of bacteria in the stored components), 2) reliable typing reagents and strict adherence to standard procedures (which minimized the risk of an ABO incompatible transfusion) and 3) laboratory testing for specific disease conditions (such as a non-specific test for syphilis and a specific test for the hepatitis B surface antigen (HbsAg) in 1972 (which dramatically reduced the risk of hepatitis B virus (HBV) from transfusion) were added as they became available. The possible immunological hazards of transfusion, beginning with the first report of graft-versus-host disease due to transfusion (TI-GvHD) in 1965 [3], were beginning to surface, but were not considered to be a major problem in routine transfusion practice. By the end of the 70's, blood bankers in the U.S. were comfortably unconcerned about any significant residual risks from transfusion. Even the occasional report (approximately 16/year) of death from an ABO incompatible transfusion was viewed as an acceptable, although unfortunate, risk (estimated as about 1 per million red blood cells concentrate transfused). Then came the first report of a new disease that would rock transfusion medicine to its foundation – the acquired immune deficiency syndrome (AIDS).

Quality measures to reduce possible AIDS transmission by transfusion focused initially on efforts to educate ; identify and defer donors whose lifestyles placed them at increased risk of acquiring human immunodeficiency virus (HIV) infection. (HIV is the virus that causes AIDS.) There was no test, specific or surrogate, that could reliable identify infected components. The question of what was the 'right thing' to do has been widely debated in the legal arena around the world in the 15 years since a specific test for detecting antibody to HIV was developed and distributed in the U.S., beginning in March 1985. (The test development depended on identifying the virus, a discovery that was first reported in April 1984.)

In the decade between 1985 and 1995, specific tests for detecting antibodies to human immunodeficiency viruses, types 1 & 2 (HIV1/2), human T-lymphotropic viruses, types I & II (HTLV-I/II), hepatitis B core antigen (HBc) and hepatitis C virus (HCV), as well as a test to detect the HIV p24 antigen, were developed and became widely used in the U.S. and subsequently throughout other countries. In addition, donor blood was tested for the enzyme alanine aminotransferase (ALT) as a surrogate indicator of liver damage that might be related to a hidden viral infection. Plasma for transfusion has undergone viral inactivation using solvent/detergent manufacturing methods and/or has been quarantined and distributed following plasma reserve protocols only after a second negative test of the donor. In1999, newer testing methods using nucleic acid amplification and detection have been added for detecting the viral genome of HIV and HCV. All of these testing and manufacturing activities have developed in laboratories with strict QC and QA monitoring.

However, both the quantity and speed of implementation of these new tests have highlighted a quality gap in the very processes that are intended to ensure that the intent and action coincide. As has become glaringly apparent in legal events that subsequently occurred, blood collection and transfusion services throughout the world were ill equipped to deal with this rapidly evolving crisis. The demand could not be met in a manner that ensured the quality of the blood being transfused, with resultant impairment in safety to the transfusion recipient. In addition, in the background (and nearly eclipsed by the public hysteria over the AIDS epidemic), the increasing importance of immunological effects of transfusion, as evidenced by the recognition of TI-GvHD in immunocompetent patients [4] in 1986, and the emerging debate over immunomodulatory effects of transfusion [5] surfaced.

Suddenly, in the late '80's and early 90's, the transfusion medicine world was confronted with the need to focus specifically on means to further improve quality. Quality improvement (beyond the QC and QA processes already in place) rests squarely on the shoulders of individual persons committed to addressing systems problems. Our understanding of the quality hierarchy (Figure 1), widely used in the manufacturing world (especially in Japan) since the 1960's, has evolved from this recognition. The language of quality has permeated the lexicon of many businesses and professional activities. (Table 1) QA was the first initiative beyond the basic QC testing emphasis of the 50's, expanding QC into the broader concept of quality as applied to personnel, equipment, processes, reagents, facilities and procedures. Responsibility for quality encompassed not just the immediate 'hands-on' events but included a broader scope of activities that supported the QC decision. Suppliers were brought into the equation, with responsibility for the validity of claims about their products. Pre-analytical preparation of samples for testing was identified as a necessary quality step. The manner of dissemination of information, including donor self-exclusion or exclusion due to prior deferral and testing data that disqualified the donor and/or the blood component from transfusion, became a new focus of improvement actions.

At about the same time the awareness of the need to increase quality measures was dawning in laboratory and collection services, the clinical practice arena became refocused on outcome measures, specifically on patient safety and the appropriateness of transfusion. In the U.S., clinical practice guidelines and practice parameters were created and analyzed. Worldwide, the concept of haemovigilance began to emerge [6,7]. The role of hospital transfusion committees (HTC) to retrospectively monitor blood use and audit wastage, a concept introduced in the U.S. in the mid-60's, was revised to emphasize the development of clinical pathways or practice protocols for transfusion [8]. Reviews were expanded to include audit by component type and included recognition of the need to limit use of blood transfusion for selected surgical procedures. Policies for lookback and notification of recipients when donors seroconverted were drafted and implemented. Guidelines for autologous practice and for use of newer modalities of therapy such as platelet crossmatching, irradiated components or virally-inactivated (or donor retested) plasma were prepared and ratified by hospital transfusion committees. By 1993, the U.S. JCAHO emphasized the need for outcome evaluation and performance improvements, using multidisciplinary approaches [9], especially for activities such as blood transfusion (that by their very nature are multidisciplinary). New questions were added to the JCAHO survey tool that emphasized the medical staff's responsibility to participate in selection and monitoring of the blood components being acquired and used for patients in their own institution. Suddenly the question of blood availability became a broader focus.

By the mid-90's, various definitions and applications of the concept of quality, as Total Quality Management (TQM), Continuous Quality Improvement (CQI), Systematic Quality Management [10], Quality Assurance (QA) [11], Quality Systems, Performance Improvement and the like, were introduced as standards within hospitals. Many hospitals created new departments or positions responsible for ensuring that performance improvement activities were in place and (usually) that they met voluntary accreditation standards.

The Quality Movement

While blood bankers were celebrating the end of WWII and bringing to the civilian medical world the benefits of technology that evolved from that era, quality mavens such as Drs Deming and Juran were quietly beginning a revolution in manufacturing philosophy, mostly in Japan. The movement away from the Taylorism [12] embedded in American and European business occurred much later, in the late 70's and early 80's, only after the obvious superiority of the Deming quality model had been demonstrated in the marketplace. However, during the same time period of the Deming/Juran revolution in Japanese industry, the European community (with U.S. participation) recognized the value of global standardization with the establishment in 1940's of the International Organization for Standardization (ISO). Working from Europe (with minimal recognition initially by U.S. manufacturers and standard setting organizations), ISO developed a series of guidance documents that provided for standardization of numerous manufacturing processes and a vocabulary for discussing quality as a unique concept.

Quality in Blood Banking in the United States – The Private Sector

Meanwhile, in the late 50's, quality concerns surfaced in two practice areas in the U.S. The College of American Pathologists (CAP) devised a system of QC, first by using local and then by providing national laboratory samples that permitted laboratory to laboratory comparisons of proficiency (proficiency testing), and then created a national system of clinical laboratory accreditation based on a few general standards. Simultaneously, the American Association of Blood Banks (AABB) published its first 'Standards for Blood Banks' and began its peer reviewed accreditation program for blood collection and transfusion facilities in 1958. Both societies believed that these programs would enhance the quality of services provided, verified through using external observers (inspectors/assessors) and peer reviewed processes.

Beginning with its 16th edition, the AABB's 'Standards for Blood Banks and Transfusion Services' has explicitly required use of QA and, ultimately (in the 20tth edition [1] to be implemented on 1/1/2001), the use of quality systems in accredited facilities.

Quality in Blood Banking in the United States – The Government's Initiatives

In 1965, the U.S. Congress endorsed the concepts of standardizing laboratory practices to improve quality by enacting the Clinical Laboratory Improvements Act of 1965 (CLIA '65). CLIA'65 required the majority of U.S. clinical laboratories to enroll in proficiency testing programs and to be certified based on inspection, either by the HCFA or by authorized entities such as certain individual states or by CAP accreditation. Broader quality initiatives were introduced into CLIA '65 by the amendments enacted in 1988 (CLIA '88) in which QA language was added (among other revisions).

In 1972, the U.S. Food and Drug Administration was made responsible for overseeing blood collection and transfusion, removing these activities from the NIH Laboratory of Biological Standards. The FDA regulations for oversight were implemented in 1976 [13], containing requirements for error and accident documentation and reporting, for standard operating procedures, use of QC at all stages of manufacturing, for reporting of fatalities and other quality-driven measures. In subsequent years, the regulations have undergone little revision and updating, making them less useful in the rapidly changing world of the next millennium. Instead, the FDA has been forced to use guidance documents that lack the full enforceability of regulations. Only the requirement to test blood for HIV has reached full regulatory stature in the past two decades, while a singularly important guideline related to QA remains a guideline only. The FDA initiated its new quality focus by issuing a draft guideline, 'Guideline for Quality Assurance in Blood Establishments' in July 1993, finalizing it on July 11, 1995, after incorporating input from a public workshop in which transfusion medicine experts participated.

The Quality Movement in Europe

The World Health Organization (WHO), working with the International Red Cross, the World Federation of Hemophilia and the International Society of Blood Transfusion (ISBT), created the Global Blood Safety Initiative (GBSI) in the mid 1980's, laying the foundation for quality systems for blood banks and transfusion services. In addition, a number of national blood transfusion organizations, such as the Netherlands Society of Blood Transfusion (NVB) and the British Blood Transfusion Society (BBTS), were organized, beginning in the mid-1980's. The European Union has fostered consideration of single standards for member states, a challenge in the transfusion medicine arena due to the very different philosophical approaches of individual countries [14]. Private initiatives in many countries began looking at outcomes as a means to understand and improve quality.

Table 1. The language of quality.

Quality	The totality of characteristics of an entity that bear on its ability to satisfy stated and implied needs	ISO* 8402, 2.1
Quality Assurance	Planned and systematic activities to provide adequate confidence that requirements for quality will be met	ISO 8402, 3.5
Quality Control	Operational techniques and activities that are used to fulfill requirements for quality	ISO 8402, 3.4
Quality Management	All activities of the overall management function that determine quality policy objectives and responsibilities and implement them by means such as quality planning, quality control, quality assurance; and quality improvement within the quality system	ISO 8402, 3.2
Quality Policy	Overall intentions and direction of an organization with regard to quality (e.g., quality system essentials) as formally expressed by top management	ISO 8402, 3.1
Quality System	The organizationa structure, resources, processes and procedures needed to implement quality management	ISO 8402, 3.6

* ISO = International Organization for Standardization.

Quality Systems: Where We Are Now

Since 1994, the concept of quality systems has entered the lexicon of transfusion medicine [15-19]. The language of quality has been established (Table 1). The AABB's accreditation program requires facilities to demonstrate their quality systems as a condition for continued accreditation, based on the current ed-

Table 2. AABB quality system essentials (QSE).*

* Organization
* Resources
* Equipment
* Supplier and customer issues
* Process control
* Documents and records
* Incidents, errors, accidents, nonconformances, and complications
* Assessments: internal and external
* Process improvement through corrective and preventive action
* Facilities and safety

* Standards for Blood Banks and Transfusion Services, 20th Edition, 2000.

Table 3. AABB quality system essentials and ISO-9001H compared.

AABB QSE	ISO-9001H clauses
Organization	4.1 Management responsibility 4.2 Quality system
Resources	4.18 Training
Equipment	4.11 Control of inspection, measuring, and test equipment
Supplier and customer issues	4.3 Contract review 4.6 Purchasing 4.19 Servicing
Process control	4.4 Design control 4.7 Control of customer-supplied product 4.8 Product identification and traceability 4.9 Process control 4.10 Inspection and testing 4.12 Inspection and test status 4.15 Handling, storage, packaging, preservation and delivery 4.20 Statistical techniques
Documents and records	4.5 Document and data control 4.16 Control of quality records
Incidents, errors, accidents, nonconformances, and complications	4.13 Control of nonconfirming product
Assessments: internal and external	4.17 Internal quality audits
Process improvement through corrective and preventive action	4.14 Corrective and preventive action 4.20 Statistical techniques
Facilities and safety	4.9b Process control

Table 4. Comparison of AABB quality system essentials with European Colloquium.

AAB QSE	**European Colloquium**
AABB standards	Ad 1. Core standards
Organization	
Resources	Ad 3. Core education and training system
Equipment	
Supplier and customer issues	
Process control	Ad 5. Core haemovigilance system
Documents and records	
Incidents, errors, accidents, nonconformances, and complications	Ad 2. Core documentation system
Assessments: internal and external	
Process improvement through conrrective and preventive action	Ad 4. Core audit and accreditation Ad 4. Core audit and accreditation
Facilities and safety	

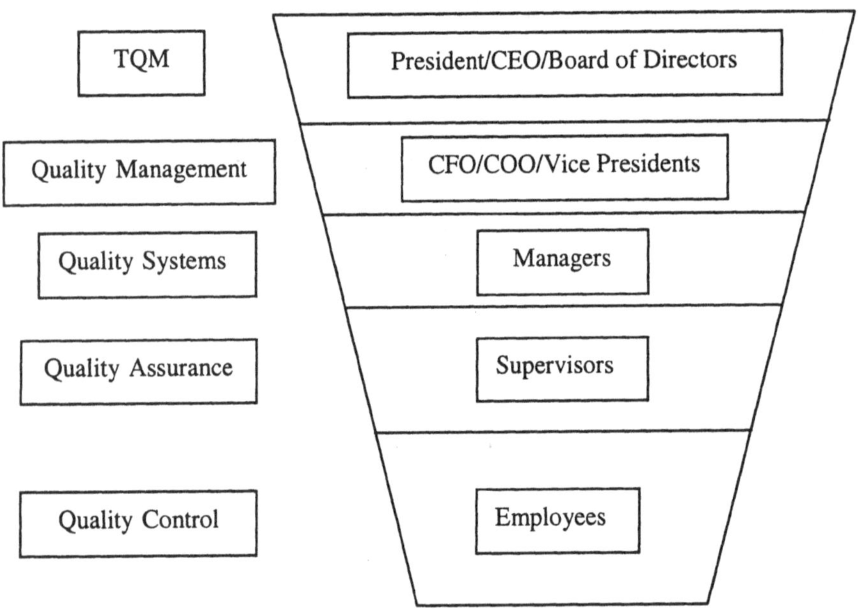

Figure 3. Quality responsibility and impact.

tion of Standards [1] The AABB's Quality System encompasses 10 quality system essentials (QSE's) (Table 2) which are consistent with, although worded slightly differently from, the ISO 9000 quality management series (Table 3). The European Colloquium on Quality System for Blood Banks [20] parallels the AABB and ISO requirements, but is organized differently (Table 4). Numerous

The central role of knowledgeable and committed people in making quality a part of all processes and measurements is fundamental to success. No organization will successfully incorporate quality systems into their operations without the commitment by the leadership, and even the commitment will fall short of actualization without the 'buy-in' of every single employee [21] (Figure 3).

Studies such as those conducted over several decades by Dr. Howard F. Taswell at the Mayo Clinics illustrate the predictability of human errors in technical and clerical activities [22-23]. An increasing awareness of human fallibility in healthcare was highlighted in the recent report from the U.S. Institute of Medicine entitled "To Err is Human: Building a Safer Health System" [24] in which an estimate that 44,000 to 98,000 Americans die each year from avoidable mistakes by healthcare providers was made. In response, the JCAHO mandated reporting of so-called 'sentinel events' [25], and the FDA reminded U.S. licensed facilities that error and accident reporting was mandatory [26]. This refocus on capturing and learning from errors [27], including 'near miss' situations, is fundamental to moving up the quality hierarchy.

In addition to detecting and responding to mistakes and accidents, most organizations recognize that ongoing audits focusing on outcomes of processes will bring information to light that has previously been known to only a few employees [28]. Audits require dedicated resources and appropriate education of personnel, as well as standard processes [29]. Properly performed, audits can prepare the organization for external assessments, as well as support opportunities for improvement. Good audits will focus on the outcome, not just the details, of a process.

Organizations committed to quality will also choose to benchmark their operations. Benchmarking is the process of comparison between organizations or practitioners to understand where opportunities for quality improvement exist. The global acceptance of haemovigilance indicates an awareness of the need for such comparisons [30-32]. Many U.S. institutions have routinely benchmarked financial activities, but only recently have we begun benchmarking health outcomes. The variation in transfusion practices reported through various published studies such as those from the European SANGUIS study [33], and various hospitals in the U.S. and elsewhere illustrate that consensus guidelines [34] and enlightened commentary [35] may be a rational solution to conserve resources (a necessary component of quality management) without impairing outcomes.

Quality Systems and Management: Where Are We Going?

Manufacturing organizations have a gold standard for quality, the Baldridge award, symbolizing having met the stringent criteria to achieve 'six sigma' of quality (practi cing total quality management). Transfusion medicine has not yet met the challenge of the Baldridge or any other equivalent criteria. To do so, there are two essential steps to be conquered beyond the quality system level to which we now aspire. The next and increasingly critical step is reaching QM, a level in which the demonstration of quality includes ensuring that 'the price is right' for the quality of goods and services provided [36]. Making certain that quality is also economical is the challenge of QM. At least in the U.S., the economics of blood collection has frequently been separate from the economics of transfusion, creating tension and adversarial situations. Within the past few months, the fiscal needs of patients has been identified as a priority for both blood collection and blood transfusion facilities who have united to heighten awareness of the inequities of the current reimbursement schema used in the U.S.

The challenge for the future is to continue to develop a QM approach to transfusion medicine, seeking solutions that benefit patients both in the quality of the product and services they receive but also in ensuring that the price for these services/products is affordable. Every establishment, whether collector, transfuser or both, must meet the QM challenge to continue improving quality for transfusion medicine.

The ultimate achievement, TQM, will be determined by the patient, whose satisfaction must reflect both the best component at the right time as well as the having those services provided at the right cost. The patient's satisfaction is the essential ingredient to achieving the pinnacle of quality. How we meet that challenge in the 21st century is yet to be defined.

References

1. Menitove JE, ed. Standards for Blood Banks and Transfusion Services, 20th ed. American Association of Blood Banks, Bethesda, MD, 2000.
2. Belanger AC. Joint Commission on Accreditation of Healthcare Organizations' expectations for transfusion medicine in health care organizations. Arch Pathol Lab Med 1999;123:472-74.
3. Hathaway WE, Githens JH, Blackburn WR, et al. Aplastic anemia, histiocytosis and erythrodermia in immunologically deficient children. N Engl J Med 1965;273:953-58.
4. Sakakibara J, Juji T. Post-transfusion graft-versus-host disease following open heart surgery. J Cardiovasc Surg 1989;30:687-91.
5. Vamvakas ED, Blajchman MA, eds. Immunomodulatory Effects of Blood Transfusion, AABB Press, Bethesda, MD, 1999.
6. Engelfriet CP, Reesink HW, Brand B, Levy G, et al. Haemovigilance systems. Vox Sang 1999;77:110-20.
7. Williamson LM. Systems contributing to the assurance of transfusion safety in the United Kingdom. Vox Sang 1999;77:82-7.
8. Popovsky MA. The transfusion medicine consultant and hospital transfusion committee. Vox Sang 1998;74 (Suppl 2):391-93.
9. Appendix B, 1994 Accreditation Manual for Pathology and Clinical Laboratory Services. The Joint Commission on Accreditation of Healthcare Organizations. Oakbrook Terrace, IL, 1994.
10. Clark GB. Systematic Quality Management. ASCP Press, Chicago, IL, 1995.
11. Guideline for Quality Assurance in Blood Establishments, U.S. Food and Drug Administration, Center for Biologics Evaluation and Research, Rockville, MD, July 11, 1995.
12. Bremer H. TQM and Taylorism: How they compare. In: Smit Sibinga CTh, Das PC, Heiniger HJ (eds). Good Manufacturing Practice in Transfusion Medicine. Kluwer Academic Publishers, Dordrecht, Boston, London, 1994: XIII-XX.
13. Title 21, Code of Federal Regulations, Parts 600-799, Superintendent of Documents, U.S. Government Printing Office, Washington, DC, April 1, 1976. (Updated annually).

14. AABB Technical Quality Assurance Committee. Robins J (eds). Quality Program. American Association of Blood Banks, Bethesda, MD, 1994.
15. Nevalainen DE, Callery MF. Quality Systems in the Blood Bank and Laboratory Environment, Abbott Quality Institute, Abbott Park, IL, and American Association of Blood Banks, Bethesda, MD, 1994.
16. Nevalainen DE, Callery MF. Applying Self-Assessment and Process Analysis to Create a Quality System. Abbott Quality Institute, Abbott Park, IL, and American Association of Blood Banks, Bethesda, MD, 1995.
17. Duckett JB, Woods LL, Santrach PJ, eds. Quality in Action. American Association of Blood Banks, Bethesda, MD, 1996.
18. Rhamy J, ed. Error Management. An Important Part of Quality Control. AABB Press, Bethesda, MD, 1999.
19. European Colloquium on a quality system for blood banks, Transfusion Today 1998;35:3-7.
20. Myers LK, Kalmin ND, Fisk MB. ISO 9002: impact on a blood and tissue center's operations. Transfusion Med Rev 1999;13:187-93.
21. Taswell HF, Smith AM, Sweatt MA, Pfaff KJ. Quality control in the blood bank – a new approach. Am J Clin Pathol 1974;62:491-95.
22. Taswell HF, Galbreath JL, Harmsen WS. Errors in transfusion medicine. Detection, analysis, frequency, and prevention. Arch Pathol Lab Med 1994;118:405-10.
23. To Err is Human, Institute of Medicine, Bethesda, MD, 1999.
24. Sentinel events in the age of performance improvement, and Sentinel events: Evaluating cause and planning improvement. Joint Commission on Accreditation of Healthcare Organizations, Oakbrook Terrace, IL, 1998.
25. Title 21, Code of Federal Regulations, Part 600.14, U.S. Government Printing Office, Washington, DC, April 1, 2000.
26. Rhamy J, ed. Error Management: An Important Part of Quality Control AABB Press, Bethesda, MD, 1999.
27. Shulman IA, Jones FS. Practice aspects of the self-assessment of the issue and administration of blood: a review of two hospitals' experiences. Am J Clin Pathol 1997;107 (Suppl 1):S17-22.
28. Smith JL, Russell JP. The Quality Audit Handbook. ASQ Press, Milwaukee, WI, 1997.
29. Menitove JE. Hemovigilance in the United States of America. Vox Sang 1998;74: 447-55.
30. Noel L, Debeir J, Cosson A. The French haemovigilance system. Vox Sang 1998;74: 441-45.
31. McClelland B, Love E, Scott S, Williamson LM. Haemovigilance: Concept, Europe and UK initiatives. Vox Sang 1998;74:431-39.
32. SANGUIS Study Group. Use of blood products for elective surgery in 43 European hospitals. EC, 1994.
33. Gabra GS, Doughty HA, eds. Rational transfusion therapy – Improving the quality of care by reducing inappropriate blood transfusion and promoting the use of alternatives. A framework for a National Blood Policy and Guidelines. Transfusion Today 2000;43 Suppl.1:1-14.
34. Allain JP, Williamson LM. How can we best achieve optimal transfusion practice? Med J Austral 1997;167:462-63.
35. AuBuchon JP. Optimizing the cost-effectiveness of quality assurance in transfusion medicine. Arch Pathol Lab Med 1999;123:603-06.

TRACEABILITY AND CODING PRINCIPLES

J. Koistinen[1]

Introduction

Tracing from a blood donor to each blood product and from blood product to each blood donor is the backbone of quality systems in transfusion medicine and must be assured by the blood transfusion service (BTS). Tracing from each blood product and component to the patient and back from patient to components is just as important, and is done by the hospital. When the blood transfusion service is part of the hospital organisation, both of those arms of tracing can be done by the same organisation, the BTS of the hospital.

If the tracing from donor to patient and back is the trunk of a quality tree, tracing of the samples and laboratory results back to the blood donors and blood products are the main branches of the same tree. It is reasonable to say that the branches do not survive if the trunk is sick.

Main weakness of the tracing systems has been the risk of human errors in information transfer. These are possible at identification of the donor, at labelling of the blood units, test tubes, intermediate and final products, at transfer and recording of laboratory results in the BTS as well as in identification of the products, test tubes, test results and patients in the hospital. As an example, labelling errors alone constitute some 6% of the errors reported to FDA in year 2000 [1].

The Process and Information Transfer

The donation and basic production procedure are illustrated as a flow chart in figure 1 showing the steps where information transfer occurs. The more products are made from a whole blood unit the more complicated the information transfer becomes (Figure 2). The laboratory procedures in a blood transfusion service also have a number of steps where information is transferred (Figure 3). The information transfer continues in the hospital starting already before the blood component arrives in the hospital laboratory and ending at the patient in the ward (Figure 4). Some of the basic information transfer steps both at the BTS and in the hospital can be done by automatic reading and recording devices as indicated in Tables 1, 2 and 3.

1. Finnish Red Cross Blood Transfusion Service, Helsinki, Finland.

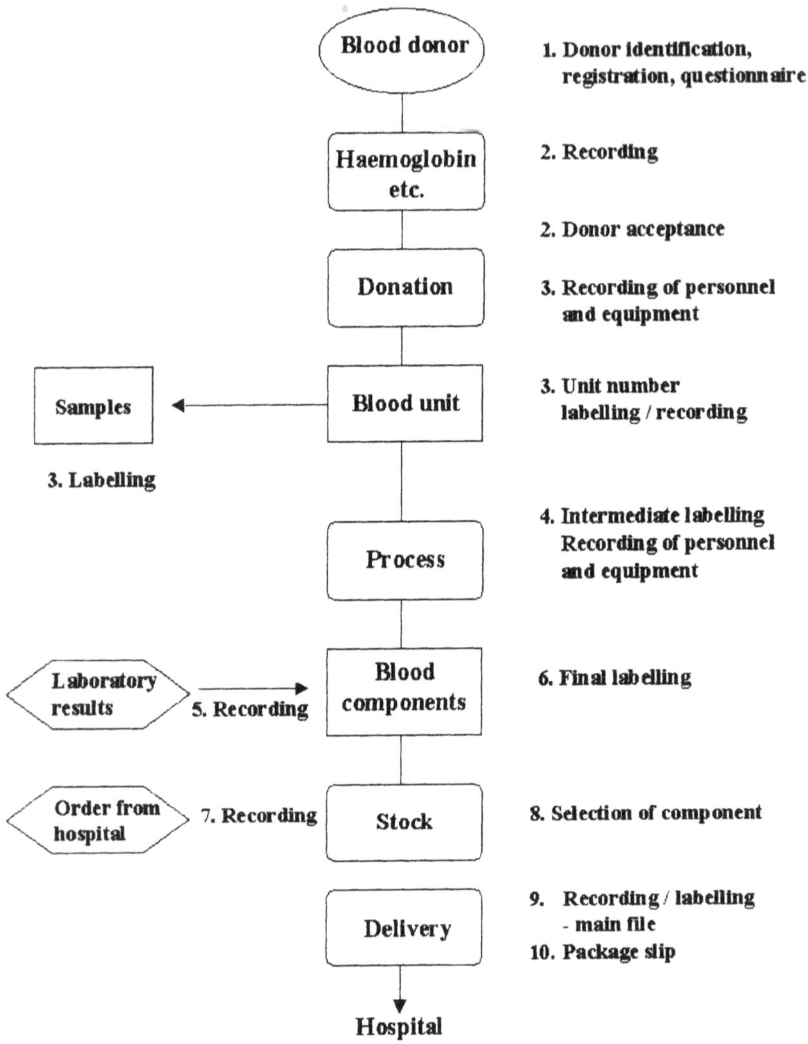

Figure 1. Flow scheme of the main steps at blood donation and processing showing the different stages where information transfer occurs. The numbers refer to the numbers in tables 1, 2 and 3.

Coding Systems and Automatic Information Transfer

Pre-printed labels and stickers with numbers eliminated at least the errors, which occurred in writing and rewriting the names and numbers by hand. Introduction of codes and computers which were able to read the code numbers added to the safety by eliminating more than half of the chances for human errors as listed in Tables 1, 2 and 3.

Optical character recognition (OCR) is a method of printing alphabetical and numerical characters so that they can be read by scanning devices and humans

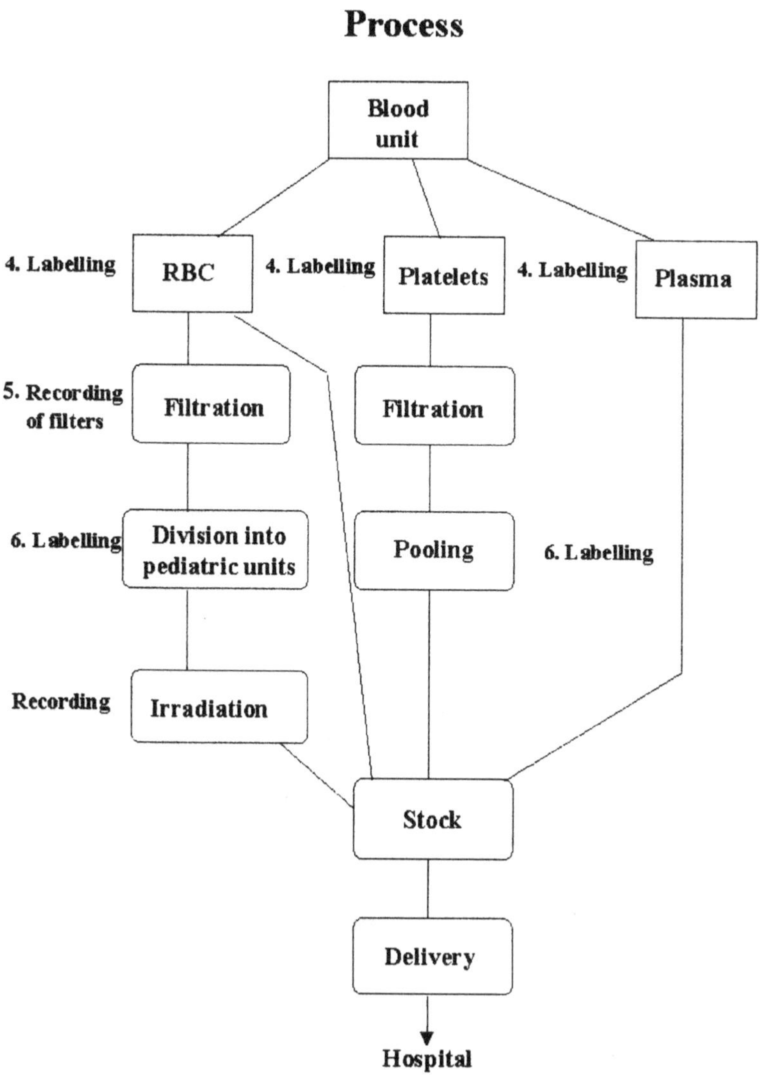

Figure 2. Additional processing further complicates the tracing and information transfer.

alike. However, OCR characters are not 'vertically redundant', meaning that the scanner beam has to pass the number fairly exactly horizontally across. Thus the physical act of scanning is much more difficult than scanning a bar code, which has led to abandoning of this code in blood bank use.

A bar code is a series of black bars and white spaces that are used to represent letters and/or numbers. The specific arrangement of these bars and spaces follows strict rules which are defined by the bar code language (known as symbology) used. They use more reliable technology that is easier, faster, and less expensive than the one used for OCR. The bar codes are read with a scanning device, which can be a hand-held wand, a fixed-beam or moving-beam laser or a

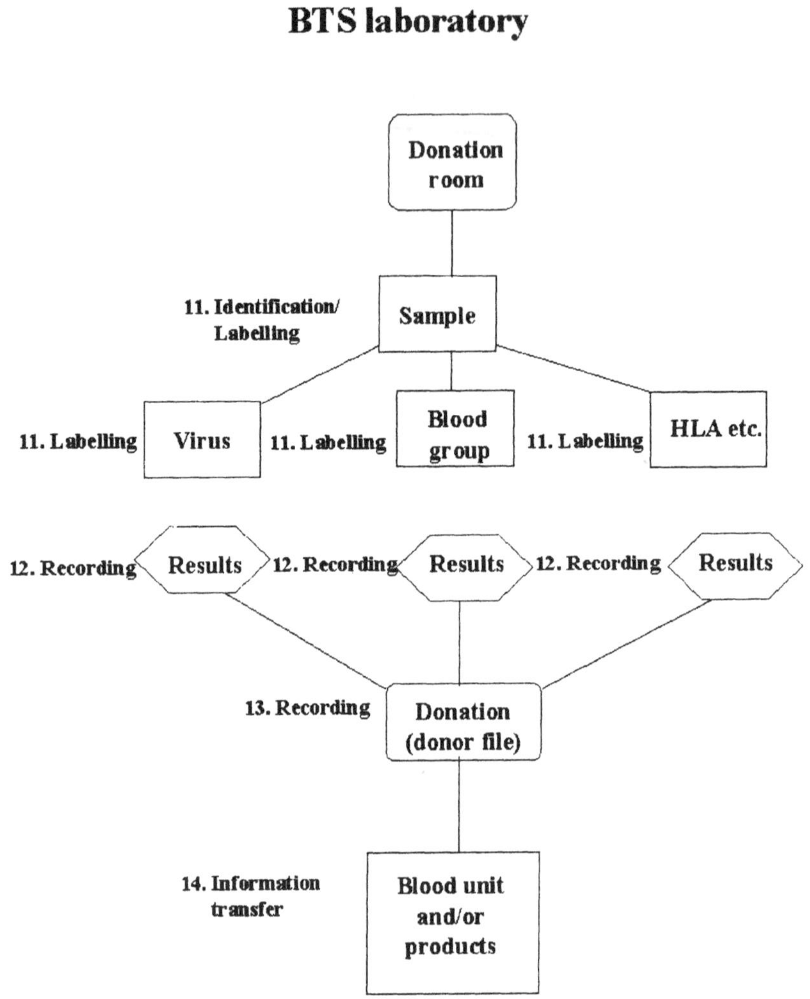

Figure 3. Tracing of samples in the BTS laboratory and test results back to the donation files and products.

charge-coupled device. The bar code symbol reflects the spot of light back into the scanner in varying amounts and the differences in reflectivity are converted into electrical signal by a light detector within the scanner. The signal is then converted into binary ones and zeros which are used in various combinations to stand for specific numbers and letters. Although the bar codes are more reliable and easier to read than OCR, they also require good printing quality. Specks on the code or voids in the printed bars may cause miss-readings.

Some bar code standards use two element widths, some, like the standard Code 128, uses four element widths. Other standards are e.g. Codabar, and Code 39. Codabar is perhaps still the most common in BTSs. It has been approved by

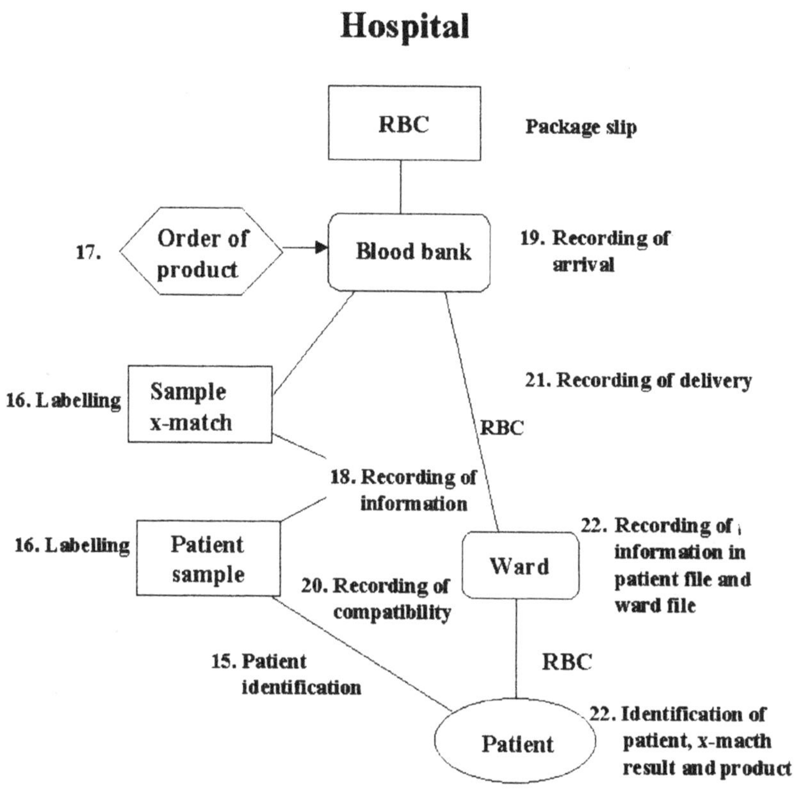

Figure 4.Tracing of the blood unit, test results, patient samples and patients in the hospital.

FDA in the USA. However, it allows more miss-readings than some other bar codes. Consequently, Code 128 which has also a check character, is becoming more common even in blood banking. It has been calculated that with a high quality Code 128 symbol, error rates can be lower than one error in every 30-40 million characters scanned [2]. This code is also able to encode the full ASCII character set and double-density encoding of numeric data is possible, conserving space on the label. It also supports concatenation, which allows the user to scan a number of symbols, hold the data in buffer memory in the scanner, then combine the data prior to transmission to the host. Thus a particular number of a blood unit can be electronically linked to its specific product code, ABO/Rh code, and/or expiration date.

Standardisation of Coded Information

Blood units have traditionally been labelled with coloured labels, where each ABO blood group has its own colour. However, there has been no success with the attempts to reach a universal standard for the colours. This and earlier computer technology have resulted in abandoning the colours in most of the BTSs

Table 1. Information transfer at blood donation, component production and product delivery.

Procedure	Can be automated/ eliminated
1. Identification of the donor, questionnaire	Yes, partially
2. Recording of the donor information, donor acceptance	No
3. Recording of personnel and equipment Labelling the blood bag and test tubes	Yes, partially
4. Transfer of the donation number on red cell, platelet and/or plasma unit, etc. recording of personnel and equipment	Yes, partially
5. Recording of laboratory results	Yes
6. Final labelling of blood components	Yes, partially
7. Reception and recording of the order for a blood component	Yes
8. Selection of the component from the stock	Yes
9. Transfer of information at delivery into the BTS files: destination of the product, donation number and product identification	Yes
10. Transfer of information onto the package slip	Yes

Table 2. Information transfer in the BTS laboratory.

Procedure	Can be automated/ eliminated
11. Labelling of eventual additional test tubes in the laboratories	Yes, partially
12. Recording of results in laboratory register	Yes
13. Recording of results in donor files	Yes
14. Recording of results in production department	Yes

Table 3. Information transfer in the hospital.

Procedure	Can be automated/ eliminated
15. Identification of the patient needing blood	Yes, partially
16. Taking and labelling the blood grouping and cross matching samples	No
17. Ordering the blood product	Yes, partially
18. Recording the samples in laboratory register	Yes
19. Recording the blood component in laboratory register	Yes
20. Recording the results of cross matching	Yes, partially
21. Recording the blood component for delivery to a patient, in blood bank and ward	Yes
22. Verification of the patient identification, cross matching results, number of the blood product to be transfused	Yes, partially

that have achieved a fair degree of automation of their processes. This development has been accelerated by the introduction of on-demand labelling, where the blood unit label is printed when the laboratory results are ready, and the unit is transferred from quarantine to the delivery storage.

There has been no success with standardisation of the bar coded information in blood banking during the quarter of a century that the bar codes have been used. This has not been considered a problem, but the rare occasions when blood components have been brought to hospitals from many different sources and have had identical numbers, have shown that standardisation would be beneficial. Plasma fractionation plants that collect plasma from many different sources and from many different countries should also find an international standard of blood and plasma unit labelling useful.

Code ISBT 128

The International Society of Blood Transfusion (ISBT) has a working party on automation and data processing (WPADP), which was created in the seventies when the first automatic blood grouping machines were introduced. At the end of the eighties, when it was realised that errors found with the use of Codabar could be eliminated by a change to another bar code symbology, it was also understood that with the change of the bar coding standard, it would be feasible to create a new and unique coding standard for blood banks. The ISBT working party undertook the task of its design and agreed to use Code 128 symbology. The standard was given the name ISBT 128, and work on the basics was completed in 1995. It is a coding system, where the donation number has a country code for each country and which allows assignment of an own code for each donation site. In addition, it has a code for the year of collection and a six digit figure for the collection number proper. There are also codes (primary data identifiers) to identify that it deals with a blood collection or with a blood product and appropriate check digits, even for manual reading [3]. All this means that the donation number is unique and the same number does not appear in any other blood unit anywhere, where ISBT 128 code numbers are used. The structure of the labels and position of the codes is also standardised.

Several different types of information are carried in the semistructured eight-character ISBT 128 product code. The first five characters of the code identify the product type (such as red blood cells or fresh frozen plasma) and attributes associated with the product (such as irradiated, leukocyte reduced). The type of donation (volunteer, homologous, autologous) is specified in the sixth character. Characters seven and eight are reserved for encoding information about divisions of products. The Technical Specification published by ICCBBA has a table for donation types and detailed information of the scheme for assigning divisions.

ICCBBA

Appropriate implementation of a universal and international coding standard cannot be done by a society like ISBT which is based on a totally voluntary function. There has to be an office which can establish databases of the collection sites and product codes and which can offer information and guidance on the implementation of the code as well as manage and distribute the technical specifications for the codes.

ISBT, American Association of Blood Banks (AABB) and American Red Cross (ARC) decided in 1994 to establish a self-supporting company for the implementation of ISBT 128. It was named the International Council for Commonality in Blood Bank Automation (ICCBBA). The BTSs which decide to use the ISBT 128 code, register in ICCBBA and get a number, which allows internationally unique identification of blood units collected by them. The registered facilities have also access to the documents and standards published by ICCBBA. The office has a database of product codes, which already has more than 3000 code numbers. Any registered facility which needs a code number for its product provides a description of the product to the ICCBBA office, which issues the code. If the description does not fit to any existing product description, the new product is given a new number. For instance, the original 3000 product numbers did not fit to the European type of products. This led in 1999 to a meeting of the European registered facilities, in which an agreement was reached for some 80 new international product numbers. National product numbers may also be given. This provides a good system, where products are described in detail by the unique product number which cannot be misinterpreted. The product coding is a considerable quality improvement in the tracing system especially when raw material and intermediate products for plasma products are transported over national borders.

In summer 2000 there were 482 blood collection facilities and 32 cord blood banks in the US, and 87 and 5 respectively, in other countries that have registered in ICCBBA. They represent collection of more than 23 million units of blood annually. In addition, 70 vendors of blood bank software, material and supplies have also registered. The ISBT 128 code is already implemented in eight countries [4]. More information on ICCBBA and code ISBT 128 is available on the ICCBBA web pages (http://www.iccbba.com).

Expansion of ISBT 128 to Stem Cells and Tissues

The ISBT 128 standard can be applied not only for coding of blood collection and blood components but also for other products. Coding for placental cells and stem cells is being worked upon and interest has been expressed for coding of other tissues as well. Since stem cells and other tissues are widely transported internationally, it is obvious that a unique coding system adds to the safety and improves the quality of these operations.

Viewing the Future

The quality requirements in transfusion medicine demand more and more documentation. Standard operating procedures (SOPs) and tracing of the donor or blood components is not enough. Additional documentation, meaning recording of the individuals, equipment, material and supplies at every step of the process, seems to become obligatory. Bar coding systems help in doing this, but each bar code has only a limited capacity to contain information and a line connection to a computer is needed from every piece of equipment and at every step of the process. The blood unit itself carries traditionally only a limited amount of information, through which connections can be drawn to the blood collection and production process proper.

Radio Frequency Identification (RFID)

Modern technology allows carriage of all information on the blood unit in a tag where information can be fed in and read by radio frequency technology. This has already many applications, but is still experimental in BTSs. There are three types of radio frequency identification (RFID) tags:

- RO (Read Only), in which information is programmed by the manufacturer and can only be read by the end user.
- WORM (Write once read multiple), in which information can be programmed by the vendor outside of the manufacturer's facility.
- R/W (Read/Write), in which information can be read and written by the end user.

Using the RFID tags on blood units means that instead of recording information into a computer with the help of bar codes, it is recorded in electronic form along the donation and production process into the RFID tag which is attached on the blood bag. This makes it possible to carry information of donor number, blood group, identification of equipment and personnel of the process, etc. on each blood and product unit. The information which is not needed in the hospital can be taken off the tag at the delivery of the product and stored at the blood transfusion service. The hospitals would then be able to insert their own information in the same tag after having received the product. Thus for instance patient name and cross matching information would be transferred in the laboratory onto the product to be transfused.

An antenna in a Read/Write unit (R/W) sets up a radio frequency (RF) signal between the R/W and the tag. The tag receives data and energy and sends a response to the R/W unit with another RF signal. The R/W unit receives the RF signal and converts it into computer readable form. The tags of today have a capacity of 8 kbits and leave 752 characters (corresponds to a full A4 size page) free for the user. They allow more than 100,000 writing cycles and an unlimited number of reading cycles, which means that they can be reused several times. Data retention time is over 10 years and the writing time for a whole tag is only one second, reading being equally fast. The tags are operational also in a harsh environment, i.e. through dust, dirt, ice, and other elements that make the visibility poor.

The Read/Write unit is a combination of an antenna and electronics. They are installed along the process at the points where the data content is, that needs to be updated. The tag gets the needed energy from the antenna energy field and there is no need for batteries (Figure 5). It can be read from a distance of several meters and the identification can be done on fly. No activity from the object to

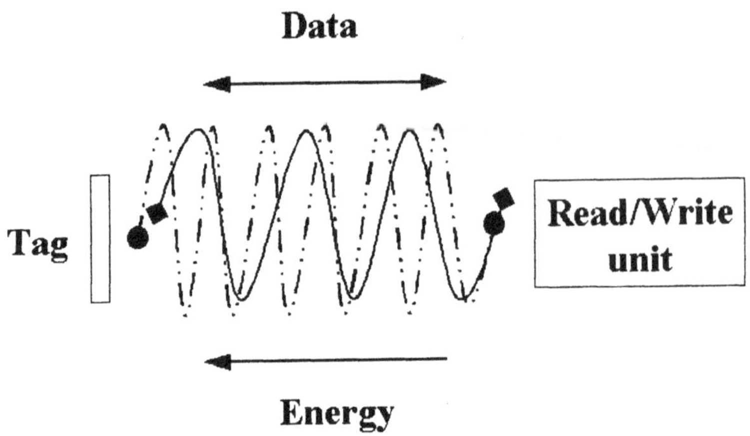

Figure 5. In radio frequency identification (RFD) the read and write (R/W) unit gives energy to the tag and both send and receive data from the tag.

be identified is needed and the target of identification may continue its normal route and speed. This means that blood bag identification e.g. in the stock of products can be done from products moving on a conveyor belt or a red cell product of a certain phenotype in the stock can be identified from a distance. The reading device can read more than 60 tags/sec.

In principle the RFID technology may offer benefits and major improvement in blood services and transfusion medicine through improved process efficiency, quality and safety. It allows thorough records from donation to transfusion with automatic data entry and collection. Data can be easily transferred with the blood product from remote collection centres to BTS, from BTS to the hospital blood bank and between the R/W units and information systems of the BTS. The R/W units can be operated either through a cord connection or by radio waves, which gives an opportunity to use handheld devices in similar fashion as cellular telephones. It may also allow easier automation of some routine operations like weighing the blood units and registration of the results.

RFID may make complete and detailed traceability of processing easier in the future, because used equipment, personnel and other information can be recorded automatically thus further eliminating human errors. The technology is reliable because the information transfer can be done also in wet and dirty or otherwise difficult conditions and the data transfer occurs without operational networking systems.

Conclusion

Development of automatic reading devices and coding systems like bar codes has improved the reliability of tracing of blood products and of blood donors thus improving considerably the safety of transfusion medicine since the time of manual labelling, bookkeeping and recording. International standardisation of the bar coding systems for blood transfusion services has finally been reached through development of the ISBT 128 code. It is now important that all blood transfusion services register in ICCBBA and start using the new code to speed up the global implementation of the unique coding of blood donations and blood products. The quality advantages offered by this code are unquestionable and it is up to the individual blood transfusion services how soon they can benefit of these advantages.

The development of new information technology is fast and there is no doubt that it will improve the safety of blood transfusion also. We must engage ourselves in research of the technology, of which the radio frequency identification (RFID) systems seem promising. Collaboration between hard ware and soft ware manufacturers, blood transfusion services, standardisation organisations and hospitals is needed to design research programs into this and to be able to evaluate whether the RFID technology is feasible and improves the safety and efficiency of the different processes in transfusion medicine.

Elimination of the possibilities for human errors is important in improvement of quality in transfusion medicine. Identification of the blood donor and of the patient remains a process that can be done only by human interaction. One could imagine that for instance if a microchip could be attached into the earlobe of donors and patients, even their identification could be made automatic. Although this would satisfy the hard quality requirements, the soft ones like the human interaction in general at blood donation and donor recruitment as well as in the ward can never be replaced by any technology.

References

1. Error and Accident Report – Summary for Second Quarter FY 2000. FDA/CBER Memorandum, May 16, 2000.
2. An introduction to bar coding. International Council for Commonality in Blood Banking Automation, 1996
3. An introduction to ISBT 128. International Council for Commonality in Blood Banking Automation, 1995.
4. Annual Report 1999. International Council for Commonality in Blood Banking Automation, 2000.

QUALITY PRINCIPLES AND RISK MANAGEMENT: AUTOMATION AND DOCUMENTATION

M. Bruce[1]

Historical Perspective

The past 25 years have witnessed remarkable technological advances that have revolutionised our life and work. Therefore, we should not be surprised to find that over this period there have been a similar number of changes in the practice of blood transfusion. These changes reflect the continuous drive:

- to increase safety for donors;
- to increase safety and efficacy for patients;
- to improve efficiency to contain costs.

Some changes have been driven by government mandate (eg the ever expanding list of infectious agents for which we need to screen; Consumer Protection legislation; increased regulation); some by blood transfusion professionals (eg component therapy, computerisation); whilst others have been driven by industry, very often working with transfusion professionals (eg automated test equipment; automated blood component separation devices; leucocyte depletion).

The net effect of these changes has been a significant increase in complexity and sophistication at the 'manufacturing' end of the transfusion chain and an acceptance that safe and effective service provision would best be achieved by managing all of these processes within a 'Quality System' that complies with the principles of Good Manufacturing Practice (GMP) [1-10].

Having an effective documentation system is, and will remain, the foundation stone of GMP compliance. However, the introduction of appropriate automation and computerisation has made an enormous contribution to facilitating GMP compliance and improving the safety and efficacy of blood components.

Indeed, the need for very high levels of process control, allied to the complexity of current practice, means that the modern blood transfusion service would find it almost impossible to operate effectively (on a routine basis) without a significant degree of automation of test procedures, interpretation and recording of results and data/information management.

How very different from 25 years ago when SNBTS had only just introduced an 'automated' instrument for blood grouping of donors (the Technicon BG 15), blood component therapy was in its infancy, barcodes were just beginning to

1. National Quality Director, SNBTS Headquarters, Edinburgh, Scotland, UK.

appear on tins of beans and we were 15 years away from understanding what GMP compliance really meant. Issues such as the theoretical risk of transmitting Creutzfeldt Jakob Disease (CJD) with blood transfusion really were the furthest thing from our minds!

The Benefits of Automation /Computerisaton

It is widely acknowledged that automation/computerisation have brought major improvements in the safety and efficiency of transfusion practice. There can be little doubt that using carefully designed and validated automated systems will reduce errors simply by removing the errors that occur through human involvement – 'to err is human'. Reducing these types of error is a fundamental benefit of automation and computerisation.

Of the more specific benefits, many represent an accumulation of improvements along a continuum which today sees the availability of blood donor management, collection and component manufacturing software, which can operate within a site on a Local Area Network (LAN) or on multiple sites over a Wide Area Network (WAN). Such systems are fully integrated, from donor management and call-up, through donor registration, blood collection, blood component production, donation testing, labelling and release into stock. Interfaces with automated test equipment and data management protocols remove the need for human intervention, thereby removing the potential for error in high risk parts of the process.

A couple of examples can be used to illustrate the significant degree of risk reduction that such fully integrated automated systems have delivered.

In infectious disease screening, an initial screening test reactive result requires confirmation by performing two repeat tests [10]. When either repeat is reactive the donation is considered 'repeat reactive' and unsuitable for use. When both repeats are negative the donation is given a negative status and can be released to stock.

Prior to the availability of fully automated equipment interfaced with integrated software, such changes had to be made manually by physically retrieving the test information and editing the database or documentation. This was clearly a high risk activity and one that required an exceptionally high level of process control.

In the fully automated system, result and donor record management issues such as setting up consequences for the donor and any future donations are actioned through carefully validated algorithms without human intervention.

'On demand' label printing [11] is another risk reduction measure which fully integrated computerisation has made possible. In this process the operator scans the donation number barcode and the computer system interrogates the database to verify that the blood component is suitable for use before printing the specific blood group label, which also carries the donation number barcode, the expiry date and other key information for that component 'on demand'.

When the component is not suitable for use, an appropriate label is printed stating eg HOLD or BIOHAZARD and the reason.

The label is attached to the pack and a concatenated barcode reading process (single sweep across two barcodes) is used. In the first step the original donation number barcode and the donation number barcode on the 'on demand' printed label are concatenated to confirm that the label has been attached to the correct pack (ie the numbers are the same). In the second step the original donation number barcode and the blood group barcode on the 'on demand' printed label are concatenated to confirm that the blood group on the 'on demand' printed label matches that of the original donation number.

This process ensures that not only is the correct label produced but also that the correct donation is labelled and represents a very significant increase in process security.

In summary, the key benefits of automation and computerisation in blood transfusion are listed below:

- reduces opportunities for error and delivers improved consistency by significantly reducing human intervention;
- facilitates effective donor management, eg donor record management, call up, management of deferrals etc;
- use of barcodes for data capture avoids transcription errors and facilitates automation;
- laptop computers at blood collection sessions greatly improve the security of donor registration;
- capacity to electronically link the blood donation, associated samples and documentation to their donor;
- access to relevant historical donor information;
- linking of the donation to the batch of blood packs into which it was collected;
- robotic sample handling;
- automated assay processing, results interpretation;
- automated results transfer by interface software;
- single database for multiple sites offers many benefits;
- 'on demand' label printing with associated verification of component suitability for release (which also brings significant improvements in the control of labels;
- control of access to specific programmes, eg no access given until training is complete; access restricted to specific menus/options within menus;
- consequences can be carried forward automatically in the donor record, forcing specific actions for future donations;
- complete audit trail of transaction logs provide a clear record of what was done, when, where and by whom;
- greatly facilitates statistical analysis and control;
- facilitates the process of reconciliation prior to release of acceptable components to stock;
- facilitates the rapid application of a 'HOLD' condition at any point in the process, eg if a donor calls back to report an illness that might affect the suitability of their donation;
- permits a rapid and accurate search of the database such as would be required when investigating a possible transfusion transmitted infection.

Documentation Systems

Earlier in this text it was claimed that an effective documentation system is, and will remain, the foundation stone of GMP. So why is the documentation system fundamental to good manufacturing practice and what does it include?

We need an effective documentation system to ensure there is absolute clarity about our processes and procedures, i.e. it defines the quality system.

This prevents errors from verbal communication, introduces formality and the basis for control. These outcomes in turn ensure consistency of manufacture and of service provision.

The records that arise from application of these principles provide confirmation that procedures were followed and followed correctly. They also permit retrospective review to take place when investigating errors, problems, complaints and so on, thereby allowing facts to be established in order that effective corrective and preventative measures can be designed and implemented. They are also essential for the 'lookback' procedures that would be initiated, eg following a transfusion transmitted infection.

The controlled document system covers many 'documents' including SOPs; specifications; forms and worksheets; policies; batch manufacturing records; labels; site master file; validation/calibration reports and a wide range of completed quality records.

The basic elements of such a system are as follows:

- the system is controlled by an authorised person;
- every page of every document, including any revisions, is uniquely identified;
- there are formal review and authorisation procedures before 'controlled' documents are issued;
- paper copy 'controlled' documents are printed on paper that is specifically designated for this purpose, eg coloured paper or paper carrying a specific watermark. This helps to emphasise the status of the document, ie that it is an 'official' controlled document, therefore not for unauthorised copying;
- a distribution list is maintained;
- superseded versions of documents are withdrawn to ensure that current policies and procedures are followed;
- strict 'change control' is enforced;
- documents are reviewed to an agreed schedule;
- an archive of superseded documents is maintained, allowing retrospective review of processes.

Managing the controlled document system is a major administrative undertaking that can be greatly facilitated by computerisation. There are many proprietary 'Quality Management' software packages which include the capacity to authorise specific individuals to perform certain tasks, eg review documents; approve documents; receive documents. Target completion dates for various activities are entered into the system. Therefore it is possible, for example, to generate a list of SOPs from the blood component production department that need to be reviewed, say next month.

That report will also show the person(s) responsible for this activity and the report (= work instruction) can either be e-mailed to that person(s) or printed and sent as hard copy. These systems can also allow SOPs and other controlled documents to be accessed electronically, making the 'paperless office' concept a reality – if only it could be so!

There is a significant benefit in this approach as the document version available 'on-line' should always be the current version. However, in practice, this approach does have attendant problems. In the author's experience many personnel feel happier reading a paper document than reading the same document from a screen; there can be problems of accessibility, i.e. SOPs are best located where the procedure they describe and control is taking place. This will not always be possible if the document is on a computer. Ensuring all staff who need to use the SOPs have access to the computer and the relevant SOP directories can also be problematic.

Finally, when initially developed, most quality management software packages did not operate over a wide area network. This limited their potential for organisations like SNBTS who function on more than one site. This position is changing and one solution is to offer a 'Thin Client Server' approach where the software is loaded onto a fairly powerful, dedicated server that can be accessed rapidly and remotely via a telephone connection.

In conclusion, the importance of effective documentation systems cannot be overstated. Documentation errors remain the single biggest source of serious errors in blood transfusion. For example, in the UK Serious Hazards of Transfusion (SHOT) reporting scheme in 1998-99 [12], some 57% of the 'incorrect blood component transfused' errors resulted from errors or deficiencies in documentation.

There is a high probability that the introduction of appropriate, computerised solutions would significantly reduce the incidence of documentation problems.

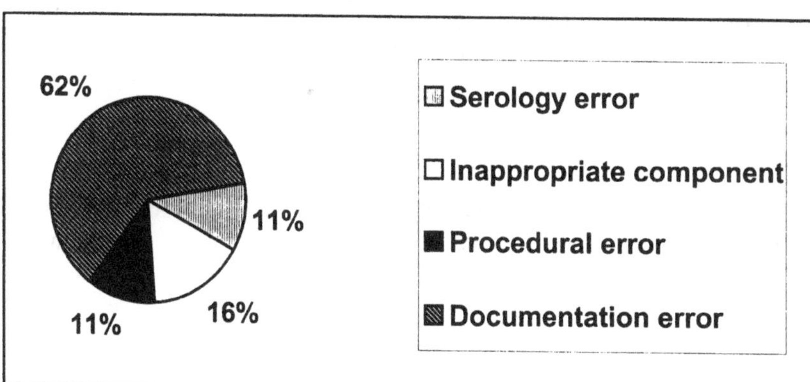

Figure 1. Analysis of the cause of 'incorrect blood component transfused errors'. Extract from the 1998-99 report of the Serious Hazards of Transfusion Reporting Scheme.

A Note of Caution

Whilst application of appropriate and carefully validated automated/computerised systems can significantly increase safety and efficiency, it must be acknowledged that such systems can, and do, fail. Most often, these 'failures' are human errors that generally result from a failure to follow documented procedures. However, very occasionally, computerised systems produce unexpected and erroneous results. To some extent, these errors give perspective to the need for very careful and comprehensive validation of automated equipment and computer systems [13], not least because these systems now very often involve data capture, computerised control and interfaces to other systems.

Planning such validation to cover all eventualities is a very difficult task and, despite the best efforts of software production companies and user organisations, software problems or 'bugs' do manifest themselves as unexpected system errors, sometimes with potentially serious outcomes.

Data Input /User Errors

User errors are by far the most common source of problem with computerised systems. These can arise from errors in the use of the system or errors in data entry.

In the case of the former, it can often take many hours of work by a highly experienced person to establish what errors were made. Transaction logs, which record who did what, where and when are of crucial importance in this situation. This is an essential tool that allows the reconstruction of events thereby permitting effective corrective and preventative measures to be put in place.

Despite our best efforts, eg requiring 'double blind' entry for test results such as anti-CMV testing or a minor blood group phenotype, data entry errors continue to occur. In this regard, it is of great concern that there is an opportunity for this to occur at what is arguably the most critical point in the entire process – the linking of donor, donation and documentation in the database. Whilst this is by no means a common problem, it does highlight the problems of human error and the absolute requirement to provide computer systems with accurate information.

Barcode 'Misreads'

The introduction of barcode technology has been fundamental to the development of automation and computerisation in blood transfusion. Listed among the many advantages of barcodes are avoidance of transcription errors and assurance of identity. Perhaps because we have come to be so dependant on barcodes we have absolute faith in them.

For the author, that faith was dented somewhat in 1996 when the investigation of a donor/donation mislink disclosed that an operator failure to replace a printer ribbon to schedule resulted in a donor identification number barcode being poorly printed. When presented to the barcode reader, the wrong number was interpreted, resulting in a linkage of the donation to the wrong donor record.

A more significant reminder that automated systems have limitations was obtained in 1998. Within SNBTS we use a fully integrated and comprehensive software package. 'On demand' label printing is an important feature of this system. When performing blood component verification and labelling, an operator noted that an error occurred when verifying and labelling red cell components. Essentially, the blood group label for donation '2' was attached to donation '1'. Although the two barcode numbers were different and the blood groups were different, the double concatenation process failed to flag up a problem. When donation '2' was presented for labelling the computer screen displayed a message that the component had already been labelled – this alerted the operator to the problem. Clearly, this was a matter of very serious concern to us that required urgent resolution.

Analysis showed there to be three key errors:

1. Labelling Error

The wrong blood group label was applied to a red cell component. This may have arisen from a barcode misread or through operator error. However, the operator was very clear that procedures were followed to the letter. Whilst barcode misreads are a very rare occurrence, we had an earlier report of a blood pack batch misread problem with the same type of scanner as was implicated in this event.

The actual donation numbers (ABC Codabar format) were:

550187 3

550168 7

and it was noted that there was some similarity between these numbers, eg if the number 6 were to be inserted at position 5 in the first number (# 550187/3), and if the last number were not read, the number # 550168/7 would be presented, complete with check digit. It is also of interest that, as a result of communicating this problem to other Blood Services, colleagues in Ireland (P. Coakley, personal communication) advised that they were using these same barcode scanners. They had identified some instances where the scanners did not read the full number, eg #192738/8 became #197388 and some where the entire number was transposed, eg #192738/8 became #689407/7.

2. Donation Number: Donation Number Concatenation Error

Investigation demonstrated that the particular barcode scanner unit being used had an 86% error rate. It was quickly established that the fault was restricted to one type of scanner when used in concatenated mode and these scanners were immediately withdrawn from use in this application.

A test script was prepared and used to test all scanners within SNBTS. This included reading the numbers #000001/9 and 000002/7 in concatenated mode (single sweep across the two numbers) 50 times and recording the results. An extract of the results of this testing is shown on Table 1 below.

These results show the extent of barcode misreads and the enormous varability in the performance between scanners. Given our absolute dependence on accurate barcode interpretation, such results were shocking for it was difficult to grasp that you could read ABC Codabar number combination 0000001/9:000002/7 50 times and obtain any errors at all let alone such frequently and wildly differing results. All of these scanners performed with 100% accuracy when used in non-concatenated mode.

Table 1. Bacode scanner validation exercise. 50 concatenated reads of the barcode numbers 000001/9 and 000002/7. The table shows an extract of the results for 6 different scanners.

Barcode scanner ID	Correct read	Incorrect read		
	000001/9: 000002/7	000001/9: 000001/9	000002/7: 000002/7	Other
# 449332	2	48	0	0
# 479321	17	15	18	0
# 299165	34	6	2	8
# 442885	15	5	30	0
# 442901	45	5	0	0
# 442930	25	4	21	1

The fault was subsequently traced to a specific revision of the 'firmware' which was supplied as a sub-component to the company who made the scanners. Eventually, this firmware was replaced. We now routinely check all scanners are functioning correctly before placing them in service.

3. Donation Number: Blood Group Concatenation Error

By preparing appropriate test scripts we were able to demonstrate a defect in the logic of our computer system during the component verification:labelling process. It emerged that at the donation number:blood group concatenation step the system checked the blood group matched that of the donation number on the blood group label. It did not check that the blood group for the original (left hand side) donation number matched the blood group barcode on the label.

A correction for this fault was provided, validated and loaded into the live system within 24 hours. However, this provides an excellent illustration of the difficulties of designing a sufficiently comprehensive software validation plan ie if the label verification system had not been in use and had not failed then this error would not have been detected at all.

Unexplained, Erroneous Test Results

It is likely that all blood transfusion services encounter erroneous test results that have been produced on fully automated systems and for which no explanation can be found. Here are a few examples from the author's experience.

On 24 April 1998, the SNBTS Blood Centre in Aberdeen reported a spurious anti-HCV test result. With a very widely used test kit and assay processing system the assay processor produced a negative result (OD 0.153 vs a cut-off value of 0.348). Visually, this test well was clearly reactive. The same tray was re-presented to the processor 11 minutes later and, on this occasion, produced a reactive result (OD 1.517 vs a cut-off value of 0.350).

The instrument was taken out of service, serviced, revalidated and reintroduced to routine use. No satisfactory explanation could be found.

On 19 April 2000, Nucleic Acid Amplification Testing (NAT) for HCV produced a positive minipool result which was resolved to a bone donor sample. On initial testing, this sample had been anti-HCV negative (ELISA) but on subsequent retesting was repeat reactive and confirmed as HCV positive.

Very detailed investigation excluded:

- low sample volume;
- inadequate volume of wash buffer;
- inadequate volume of substrate or conjugate;
- an uncoated microplate well;
- equipment problems.

Addition of insufficient acid at the end of the assay process (due to a blocked probe, air bubble or insufficient reagent) was considered extremely unlikely.

No satisfactory explanation could be found. However, this finding demonstrates that the benefits of introducing NAT extend beyond the detection of 'window' donations. In this instance the NAT has successfully 'failed safe' against a technical failure in the routine serological assay. Previously, using SNBTS data, McClelland et al [14] estimated that the residual risk of infection with HBsAg attributable to laboratory error was less than 1 in 750,000. This observation confirms that technical failures (which will include laboratory errors) still occur – in this instance the frequency of the event is around 1 in 750,000 donations tested to date.

On 06 October 1999, a donor with a historical group of O Rh D Neg was tested on a 'state of the art' automated blood grouping system and found to be a clear O Rh D Pos. All repeat tests (including the automated system) were O Rh D Neg.

A number of other 'machine' errors and discrepancies have been found. Almost all of these tend to be detected by the robust nature of the quality system. Conversations with colleagues in other Blood Transfusion organisations confirm that they identify similar events. These cases serve as a reminder that automated systems do have an inherent error rate, albeit very small.

Automation, Computerisation, GMP and the Challenge of Being at the Leading Edge

As has already been alluded to, the drive to improve transfusion safety, efficacy and efficiency is relentless. For those Blood Transfusion Services who wish to stay on the leading edge of such improvements (and for very good reasons, there are very few who are content to fall behind) then they will be confronted by an interesting dilemma. Very often the leading edge processes and/or equipment lack the level of sophistication and control we have come to expect and we have little option but to accept manually operated/controlled practices which we thought were left behind long ago. That observation is a real measure of the extent to which our attitude to quality has progressed over the past 10 years or so.

From the author's experience, this is amply illustrated by the introduction of NAT for HCV. At a fairly early stage in this process, SNBTS were using sophisticated robotic technology to construct minipools with manual entry of minipool results into a computer database which transferred individual results into individual donation/donor records via interfacing software.

However, initially, in contrast to the theoretical elegance that underpins the method, the entire test process was a step back in time, for this was entirely manual and used reagents that were produced in-house. Those familiar with the technique will understand the significant number of manual transfers between tubes and the often tiny volumes of sample being processed. End point determination was by visual inspection of a gel. The potential GMP deficiencies were many and obvious.

Before approval was granted to proceed to live testing, all of these variables had to be brought under an acceptable level of control. As a result of on-going development, and an appreciation of the 'GMP' philosophy by our NAT team, one year down the line we have automated extraction and automated second round amplification/results reading via a lightcycler. It is hoped that direct download of results into the donation/donor record will be achieved by the end of 2000.

Clearly, we must anticipate that such technological advances will continue with ever increasing speed. Against this expectation, public, media and political demands for a 'risk free' blood supply will create continuing pressure to introduce these technologies before their development is complete. Ironically, in those countries where the regulatory process is more stringent, approval to implement is likely to take longer. In those instances where a delay is a result of demonstrating product safety eg through a clinical trial, a delay is likely to be accepted. However, when the improvement is perhaps an assay for a new transmissible disease or a more sensitive assay for an existing disease marker then any delay beyond the first date of implementation by any organisation introduces the possibility for criticism and claims for damages. Similarly, introduction by one regulatory authority of measures that confer even marginal enhancements in safety makes it difficult for other regulatory authorities to follow suit. Introduction of HCV NAT illustrates this point very well [15].

Virus inactivation of cellular components is currently a prime contender for the next major development. However, undoubtedly the most exciting development on the horizon is microarray technology (J. Petric, unpublished observations). This has the potential to provide an integrated platform on which Blood Centres and Blood Banks could perform all their tests. This might mean infectious disease screening (viruses and bacteria) and blood group serology (red cell, platelet and granulocyte antigens and antibodies) in a single test – a truly remarkable prospect!

Automation and Computerisation in Clinical Transfusion Practice

A multitude of 'drivers' have forced Blood Transfusion Services to assure the quality of their processes and thereby ensure product safety and efficacy. These drivers have included:

- the potential to transmit serious infectious diseases with blood transfusion;
- regulatory requirements for GMP compliance;

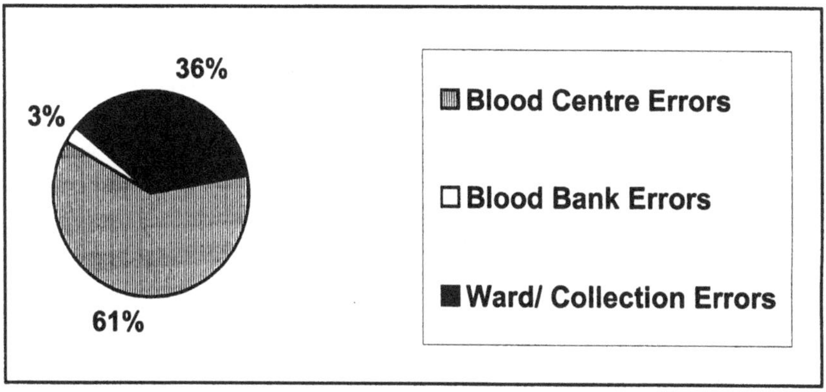

Figure 2. Analysis of the source of 'incorrect blood component transfused errors'. Extract from the 1998-99 report of the Serious Hazards of Transfusion Reporting Scheme.

- litigation;
- public (and media) demands for a risk free blood supply.

As a result, the manufacturing 'end' of the blood supply chain has invested heavily in automating its processes and this has done much to ensure blood components are of a consistently high quality. However, as the blood supply chain extends outward towards the patient, in general the extent and level of the quality system diminishes; the level of automation decreases; the simplicity of the management structure diminishes; the level of direct human intervention increases, as does the error rate.

This is amply illustrated in the 1998-99 SHOT Report [12]. There were 239 errors for the category of incorrect blood component transfused and the analysis showed (8) 3% of these to be Blood Centre errors; (85) 36% were Blood Bank (hospital transfusion laboratory) errors and (146) 61% of errors were made either at collection from refrigerators or in the ward.

In the UK, almost all Blood Banks have a computerised system to manage stock transactions, patient histories, record test results and product issues. A significant number now use semi-automated test equipment and of those, a few have direct transfer of automatically interpreted results from the test equipment into their patient database.

Whilst progress is being made in automating Blood Banking, in general, GMP principles are not applied with the same rigor as they are in the Blood Centre environment. This tends to be reflected in the blood bank software which often is a module that has been 'bolted on' to the end of a multidisciplinary Laboratory Information Management System. On occasions, Blood Bank equipment and computer systems have deficiencies which would rule out their use in the blood component manufacturing environment. However, more often Blood Bank systems lack the sophisticated, GMP compliant features that have been carefully designed into automated/computerised manufacturing systems over time. Therefore, not only is there a gap in the level of automation and computerisation between Blood Centre and Blood Bank, there is also a significant difference in the philosophy which underpins system design and use.

Clearly there is an opportunity to accelerate progress in this area of blood banking by transferring existing systems and solutions from Blood Centre to Blood Bank. Indeed, it can be anticipated that regulation/accreditation of blood banking activity will, in time, demand a much more rigorous approach to Quality Assurance. The real challenge for this will be to create sufficiently strong 'drivers' to force a change in culture.

Whilst most Blood Banks have a computer system and many use semi-automated equipment, computerisation in the hospital ward is the exception rather than the rule. This is indeed unfortunate as the available evidence indicates that this is the part of the transfusion process where the greatest proportion of errors occur. Once again this can be illustrated from the 1998-99 SHOT Report 'incorrect blood component transfused' errors [12]. Failure of bedside checking was a factor in 44% of the incident reports and collection of the wrong component from the storage location featured in 22% of incident reports (n=136).

Computerised systems which would significantly reduce the frequency of such errors have been available for a number of years and some of those currently available are very good. However, they are at present relatively expensive and require the active and effective participation of a much broader group of personnel than are presently involved in the clinical transfusion process. Nevertheless, some hospitals do use these systems and find them both helpful and effective. The challenge for the manufacturers of such systems is to make them easily affordable and simple to use.

Conclusions

It could be argued that blood transfusion has changed very little in the past 25 years. We still recruit and select donors, collect, test and process donations, store those that are suitable for use and perform testing and checking to ensure the blood is suitable for the patient before transfusing it.

However, the underlying detail tells a very different story. The blood transfusion system can be divided into three major types of activity:

- those concerned with the procurement and provision of blood components (= Blood Centre/Bank Activity);
- those concerned with the provision of blood components that are suitable for specific patients (= Blood Transfusion Service Activity);
- those concerned with the ordering, collection and transfusion of blood components (= Clinical Transfusion Process).

From a UK perspective, the pace and extent of change on these three parts of the blood transfusion system has been very different. Therefore, it should be expected that the outcomes of the changes will also be different.

Blood Centres/Banks

Universally, Blood Centres have been forced to change to meet very powerful drivers, eg steps to prevent transmission of HIV, Hepatitis; and other infections (increasingly more tests, more sensitive tests and virus inactivation); Consumer Protection legislation; increasing regulatory constraints; universal blood component leukocyte depletion. Underpinning all of these issues is the political expedient to deliver public (media) demands for a 'risk free' blood supply.

Collectively, and over time, these drivers undoubtedly have generated an increase in blood component safety and efficacy and contributed significantly to reducing the inherent risk in receiving a blood transfusion.

A significant proportion of that risk reduction has arisen from the development and implementation of quality systems that are compliant with the principles of GMP. Integral to the success of such systems has been the development and introduction of a high degree of automation, linked to sophisticated computer systems. Indeed, such is the importance of these aspects of the quality system that it must be conceded that, were they not available, then risks undoubtedly would increase.

Blood Transfusion Services

Drivers for risk reduction in Blood Transfusion Services (hospital transfusion laboratories) have been very limited. Whilst, in the UK, the development of a voluntary pathology laboratory accreditation scheme and voluntary participation in the SHOT reporting scheme are very welcome, there is no regulatory control.

Against such a background it is not surprising that the uptake of automation and computerised systems is highly variable. Furthermore, as there has been only limited exposure to the rigors of regulatory control then the philosophy that underpins the development of automated equipment and computer systems for use in this environment will often only reflect customer experience/requirements.

Therefore, the degree of risk reduction in Blood Banks that can be attributed to computerisation/automation is dependent on the extent to which such systems are deployed and effective. Certainly, it would seem that an enhanced degree of risk reduction could be achieved if there was an effective mechanism for transferring Blood Centre/Bank experience to Blood Transfusion Service operations.

The Clinical Transfusion Process

Once again, drivers for risk reduction in this part of the transfusion process have been very limited. This is unfortunate as this is a critical part of the process, but is almost entirely dependent on human intervention and, not surprisingly, is most prone to errors. Whilst there are devices which will prevent errors, these are not widely used, mainly on the grounds of cost.

Over the next five or so years it is hoped that attention will focus on introducing affordable automated/computerised systems all the way to the bedside where these are appropriate and effective process control steps where they are not.

Technological Change

As it is anticipated that the current drivers in the global blood transfusion environment will continue to force the agenda towards a 'risk free' blood supply then further safety improvements in the Blood Centre/Bank end of the chain are anticipated. Similarly, technology must be expected to continue to progress at its current remarkable rate.

Whilst looking into the future carries the risk of 'retrospective ridicule', here are a few developments that are likely to have a major impact over the next 5-10 years:

- technology will deliver improvements in the security of donor identity and recognition;
- 'smart' chips will replace multiple barcodes on blood bags, probably recording manufacturing and storage history including temperature, time and location;
- affordable technology will deliver significant safety improvements to the Clinical transfusion process;
- microarray technology will revolutionise testing procedures in Blood Centre/Bank and Blood Transfusion Service;
- the current trend in miniaturisation of record databases will continue.

'System' Limitations

Finally, it should be borne in mind that automated/computerised systems have limitations. The most obvious limitation relates to the knowledge and experience of the person(s) specifying what is required. That observation equally applies to those designing and to those performing validation exercises.

The difficulty of getting these elements right is reflected in the acceptance and appearance of software 'bugs'. Therefore, it is important that staff record and report problems rather than concluding they must have done something wrong. There also are occasional and unexpected hardware or 'firmware' defects and very unexpected and worrying test result errors.

Last of all there are people. Perhaps if we said *'To err is inhuman'*, then people would stop making mistakes. However, even with highly sophisticated, fully automated, carefully validated processes, people always find a way around the system. Furthermore, many equipment/computer system problems arise because procedures simply have not been followed. Finally, somewhat juxtaposed, is a reminder of the absolute necessity for accurate data entry.

Acknowlegements

The author wishes to acknowledge support received from S.R. Houston and C. Lofthouse in preparing this manuscript.

References

1. Quality assurance of blood components prepared in the blood transfusion centre/blood bank. International Forum. Vox Sang 1994;67:99-111.

2. Food and Drug Administration. Guidelines for quality assurance in blood establishments (July 11, 1995). Rockville, MD: CBER Office of Communication, Training, and Manufacturing Assistance, 1995.
3. Buckman JF. Quality is not optional. Transfusion 1994;34:842-45.
4. Zuck TF. Current good manufacturing practices. Transfusion 1995;35:955-66.
5. Sazama K. Current good manufacturing practices for transfusion medicine. Transfus Med Rev 1996;10:286-95.
6. Callery MF, Nevalainen DE, Kerst TM. Quality systems and total process control in blood banking. Transfusion 1994;34:899-906.
7. Medicines Control Agency. Rules and guidance for pharmaceutical manufacturers and distributors 1997. London, The Stationery Office, 1997.
8. European Commission. The rules governing medicinal products in the European Union. Vol 4. Good manufacturing practices; medicinal products for human and veterinary use. Luxembourg: Office for Official Publications of the European Communities, 1997.
9. Guide to the preparation, use and quality assurance of blood components. 6th edition. Strasbourg. Council of Europe Publishing, 2000.
10. Guidelines for the blood transfusion services in the UK. 4th edition. London, The Stationery Office, 2000.
11. Houston SR, Muircroft JH, Barr A, Mitchell R. Print on-demand blood group labels. Transfus Med 1993;3:243-45.
12. Love EM, Williamson LM, Cohen H et al. The Serious Hazards of Transfusion Steering Group. Annual report 1998/99. Manchester, 2000. ISBN 0 9532 789 2 1.
13. Stokes T, Branning RC, Chapman KG, Hambloch H, Trill TJ. Good computer validation practices. Common sense implementation. Interpharm Press Inc, Illinois. 1994
14. McClelland DBL, McMenamin JJ, Moores HMM, Barbara JAJ. Reducing risks in blood transfusion process and outcome. Transfus Med 1996;6:1-10.
15. Dodd RY, Stramer SL, Aberle-Grasse, Notari E. Risk of hepatitis and retroviral infections among blood donors and introduction of nucleic acid testing (NAT). Dev Biol Stand 2000;102:19-27.

HAEMOVIGILANCE[1]

N. Drouet[2]

The word 'hémovigilance' was first coined in France in the early 1990s. The first paper in the world medical literature that used this key word was French and was published in 1994 [1]. Since then, the English equivalent, 'haemovigilance' or 'hemovigilance', has been used in 33 publications indexed by Medline(r). 'Haemovigilance' is still a European concept and word. Americans do not use this word much, although they do monitor transfusion related morbidity [2]. The word 'haemovigilance' has not yet appeared in any of the standard dictionaries, either. It is obviously a new word for a new concept. But, just how new is this concept?

Table 1. Number of publications indexed by Medline(with the key word 'haemovigilance' or 'hemovigilance'.

Year	Number of publications	Country of authors						
		F	NL	UK	DK	L	B	USA
1994	1	1						
1995	1	1						
1996	2	2						
1997	1	1						
1998	14	10	1	1			1	1
1999	8	4	2	1	1			
2000	6	5				1		

F = France, NL = Netherlands, UK = United Kingdom, DK = Denmark, L = Luxembourg, B = Belgium, USA = United States of America.

Introduction

The very first reported instance when vigorous preventative measures were taken because of a transfusion related accident occurred in the seventeenth century, in France [3-5]. This was a time when animal-to-man transfusions were

1. The contents of this paper do not necessarily reflect the views of the Société Française de Vigilance et de Thérapeutique Transfusionnelle.
2. Société Française de Vigilance et de Thérapeutique Transfusionnelle.

being experimented. One of King Louis XIVs physicians, Jean-Louis Denis, performed successful sequential transfusions of blood from a live calf to a patient suffering from mental illness, probably tertiary syphilis. Of course, he developed severe intravascular haemolysis, but survived. He was found to be saner after the transfusion. Following this apparent success, doctor Denis tried blood transfusion as a treatment for many other ailments, such as leprosy, ulcers, St. Anthony's fire, cancers, dementia, with varying degrees of success. Denis' colleagues did not at all approve of this, calling blood transfusion 'a form of satanic cannibalism'. However, the first patient relapsed. He was due to be transfused again, but died just beforehand. Doctor Denis was brought to court for murder. At the trial, although he was found not guilty, the judges decided on April 17th 1668 that any further experiments with blood transfusion would require a prior authorisation from the Faculty of Medicine of Paris. No authorisation was ever actually grant and, in 1670, Parliament forbade all blood transfusion practices. Other countries, like Britain, followed the outcome of the suit.

This episode from the early history of blood transfusion shows that, from the start, clinical blood transfusion has been the victim of various myths, rumours and misunderstandings. In order to protect both physicians and patients, judges and parliamentarians of the time took very strong preventative measures, albeit not evidence-based!

Haemovigilance

Modern haemovigilance has been developed along the same lines. As a result of various difficulties concerning blood transfusion in the 1980s and early 1990s, French parliamentarians under pressure of public opinion created a complete surveillance system for blood transfusion. A decree was passed on January 24th 1994 [6] defining haemovigilance as an essential part of transfusion safety. Its official definition is as follows: *"All the surveillance procedures, starting with the collection of blood and its components up to and including the follow-up of transfused patients, which aim to collect and assess information concerning the unexpected or adverse effects due to the use of labile blood components and to prevent their taking place."* Basically, three surveillance procedures are mentioned in this definition:

- notification of adverse or unexpected effects related to transfusion,
- traceability of blood components, so that the complete transfusion chain can be pieced together for all blood components. Without this element, adverse effect reports are no more than simple observations and case histories.
- prevention of adverse effects, which depends on both of the previous procedures.

Haemovigilance covers the whole field of transfusion medicine, from the donor to the patient. Indeed, the transfusion chain is a whole, which cannot be separated into different elements. This is one of the major assets of successful haemovigilance: it crosses the borders that exist between establishments. All events occurring somewhere in the chain will necessarily have consequences further along this chain. These effects will also tend to accumulate. Quality managers know that errors or system malfunctions are only rarely due to a single factor, but are the result of the accumulated effects of several minor disfunctions. This is also true for blood transfusion. This cascade effect of adverse events needs to be monitored closely. Haemovigilance gives a systems approach to the surveillance of blood transfusion. Such a surveillance system cannot just observe events and their effects. This would be insufficient to improve the safety of blood transfusion. Surveillance needs to be interactive, i.e. observing an adverse effect must set off corrective and preventative measures. This interactivity means that haemovigilance interferes, in a positive manner, with the organisation of the transfusion chain. Quality systems generally organise production, whether of a product, like labile blood components, or a service, like transfusing a patient. They aim to increase reliability, both in the production process and in the product or service being produced, and to cut the cost of production. This unavoidably includes correcting, and avoiding, events that could disrupt the production tool more or less seriously. By interacting with the production processes, haemovigilance is a key element of quality systems in blood transfusion, whether in the manufacturing setting, or in the clinical setting. Indeed, we can no longer accept that quality and surveillance systems only concern the manufacturing of blood components, and that once within the walls of a hospital, surveillance is random or greatly reduced?

Nevertheless, haemovigilance does not just concern possible errors in the transfusion chain. Adverse effects can also have their origin in any one of several interfaces, without any error having been made; these interfaces concern the donor blood, the patient, the patient's disease process, the material in which the donor blood is stored, the manufacturing process, the storage process, the transport process. All the interest with haemovigilance lies not just in discovering possible errors in the transfusion chain, but also in discovering sources of adverse effects that can be dealt with so as to prevent them in the future.

Haemovigilance world-wide

Many countries have developed their own haemovigilance systems using definitions that often differ in some details from the French one [7]. The differences lie in the type of notification, whether voluntary or mandatory, in the range of adverse reactions to be notified, and in the body to which these reports are made.

Most countries have adopted a mandatory approach. However, this is not necessarily a guarantee for efficiency. In Germany, where blood components are considered licensed drugs, there are relatively few notifications although reporting is mandatory: 1488 suspected serious adverse effects between January 1st 1995 and January 1st 1998 [8]. On the other hand, the United Kingdom has opted for a voluntary reporting system, the SHOT initiative, to which 366 reports were made in a 24 months period between October 1966 and September 1998 [9].

Underreporting is of course a major drawback of all existing systems, including the French network. It would be of the greatest interest to estimate the degree of underreporting in each country. This would, of course, require a very

Table 2. Differences in haemovigilance systems.

Country	Type of notification				Notification to	
	Voluntary		Mandatory		Govt body	Other
	Type of adverse reaction notified					
	All	Only serious	All	Only serious		
Austria				×	×	
Belgium	×					×
Canada (Quebec)			×		×	
France			×		×	
Germany				×	×	
Ireland		×				×
Italy			×			×
Luxembourg			×		×	
Netherlands				×	×	×
Sweden			×		×	
Switzerland				×	×	
UK		×				×
USA				×	×	

Table 3. Number of adverse reactions notified to the French haemovigilance system as of end of August 2000 (unpublished data, Agence Française de Sécurité Transfusionnelle des Produits de Santé, Paris).

Degree of involvement of blood transfusion	Severity score				
	Score 1	Score 2	Score 3	Score 4	Total
Degree 0	1458	772	131	59	**2420**
Degree 1	4482	269	145	56	**4952**
Degree 2	9350	2356	218	54	**11978**
Degree 3	7573	2336	306	25	**10240**
Degree 4	2786	2761	307	34	**5888**
	25649	**8494**	**1107**	**228**	**35478**

strict, accurate and common definition of the events and effects that are to be reported.

Another major difference between existing haemovigilance systems concerns the range of adverse reactions that are to be notified. About half the systems only require serious adverse events to be reported, whereas for the other half, all events are to be notified. This debate is far from closed. The reasoning underlying this is obvious, especially when one looks at the French data. This database is the most comprehensive in the world, with more than 36,000 adverse reactions notified to date! The proportion of life-threatening and fatal events with respect to the total is 3.8 %. However, if we take into account the fact that, for example, some bacterial accidents and some ABO errors can present as relatively benign reactions, how many of these are being missed? This question holds, whatever the reporting system is in place, precisely because of underreporting. Are we not more likely to miss such an event if reporting is selective from the start? The underlying question is whether it is considered important that all adverse effects be known about. The answer lies in the corrective and preventative actions that can be undertaken as a result of an adverse effect report. A clinically benign bacterial accident may lead to finding a faulty donation procedure, for example, or a clinically benign ABO accident may reveal a major transport dysfunction. The objective of reporting all transfusion related adverse effects is that the system is less likely to underreport serious effects, even if they are clinically benign. It is very delicate to consider cost-effectiveness here, at least for France: individual patients, individual donors, and public opinion would not understand that no action had been undertaken to treat and prevent an adverse effect because of a deficit in reporting.

The last main difference between existing systems is the body to which adverse effects are reported. Most countries have set up government bodies to which reports are sent: the Food and Drug Administration (FDA) in the USA [10], the Agence Française de Sécurité Sanitaire des Produits de Santé (AFSSPS) in France, the National Board of Health (NBH) and the Welfare and Medical Products Agency (WMPA) in Sweden. On the other hand, in the UK, the well-known SHOT initiative (Serious Hazards of Transfusion) is not a government programme. In Ireland, the National Haemovigilance Office is a part of the Irish Blood Transfusion Service [11]. In Italy, adverse effects are reported to the local blood establishments.

The French system

Like all surveillance systems, there cannot be any surveillance at all without an active participation from the medical and nursing teams in the wards. They are the people who transfuse blood components to patients, and they are in the position to immediately detect any clinically obvious adverse reaction related to the transfusion. This is necessarily the starting point for the haemovigilance process, which cannot be set off without any adverse or unexpected effect of blood transfusion. However, adverse effects need not all be clinically obvious (post-transfusion irregular antibodies), or even immediate (post-transfusion hepatitis C). Whatever the kind of adverse effect, it will always be the medical and nursing staff caring for the patient who will make the initial report.

However, once the initial report has been made, it should not be their responsibility to decide whether the adverse effect is really due to the transfusion, and to what degree. In France, this is the responsibility of the haemovigilance officers. All State and private hospitals, as well as all transfusion establishments, are required to have a haemovigilance officer. Moreover, all State hospitals are required to have a haemovigilance committee, which acts as the official interface between the hospital and the transfusion establishment. The whole system is overseen by a regional co-ordinator, who acts as the link between the local haemovigilance officers, and the national authorities, i.e. both the government agency and the haemovigilance unit of the head office of the French blood transfusion establishment.

The local hospital and transfusion centre haemovigilance officers have very similar duties. They register, investigate and report transfusion reactions. They also manage traceability, by ensuring that transfusions are confirmed back to the supplying transfusion establishment. They also have a major role in the writing of standard operating procedures (SOP) for blood transfusion in the hospitals. Of course, they are involved in preparing the haemovigilance committee meetings, which they are bound to attend. Lastly, but certainly not least, they are involved in preparing continuing educational programmes in blood transfusion, transfusion safety and haemovigilance for both medical and non-medical staff.

The first role of the haemovigilance committees is to organise transfusion within the hospital. This includes checking and approving SOP, and finalising continuing education programmes. They also monitor transfusion reactions, which have been investigated by the haemovigilance officers. These committees report to the hospital medical authority and management about the state of blood transfusion within the hospital.

Regional co-ordinators oversee the whole system, based on administrative regions. They organise haemovigilance in the regions, by ensuring there are haemovigilance officers and haemovigilance committees everywhere there should be one. They of course monitor transfusion related adverse reaction reports, by ensuring their coherence and completeness. They can ask for further investigations for particular reaction reports. They also monitor the degree of traceability in the various establishments under their responsibility. Being at the centre of the system, they inform the regional and national health authorities about the state of haemovigilance in their region, as well as acting as technical advisers for the regional administrative authorities.

What has haemovigilance achieved?

There are about 2000 haemovigilance officers in France, some of whom are fully dedicated to haemovigilance. Whilst most are physicians, some are hospital pharmacists. Most of those working in the private sector, the large majority of whom are consultant anaesthetists, have taken this responsibility on top of their own work. State budgets were given to help State hospitals to increase their levels of transfusion safety. An estimated 100 million Euros have been spent on haemovigilance in France since 1993. This is enormous, and not all countries can afford to spend such sums on surveillance of a small part of the health system. This is an indicator of the amount of pressure exerted by public opinion and media on blood transfusion in France. What is the return on the investment that has been made?

Traceability

Traceability is the faculty of being able to know precisely what has become of a blood donation. It therefore enables the piecing together of the transfusion chain for each blood donation. In fact, traceability is more than just a chain; it is a loop. Hospitals must confirm to blood establishments that they really have transfused or destroyed blood components that were delivered to them, when and to which patients they have been transfused. Looping the loop in this way enables 'look back procedures', i.e. from the patient to the donor, as well as the simpler 'look forward procedures', i.e. from the donor to the patient.

In France, because of the legal impetus given to traceability by various laws and bylaws, and the work done by haemovigilance officers throughout the country, the number of blood components for which the has been completed has progressively increased over time. In 1996, it was estimated that half the administrative regions had a level of traceability greater than 70%, i.e. the transfusion or destruction of blood components had been confirmed for more than 70% of all blood components. This figure reached more than 90 % for three quarters of the administrative regions in 1997. The estimated national figure is now thought to be more than 94 %. Sixteen out of twenty-one regions had an estimated traceability greater than 95%. This means that most hospitals in France have between 80 and 100 % traceability. This is a crucial prerequisite for improving surveillance of blood transfusion.

Transfusion related adverse effects

Transfusion related adverse effects started being reported towards the end of 1994. In the four years from 1996 to 1999 28,547 reports were made. This means that about 600 reports are made a day. This corresponds to 2 to 3 reports per 1000 components transfused. The database now holds 35,478 reports (as of end of July 2000).

Among these adverse effects, two types of reaction have been particularly well studied, ABO incompatibility, and bacterial contamination.

ABO incompatibility

About 30 adverse reactions due to ABO incompatibility are reported a year in France, where more than 2 million blood components are transfused annually. In France, red cell concentrates are transfused after checking compatibility between the donor blood and the patient with a bedside test. This test, which has been legally required since 1965, aims to be an ultimate check that the patient is going to receive ABO compatible blood. For most of the reported accidents, it has been shown that this bedside compatibility test did not fully play its role. This was mostly because of inappropriate technique by nursing staff carrying out the test [12, 13]. Moreover, in several cases, the patient's identity had not been checked properly before carrying out the bedside test, often because of overwork and routine. The overall conclusion is that the bedside test can be useful, but is not sufficient. A more formal check of the patient's identity is required beforehand. Another problem is the lack of standardisation of the bedside compatibility test cards. Although the reagents used are high quality antibodies, different suppliers have a different format for the cards. This can be confusing for nurses. A national standard for checking the identity of patients before carrying out the bedside compatibility test and starting the transfusion, and the standardisation of the supporting material for the test cards, are both going to be essential projects in the near future.

Bacterial accidents

One of the earliest and worrying results of the French reporting system was the large number of reports made concerning suspected bacterial contamination of the components transfused. This led the then National Centre for Haemovigilance, at the University of Bordeaux, to carry out an epidemiological study, which remains to be published, to try to understand this phenomenon. This case control study showed that, although confirming bacterial contamination was a problem, it was by far not as frequent as the first reports seemed to indicate [14]. Two practical preventative measures have since been adopted on a national scale: a national SOP for disinfection of the donor's skin at the point of venepuncture was written, and included in the criteria for inspection of donation centres, and the discarding of the first 30 ml of all donations [15]. This blood, which is contaminated with skin bacteria in 2 to 4% of donors, is used to fill the sampling tubes, before filling of the bag starts. It is too early yet to say if both these measures have had a serious effect on the number of cases of transfusion reactions due to bacterial contamination.

Other results

Universal leukocyte depletion was carried out nationally as from April 1st 1998. It was, and still is, an expensive measure, which is partly paid for by the hospitals. There would seem to be a fall in the number of cases of fever and rigors. There are of course other advantages to leukocyte depletion. It is, here again, too early to assess the efficacy and the cost-effectiveness of this measure.

The Future of Haemovigilance

It is common sense to say that systems need to evolve to maintain their appropriateness. Despite its youth, haemovigilance already needs to develop. There are two strategic directions for this change: haemovigilance must now work in synergy with other surveillance systems involved in blood transfusion, and it must become international.

Co-operating with other surveillance systems

Blood transfusion does not just concern donor blood and its components transfused into patients. When stable blood derivatives are transfused at the same time as labile components, a combined haemovigilance and pharmacovigilance enquiry is required, in France, to determine the relative responsibilities of the products during a possible transfusion related adverse effects. Various materials are also concerned in the storage and manufacturing processes: different substances which can interact with the donor blood, or diffuse into the blood, and thus be responsible for transfusion related adverse effects, as in the red eye syndrome. This material may also be deficient, due to faulty manufacturing processes (micro holes, for example), or contaminated [16]. Various reagents are made from donor blood, and surveillance of these, not just from the point of view of their biological efficiency, is also necessary. There are close relationships between tissue and organ grafting, and blood transfusion. The future French surveillance system for tissue and organ grafting, called 'biovigilance', will therefore have close links with haemovigilance. It is likely that some of the haemovigilance officers and regional co-ordinators may be involved with the setting-up of the new French biovigilance network.

All these different surveillance systems need to co-operate, and exchange data and information about individual adverse reactions to obtain as clear a picture as possible, and therefore develop adequate preventative strategies. Not one individual can be an expert in everything: blood transfusion, blood biology, materials science, pharmacology, and so on. Medical surveillance needs to be multidisciplinary, and developing synergy between all the branches of surveillance systems can be beneficial to the patient.

Internationalising haemovigilance

Blood donors travel world wide. They may give blood in a country that is not their own. The question of accepting, in countries other than Great-Britain, donations from British people or from people who have lived in Great-Britain for some length of time is a good example of questions that may arise from this mobility of donors.

Blood components are exchanged world wide. Some countries export blood components, others import them, some do both.

Patients also travel world wide. They made be transfused in a country that is not their own, such as tourists who have had trauma in a country they were visiting.

In the advent of a delayed transfusion related adverse effect in a tourist who received blood imported from another country, where another tourist made the donation, how does one unravel such a complex situation? Perfect traceability is required of the donor, of the donation, of the blood components, and of the patient, all this in four different countries. Who are to be contacted in each country? Who knows whom to call? Who calls the donor for a look back procedure? On the other hand, who calls the patient for a look forward procedure? Such a situation is waiting to happen, or has already happened. In the case of an alert due to a manufacturing problem, for example, a batch of contaminated bags used for donations, some of which have been exported to another country, the question is how to find rapidly the patients who have received this blood.

An answer can be found on a case-by-case basis. For the moment, it mostly consists in making series of telephone calls. All this takes time, too much time when people's safety and health are at stake. Managing such situations depends entirely on the easy access to information. The information technologies could be of use here to make it easier and quicker.

The European Haemovigilance Network (EHN) [17] is making a first attempt to bring an answer to this international question. This network, first set up in 1997, concerns for the moment five countries, Belgium, France, Luxembourg, the Netherlands, and Portugal. Switzerland and Denmark have now joined the network. Its aims are to exchange information about blood transfusion through an Internet web site [18], hosted for the moment by Liege University. The languages used are French and English. Most of the web site is still under construction. Confidential transfusion related alerts could then be dispatched very rapidly in these countries through the national co-ordinators for haemovigilance. The information given in this web site is for each country: News and scientific information, Haemovigilance system, Alerts, Statistics, and Legal framework.

Conclusion

Haemovigilance is still a very young surveillance system. Therefore it does not seem possible to make any worthwhile conclusions for the moment. Nevertheless, it is an essential tool for ensuring the best quality of blood transfusion to patients. It is comprised of a system involving a network of haemovigilance officers whose task it is to ensure that all blood components are traceable from end-to-end of the transfusion chain, that transfusion related adverse effects are investigated, and that the conclusions of these inquiries are acted upon to prevent as far as possible occurrence or recurrence of these events. To go further and increase the overall efficiency of this surveillance work, haemovigilance needs to work with the other surveillance networks that touch upon blood transfusion. Moreover, the international aspects of haemovigilance really need to be addressed, so as to guarantee the same quality of monitoring of transfusion throughout the world.

Acknowledgements

The author would like to acknowledge:

- the staff of the national haemovigilance unit, headed by doctor Bernard DAVID, at the Agence Française de Sécurité Sanitaire des Produits de Santé, in Saint Denis, France, who provided the data concerning traceability and numbers of transfusion related adverse reactions, as well the cost figures,
- the French national conference of regional co-ordinators for haemovigilance, presided by doctor Gérald DAURAT, who calculated traceability figures for 1996 and 1997,
- the teaching hospital of Grenoble for material support of this contribution

References

1. Baudelot J and Djoudi R. De la carte d'information transfusionnelle à la traçabilité des produits. [From the transfusion information card to the tracing of blood products.] Cah Anesthesiol, 1994;42:379-83.
2. Menitove JE. Hemovigilance in the United States of America. Vox Sang 1998;74 Suppl 2:447-55.
3. Denis J. Concerning a new way of curing sundry diseases by transfusion of blood. Philosophical Transactions of the Royal Society of London. 1667;3:489-504.
4. Denis J. An extract of a letter written by J. Denis, Doctor of Physics and Professor of Philosophy and the Mathematics at Paris, touching a late cure of an inveterate phrensy by the transfusion of blood. Philosophical Transactions of the Royal Society of London. 1668;4:710.
5. Bernard J. La légende du sang. Flammarion: Paris, 1992. ISBN 2-08-035152-4.

6. Décret n° 94-68 du 24 janvier 1994 relatif aux règles d'hémovigilance. Official journal of the French Republic, 26th January 1994, pages 1346-49.
7. Haeman Consortium, for the European Commission. The establishment of a haemovigilance network in the European Community. A feasibility project. Luemburg, December 1998.
8. Keller-Stanilawski B. in "Le risque sanitaire en Europe: les systèmes d'hémovigilance" – meeting of the Assistance Publique – Hôpitaux de Paris, Paris, January 23, 2000.
9. Williamson LM, Lowe S, Love EM, et al. Serious hazards of transfusion (SHOT) initiative: analysis of the first two annual reports. BMJ 1999;319:16-19.
10. http://www.fda.goc/cber/transfusion.htm.
11. National Haemovigilance Office. Annual report, 1999. http://www.ibsts.ie.
12. Rouger P, Le Pennec PY, Noizat-Pirenne F. Analyse des risques immunologiques en transfusion sanguine: période 1991-1998. Transfus Clin Biol 2000;7:9-14.
13. Ingrand P, Surer-Pierres Houssay D, Salmi LR. Reliability of the pretransfusion bedside compatibility test: association with transfusion practice and training. Transfusion 1998;38:1030-36.
14. Morel P, Leconte des Floris MF, Bardiaux L, Pouthier F, Hervé P. Transfusion sanguine et risque bactérien. Transfus Clin Biol 2000;7: 5-23.
15. Vassort-Bruneau C, Allouch P, Audurier A, et al. Efficacité d'une procédure de prélèvement sur les contaminations bactériennes lors de la ponction veineuse. Transfus Clin Biol 1998;5:95S.
16. Heltberg O, Skov P, Gerner-Schmidt H, et al. Nosocomial epidemic of Serratia marcescens septicemia ascribed to contaminated blood transfusion bags. Transfusion 1993;33:221-27.
17. Faber JC L'hémovigilance en Europe. Transfus Clin Biol 2000;7:5-8.
18. http://www.ehn-org.net.

HUMAN RESOURCES: TEACHING AND TRAINING IN TRANSFUSION MEDICINE

J.F. Harrison[1]

Introduction

Education and training are vital to the provision of a safe blood product, delivered in a timely manner and administered appropriately to the correct patient. Workers will not consistently perform tasks to a high standard unless they not only know what needs to be done, but why a task should be performed in a certain way. Three groups of people require education in order to achieve the highest possible standards of transfusion practice. These are transfusion service staff, hospital staff and the general public (both donors and patients). Educating staff with such a wide range of educational backgrounds and abilities, presents an enormous challenge.

Because of the author's experience, discussion in this chapter will be largely confined to the situation in the United Kingdom.

History

Until recently, the issue of training in transfusion medicine was not taken very seriously. Indeed, few have taken transfusion medicine seriously as a discipline. When I announced my intention to join the National Blood Service in England 20 years ago, colleagues remarked that it would be easy because all I would have to learn was how to say 'no' to requests for platelet concentrates!

At the beginning of the 20th Century a few pioneers endeavoured to establish standards to educate colleagues into adopting good transfusion practice. Geoffrey Keynes, a surgeon working at St Bartholomew's Hospital, had difficulty persuading his surgical colleagues to use blood transfusion as a means of replacing blood lost during surgery. They felt that the transfusion apparatus 'got in the way' of their operative field.

Mr Percy Lane Oliver, who set up the first volunteer blood donor panel in London in 1921, laid down a number of standards which he insisted hospitals should strictly follow [1]. Some of these have a familiar ring, such as the requirement that hospitals should give group specific blood to their patients, rather than using universal donor (group O) blood without establishing the patient's blood group. He was also concerned with donor welfare and if hospitals kept

---

1. National Blood Service, London, UK.

donors waiting or treated them badly eg by performing 'cut downs' to obtain venous access, he would send a medical officer to try and 'educate' the hospital staff. If the hospital still failed to comply then the London Red Cross Blood Transfusion Service would refuse to send further donors.

The general public have always been greatly influenced by the press despite the efforts of transfusion specialists to educate them about blood donation and transfusion. In the 1920's and 1930's there were:

'occasional articles in the Press which lauded highly the 'heroic' nature of blood donation, particularly where the recipient was a lady around whom the journalist could weave his romance. The underlying suggestion that here was a noble hero risking his life for a beautiful but distressed maiden inclined well meaning associates of a donor to think that his continued donations would seriously impair his health.' [2]

Now frequent Press articles imply that the receipt of blood is dangerous.

Medical Staff Training

Tutorials, lectures and practical classes have been used for the training of Haematology Registrars in transfusion for many years. In the South of England, trainees currently attend a one month course and a one week revision course prior to their MRCPath part 1 examinations. The aim of the one month course is to provide the student with sufficient knowledge of Transfusion Medicine to enable him/her to manage a hospital blood bank and use transfusion services intelligently and safely when he/she becomes a Consultant. The revision course is to help with passing the exam, where there will be a compulsory written question, data interpretation and vivas. For the MRCPath part 2 students, there are 2-3 day courses for each of the relevant disciplines within Transfusion Medicine eg immunohaematology, histocompatibility and immunogenetics and platelet immunology. Students appear to be enthusiastic and committed throughout these courses and the majority do well in their examinations. Occasionally a student will express an interest in specialising in Transfusion Medicine. An MRCPath examination in Transfusion is available and such students are encouraged to spend more time working and studying at the Transfusion Centre.

Some overseas students attend these courses before taking the MRCPath exams, usually successfully. In some cases, neither the training nor the examination would appear to be entirely relevant to the situation in the student's own country. Nor is there much update training in transfusion for Consultant Haematologists, for Immunologists or Microbiologists who might be interested in working in the field.

Medical undergraduates have traditionally received little training in transfusion medicine. They usually receive just 2-3 lectures during their three years of clinical training. But the situation is improving with the advent of personal computers, enabling private study of published papers, the use of video and of interactive web sites for performing data interpretation.

Hospital doctors receive little instruction in the practical aspects of sample collection, prescription of blood and components and their safe administration. The main forum for training is the induction period at the beginning of a new job. This is usually a one day lecture course, but such courses are now so crowded with information that transfusion training may be almost squeezed out. This is an area of serious concern. Many junior doctors are unaware that mistakes in blood administration are the major cause of serious transfusion hazard.

Scientific Staff Training

There are two categories of scientific staff employed within the UK Transfusion Services, Clinical Scientists and Medical Laboratory Scientific Officers (MLSO's). Hospital Transfusion Departments employ MLSO's. Clinical Scientists enter at graduate level, with an appropriate science degree. They undergo in service training and pursue specialist courses, depending on their chosen area of work eg the British Society of Histocompatibility and Immunogenetics (BSHI) diploma, or an MSc in microbiology. Clinical Scientists tend to be employed in research orientated posts.

MLSO's also enter the field of Transfusion Medicine at graduate level. If their degree is in a subject other than Biomedical Science, then they will need to undertake a conversion course. Practical training is provided at the place of work. The MLSO's have to fill in a log book detailing their training and its satisfactory completion. When this has been done, the log book is presented to examiners and the student undergoes an oral examination before qualifying as a State Registered MLSO.

From October 2000, Clinical Scientists will also be required to undergo assessment to qualify for State Registration.

One disadvantage for Hospital and Transfusion Service MLSO's, is that the two groups do not have much knowledge of each other's problems, as there is little opportunity to work in each other's environment. Hopefully more 'exchanges' can be organised in the future.

In the past, there have been insufficient opportunities for update training and no regular formal appraisal of the work of each member of scientific staff. But there are now occupational standards and participation in Continuing Professional Development (CPD) programmes will soon be mandatory for all scientific staff.

Nurse Training

Until the mid 1980's, few nurses were employed within the UK transfusion services. There were some that assisted with plasmapheresis or helped doctors at blood donor sessions.

In the mid 1980's a project was piloted in Brentwood, Essex to extend the role of nurses so that they could manage mobile blood collection sessions in the absence of a Medical Officer. There was resistance to this change by the Medical Consultants in the Transfusion Service and there was genuine anxiety that donors would be put at risk and would not accept the change. But these fears proved unfounded, the pilot study was successful and the scheme has been extended throughout the UK [3].

The success of nurse training to conduct donor sessions, depends on thorough training of the nurses concerned and regular updating to maintain skills. The nurses serve a type of apprenticeship, working at donor sessions under the supervision of an experienced nurse or doctor and attending the Transfusion Centre for courses in donor selection, venepuncture, information about the various departments at the Blood Centre, First Aid training and management training.

It is vital that training is adequate and that there is regular updating. The danger is that training can be compromised at times of staff shortage and then donors and blood safety can be put at risk.

Hospital nurses have a crowded training programme and training in sample collection, checking, administration and monitoring of transfusions, may be neglected. Like junior doctors, nurses may be unaware that the majority of major adverse events in transfusion are the result of mistakes in blood administration. The setting up of Hospital Transfusion Committees which has become mandatory following issue of the Department of Health paper "Better Blood Transfusion" [4], will mean that all hospitals must develop local standards for sample collection and blood administration. Some hospitals have appointed Transfusion Nurses or designated a nurse as responsible for training staff in this essential area.

The Serious Hazards of Transfusion (SHOT) report [5] (an annual report summarising the serious hazards that have occurred in UK hospitals in the past year), is now being used in hospitals as part of the education process. By informing staff about mistakes that have been made leading to the administration of the 'wrong' blood products to patients, they will develop an understanding of the reasons why meticulous checking of sample and patient identity are so important.

This training and understanding is essential not only for hospital doctors, scientists and nurses but also for phlebotomists, porters, drivers and anyone else involved in collecting samples and supplying blood to patients.

Other Transfusion Service Staff

Within the Transfusion Service, the majority of staff are neither doctors, nurses nor scientists and they perform a wide variety of tasks from recruiting donors to delivering blood to hospitals. Such staff undergo in service training. This is a successful training method provided that the training is adequate and not compromised by staff shortages or rapid staff turnover. Staff training records must be kept and at each stage it is important to ensure that the member of staff agrees that he/she has completed the training satisfactorily. There must never be a culture of blame – staff must feel free to admit and report mistakes and understand that failure to report errors could harm a patient.

Standard operating procedures are not only important to ensure that tasks are performed to the same standard by everybody but also form a useful teaching tool for all grades of staff.

Whilst training of individuals is vital, it is important that people are encouraged to work as a team, both within the various departments and in the organisation as a whole. This can be achieved by developing a number of educational programmes which can be made available to all staff and indeed should form part of a mandatory training programme.

In the Transfusion Centres in South East England we have one day Induction Courses. All members of staff, whatever their grade or training, must attend an Induction Course within the first month of their appointment. The aim of the course is not only to present the scope of the work of the Transfusion Service but to point out the importance of the role of every individual within the organisation and how vital team work and good manufacturing practice are to the supply of high quality blood components and services to hospitals.

When staff have been working for the organisation for more than 6 months, they are required to attend a one day Core Knowledge Course [6] for more information about the work of various departments of the Transfusion Service. In order to consolidate knowledge obtained by staff during the course, they are asked to complete a question paper, which is sent to them following the course. Only when this is completed satisfactorily will they receive a certificate of course completion.

Other compulsory training courses are held for all staff. These include fire safety, risk assessment, manual handling and good manufacturing practice (GMP). All these courses are attended by a variety of staff and provide an opportunity for staff of different grades and departments to meet and work together. A good example is the GMP Course where 'role play' is used to good effect to illustrate problems and solutions:

Course participants are divided into 'doctors' and 'patients'. 'Doctors' are issued with boxes containing 5 doses of medication (yellow sweets) and are instructed to give the medication to the 'patients'. But some boxes contain more or fewer than 5 'doses'. Others contain some discoloured or broken sweets and for others the date on the box indicates an outdated product. The consequences of issue of faulty or outdated products are discussed.

Training of Visitors from other Countries

Medical, nursing and scientific staff from other countries, usually outside Western Europe, regularly visit and stay for training in South East England. It is a pleasure to provide training for such staff. There are pitfalls however, to providing training which may prove to be inappropriate when a student returns to his/her own country with a different culture and perhaps very limited resources. I am reminded of the situation I found in South India where medical students were learning about the incidence of chronic bronchitis from English text books.

Many countries have now recognised these problems and have set up their own training programmes and examinations, adapted to local conditions and disease incidence. Transfusion specialists from the UK are participating by acting as external examiners.

Training of visiting staff from abroad can be extremely beneficial if the staff sent for training are able to adapt the information they have gained to the situation in their own country and then act as local trainers.

The European School for Transfusion Medicine (ESTM) is playing a valuable role in setting standards for training, holding meetings of experts from various countries so that training issues can be discussed [7] and holding workshops and conferences in various countries so that local students can attend.

The World Health Organisation (WHO) has set up an excellent distance learning programme [8] to facilitate training for the large numbers of staff who work in remote locations. A series of interactive learning materials have been produced so that staff can study in their own locations (Distance Learning Materials or DLM). But it is emphasised that tutorial support must be provided by experienced trainers via regular contact by post, fax or e-mail, group tutorials and practical training sessions at designated study centres.

Education of the General Public

Unfortunately the general public continues to obtain almost all information about transfusion issues from press reports, which give an exaggerated view of the dangers of transfusion with little mention of the benefits.

It is unlikely that the transfusion services will ever be able to completely counteract the effect of 'bad news being the only news'. But a great deal can be achieved through the use of well trained transfusion service staff in their daily work in donor recruitment and blood collection, and by hospital staff in contact with patients requiring transfusions.

What Have We Achieved? – What Can We Achieve?

I have described the UK experience, which I believe to be similar to that in the rest of the developed world.

We have good training programmes for doctors specialising in haematology and transfusion, but their continuing education after qualification could be improved. This should be achieved by the Continuing Professional Development (CPD) programmes organised by the Royal Colleges or their equivalent. But this training must be regularly appraised. Statutory attendance at lectures is not necessarily a learning experience.

Medical student training in transfusion will be greatly improved by the use of modern interactive learning techniques, but proper assessment is essential.

Hospital doctors, nurses and all other staff involved in the transfusion process, must be properly trained and regularly assessed if mistakes are to be avoided in future. The use of transfusion nurses as trainers, the dissemination of information from the SHOT reports, regular audit of practice and the use of new technology (video, interactive web sites), should be employed. It is most important not to neglect the training of staff such as porters and drivers whose contribution to the transfusion process is vital, but whose educational level may be low. Above all, this training and assessment must be supported and appropriately funded by Hospital Management Boards.

Excellent training programmes in Transfusion Medicine have been developed for Scientists and Nurses. But it should be remembered that training takes time and is only effective if properly completed to the satisfaction of both trainer and trainee. It must not be compromised as the result of staff shortages and it must be properly funded.

The same is true of training for non-professional grades of staff. Regular updating, audit and appraisal of all staff training, has been neglected in the past, often as the result of staff shortages and inadequate funding. All managers should be held responsible for maintenance of staff training, keeping training records up to date and conducting regular appraisal.

General training must not be neglected. Induction and Core Knowledge Courses are an excellent way of providing this and of generating a sense of identity and the idea of team work within each Transfusion Service as well as raising morale. Updating of essential training, Health and Safety, GMP etc must not be forgotten and there should be an opportunity for all staff to attend lectures on subjects of general interest in the field. A lunchtime lecture programme can fulfil this function. To assist in the co-ordination of all training activities and to organise general training, courses for visitors (from home or abroad) and to arrange for staff to attend outside courses, an appropriately funded Training Department is essential. Library, computer and video conferencing facilities are also valuable assets for Transfusion Centres.

The assistance provided to our colleagues in the less developed world should continue with the excellent programmes developed by ESTM and WHO. But the focus should be on 'training the trainers' and helping countries to develop their own training programmes and examinations, rather than training a few individuals within one country and then sending them back to work in a completely different environment.

Conclusion

There have been enormous improvements in transfusion training in the last 20 years, largely in response to the enormous increase in complexity of the subject.

There is much still to be done. Discouraging signs include the following recent cases:

- A porter (newly appointed) who, when sent to collect a unit of blood for a patient, took the nearest unit on the fridge shelf (he thought collecting a unit of blood was like collecting a pint of milk!).
- A phlebotomist who collected a blood sample for cross matching from a patient who was aphasic and had no identifying wristband (it was the wrong patient).
- An anaesthetist who transfused a unit of blood designated for the first patient on an operating list, to the first patient in theatre that day without checking patient identity (the order of the operating list had been changed and the patient died).

Encouraging signs from recent cases:

- The clerical officer who queried the prescription of group A platelets for a group O patient.

- The nurse who reported the fact that a patient said she had not had a blood sample taken when the nurse knew that blood had been cross matched for the patient.
- The MLSO who made sure that HLA matched platelets for a lymphoma patient were irradiated when the doctor had omitted to prescribe this.

With adequate training and regular updating, auditing and appraisal of the skills of all staff involved in transfusion from the selection of donors to the transfusion of the product, the provision of a safe and appropriate blood service should be ensured.

References

5. Mills F. W. The London Blood Transfusion Service and the Psychology of Blood Donors. In: Geoffrey Keynes, ed. Blood Transfusion. Simpkin Marshall, London. 1949: p348.
6. Ibid p352.
7. Harrison J. F. Nurses in the Transfusion Service. Lancet 1987;ii:1136-38.
8. Department of Health. Better Blood Transfusion. London: Health Service Circular 1998:224.
9. Serious Hazards of Transfusion. Annual Report 1998-1999. Manchester : SHOT Steering Group April 2000.
10. Teesdale P, Devenish A. Core Knowledge – the glue that enables Blood Service staff to interact well with donors, hospitals and colleagues. Transfusion 1999; 39 (Suppl): A119-P (abstract).
11. Rossi U. Contribution of the European School of Transfusion Medicine (ESTM) to the building up of an integrated European teaching of Transfusion Medicine. In: Proceedings ESTM residential course – Castellanza (Italy) 2000. Milano, ESTM 2000: 441-53.
12. Fordham J. Distance learning in Blood Safety. An initiative by the World Health Organisation. Africa Sanguine 1999;2:9-14.

DISCUSSION

F. Canal (Madrid, E): I would like to start the discussion with a provoking thought. There is kind of a golden thread, 'cost-benefit', around technology, around creative ideas, things that could be achieved.Mr. Bruce, with regard to the role of documentation technologies how would the use of new technologies help elevate the quality and safety and the level of training to get more efficient processes by always reducing costs.

M. Bruce (Edinburgh, UK): At the present time we have a very developed and highly sophisticated system, where we are continually poring more money in to achieve very little, but in fact we could invest that money elsewhere in the process. So, in terms of automation with current generation equipment we have gone I would suggest almost as far as we can. We need to change the approach somewhere and perhaps there might come area approach for delivers some of these types of changes. In terms of increasing the technology, you must increase the training to cope with that. One of your concerns we have is that we will deskill to the extent of we do not have anyone who understands how the process is working anymore. So, the risk stands there as well as the potential benefits.

K. Sazama (Houston, TX, USA): An observation to share is that I think that another way of stating it is we focused on what I would consider to be the easy problems. We can go to the laboratory and keep devising new ways of doing things in vitro, looking for more sensitivity and more specificity, better chemicals and better bags and so forth, but the real issues I think we illustrated wonderfully. The real problem is we have not met the patients' needs. We do not have a system to ensure that the right patient gets the right blood. In today's world 'developed or developing, that is the question'. I often say that I hope I live long enough to be in a country where the importance of absolute positive identification of patients becomes the quality monitor not just for transfusion but everything we do to patients in the healthcare system. It is shocking to me that we live in a world where we pay so little attention: 61% of the errors that have occurred had significance related to a failure at the patient's bedside. Those data are very similar to the fatality data in the United States. It is amazing to me we, have known that now for close to 25 yeas and we have not done anything to solve that problem.

S. Moeslichan (Jakarta, IN): Dr. Harrison, what is the name of the medical doctors after finishing the transfusion medicine education. Do you call them a specialist or blood bankers or something else.

S. Moeslichan (Jakarta, IN): The doctors I was talking about are trained in haematology. They become consultants in hospitals and they usual manage hospital blood banks and hospital departments of haematology. A few of them, when in training, become interested in blood transfusion and then they can enter the transfusion service, but they become transfusion medicine consultants.

S. Moeslichan: Do you mean that the consultant after finishing the haematology training or just from GP to the transfusion medicine.

J.F. Harrison: No, after finishing haematologist training.

S. Moeslichan: So, the second step after haematology. Because in my country there is internist-haematologist; there is paediatric haematologist. But the persons that look after transfusion what would we call them.

J.F. Harrison: The person who looks after a hospital blood bank or transfusion service is usually a consultant haematologist: Haematologist-transfusionist.

J-P. Allain (Cambridge, UK): Dr. Drouet, two questions. The first - clearly the haemovigilance system in France came after the issue of viral transmission to blood recipients and in your report of the first 5 years of haemovigilance you did not mention anything about viral transmission. So did you not have any or not enough to tell us about?

N. Drouet (Grenoble, F): Well, there is virtually no viral no transmission at all reported at the moment. For the last three years I think there has been no transmissions of HIV or hepatitis C

*J-P. Allain:*But could it be that people were so afraid that they did not report at all?

N. Drouet: No, there are many reports; I don't have the figures with me, but there are several hundreds reports a year about suspected viral transmission. However, in the last three years none have been confirmed as being related to the transfusion.

J-P. Allain: My second question has to do with the results of the haemovigilance in general. How transparent is it to the public, because if you remember one of the main things that the public, that the media and so on reproached the medical profession is not to be transparant and not to give the right information.

So, my question is what is the degree of transparency and awareness and giving the information to the public in France?

N. Drouet: I feel there is still an awful lot of improvement to be made. Well, the adverse reaction reports leave the hospital anonymously and figures are more or less available. But there is not enough information made public in a formal way.

J-P. Allain : That could be very dangerous, because if something comes out of the blue then you can be in deep trouble after all these efforts.

N. Drouet : Absolutely, I quite agree.

A. Brand (Leiden, NL): Dr. Drouet, I was amazed that the Netherlands is reporting in an international system where they have no national system at all. But, my question addresses the point of co-ordinated vigilance. You suggested it does prove indeed that blood transfusion is not an isolated event, it is always in the midst of a clinical, often hectic situation. The reports you mentioned are tops of an iceberg with clinical symptoms and in fact low oxygen perfusion or delivery may have far more consequences. I wonder if you have such a co-ordinated system, what kind of endpoints do you have in mind that will learn anything about such a system. Because it cannot be built like it is built now: simply looking at temperature without reasoning or no clinical endpoints that can be used in such a co-ordinated system.

N. Drouet: Your first question that the Netherlands should report to an international system - this system is still being built, it is not yet operational as such, but they have been working on it for three years now. So, it will probably become operational some time soon.

I am afraid my answer will be the same for the second part of your question, because the convened vigilance system is being built at the moment in France. Some hospitals, five teaching hospitals in France have just been given money to have people to set up this system. It is a start, but there is not an active system yet. So, this is an ongoing project that is being built but not ready and operational before next year.

P.M. Ness (Baltimore, MD, USA): We heard yesterday that there is an ongoing debate certainly in the US and also obviously in the Netherlands about whether we should implement leukocyte reduction on a selective basis or whether we are to do it universally for everybody. It seems to me that a question about this would have some value to be addressed to this panel. If we are really serious about reducing errors which start from the donor centre and go all the way to the patient.

If we really have education systems such as dr. Harrison suggested, which is typical in the US where medical students and doctors have very little training in blood transfusion, than we could presume that our physicians can identify those patients who need leukocyte reduction or our blood banks could somehow find them and make sure that they get the leukocyte reduced blood. I agree, really we are just inviting more errors. Our ultimate transfusion system with any kind of a selective leukocyte reduction protocol or irradiation protocol could not even reduce AB0 errors.

K. Sazama (Houston, TX, USA): Thank you Dr. Ness for that question. Take it purely from the quality systems approach, obviously the more complex the system the more safeguards you have to build in. Just as I mentioned it is very compelling to think of a world in which you have red cells with no antigens on it, platelets that have no transmissibility of any kind and the leukocytes are gone so no adverse events from the cytokines and so forth. In that ideal world it would be easy to manage the processes, because you would have one inventory so to speak of products that you would use. I think it is safe to say, and everyone here who practices knows, that it is a lot more complex to manage multiple inventories. We have lived through this in the US and learned our lessons about not meeting public expectations or customers' expectations when for a time we did not permit the possibility of directed donations, meaning donations where patients themselves chose the donor and having the multiple inventories of a target directed regular allogeneic units and then the subset of leukocyte reduced units. It becomes increasingly challenging and difficult and the resources are enormous to manage this variety of blood products. So, if you take it further to the point that you are making about identifying the proper patient to get the proper component and not every red cell and not every platelet is identical for that recipient; that just multiplies and confounds the problem. So, I think that the preference for me would be to try the simple variety, the systems to the extent that we can focus on where the problems currently are. We do not have the right quality systems in place currently. As I said before, the AB0 is a far greater challenge to us now than the disease transmission problem in terms of the likelihood of error. So, if we are going to have multiple inventories we got to have very good processes that will manage them correctly and we are not there yet.

J. Koistinen (Helsinki, SF): Dr. Ness, your question then is very relevant there. Of course, the more procedures we have the more difficult it is to control everything and to keep track of what we have done. But, if you can imagine that you have the information on the blood unit which has gone through all these processes and if you can automate the information input into the blood unit or into whatever registry device there is, the more automated it is the more safe it may become. In other words you can have several different stocks and all in the same storage and then you just read the products there are and the product tells you what has been done to it. If that could be automated maybe it could increase the safety.

P.M. Ness: I think you are both right on both of your points, but we are still depending on the doctor in the hospital to tell us his patient there needs a specific product and I am very concerned that that often does not happen.

F. Canal: In Europe the mandate comes from the blood authorities or from the government as such. So, the trend is clearly towards 100% leukocyte reduction. We have made some studies in terms of the economy associated. You do not only get better quality but you reduce costs when you go over 40 or 50% leukocyte reduction in the laboratory. So, you tend to simplify and also get better economies by doing that. The other question is that you are implying also that some patients will receive better care than other patients. In Europe that is a question that is quite a difficult. If you look at the landscape today five or six of the European countries are already 100% leukocyte reduced and for the most part the other ones are - that is my understanding - thinking about this conversion.

J. C. Emmanuel (Geneva, CH): First I like to complement all the speakers, I think what you said is absolutely right; there is this golden thread going all through and it is a great compliment to Dr. Smit Sibinga for having put together such a nice sequence of lectures. It bakes a thousand questions, which obviously we are not going to ask, but I just wanted to follow up what Dr. Harrison was saying and dr. Drouet was saying.

On the questions sometimes we are fortunate in developing countries, because the system being the mother of invention 20 years ago. On the question of who could staff the donor clinic, it was nurses, intensive care sisters, who got tired of doing intensive care, had children, but were wonderful in blood donation and looking after donors. So, that was something 20 years ago and so I think you were right in saying it is a shared experience.

It is not so much only what you can teach developing countries, but I think by having people in your unit sometimes they can share experiences with you, which really brings us to haemovigilance and how we can spread the information. Just to give an example, the distance learning material (DLM), which is now in 9 major languages and a few minor languages; i.e. it is in Chinese and every single province in China was trained; in China there were to train a 100,000 technicians. So, when you ask the question how can we help, I think it is evident and there is a lot of experience there that is needed to get out. You cannot take out a 100,000 students to the UK but you can go out there and help train a 100,000.

Dr. Koistinen, what is ISBT doing about code 128. You said there is a code for every country and I presume that means also every developing country; how can those countries that have started trying to get some kind of computerised system within an organisation get access. How can that be promoted to fit in with the haemovigilance that Dr. Drouet was talking about.

J. Koistinen: Well, Dr. Emmanuel we have discussed this several times and ISBT really has been the organisation that has initiated and created the code and that is all that does. Unfortunately, today the global organisation of the system has to be run with some minor funds and that is why people have to pay for licences. The license fee today is 1.5 American cents per unit of blood taken. This means for instance for the whole country of Finland it costs 4,875 dollars a year, which we consider a small amount of money, but I know very well that even this money is difficult for developing countries to achieve and to get to become licensed and registered in ISBT128. I do not have any solution on how to do that. There are different proposals we have set out and many of them have not really been accepted. But we have to find a solution for the developing countries to come along and join because it definitely improves the quality; there is no doubt about that.

H.J.C. de Wit (Amsterdam, NL): Could there be a role for the industry?

F. Canal: Thank you for the question. I think there is definitely a role. Typically industry tends to make investments in terms of products. It is product driven investments that the industry makes and out of what I have heard today I think time has come to start looking forward 3 to 5 years and looking at investments that are more on the systems how to get closer to the patient in the hospital. Frankly, I do not think industry alone will get to those conclusions. It needs a kind of debate that needs to be brought up at the right instances both on the transfusion and blood banking side and the industry itself. But clearly, if that is small money for the transfusion centres particularly on the ISBT one, it would be also very good way to standardise and have also some quality issues out on the table for the industry. That is something that should be considered.

J.F. Harrison: About his training programme and the role of WHO. Well, interesting enough I know you are referring to Zimbabwe when you mentioned about the nurses and how excellent they were. Of course the time when we were setting up the nurses I was fortunate enough to go to Harare and talk to the nurses there about that training. I agree we can learn a lot from each other, but I think we must always be careful. For example our nurses have to question people about whether they have been to countries which have malaria which is clearly totally inappropriate to train people who come from countries where there is malaria. So, I think we must make sure that we are training people in an appropriate way. The distance learning programme is an excellent example of how can help setting up something which can then be rolled out to our colleagues in the less developed world.

C.F. Högman (Uppsala, S): Dr. Harrison, in our country transfusion medicine has been related to hospitals all from the beginning, which can be criticised particularly in these days when we have to centralise from a production point of view. But it has had one virtue and that is that the specialists in transfusion medicine have been connected to hospitals, quite often university hospitals, where they have been able to get a certain status of transfusion medicine versus the other specialists. So, there has been quite some communication between transfusion medicine and for instance surgery, forensic surgery, different specialities which I think has been rather important in order to get a respect from the clinical side about the problems that are connected to transfusion. I think that transfusion medicine in this way we also became aware of the clinical problems in a fairly good way and according to my experience we actually have improved very much the situation concerning getting the right blood to the right patient. Although I think the problem that we cannot face today is when there is a very stressing acute situation. Because then it is likely to go wrong and there we would like to have some kind of very strict rules with some kind of mechanical devices for instance readers or something that could give an alarm when something is getting wrong. So, in my view for the future this is the type of equipment which is already available and that should be instituted as has been stressed by several of the speakers.

J.F. Harrison: You are entirely right about the connection there should been between transfusion medicine specialist and hospitals. In fact there was not time to go into it, but that is something that we are adopting far more in the UK now. We have quite a lot of our consultants in the blood transfusion service that are actually in joint appointments. So, they are the transfusion specialists for a particular hospital, usually a teaching hospital as well as working some days in the transfusion service. This is one way to spreading the message if you like. The other thing is that every consultant in transfusion in the UK is allocated to a number of hospitals. So that we all sit on the hospital transfusion committees and there is always a transfusion specialist on those committees.

C.F. Högman: Yes, this is also what we have: a transfusion specialist who actually is in charge of a number of hospitals where good manners can be instituted.

J.D. Cash (Edinburgh, Scotland): I think this was a super session. What is demonstrated is that if you take the laboratory side as the factory side, the manufacturing side of blood transfusion, I am sure Dr. Sazama will agree looking back over the last 20 years how many things have just changed fantastically. I hate what has been demonstrated again today if you look at the clinical interface with those same quality spectacles Dr. Sazama said, it is an unmitigated disaster area. I think if patients, the customers they are not for much longer going to be worried about AIDS. and goodness knows what it is going surely sink in. The really haunting message of this afternoon, not withstanding Dr. Högman's good news from Sweden, is that some of the best clinical interface transfusion medicine I have seen practised is in the developing world, because they are short. They get up there and sit with the surgeons and the anaesthetists and role it out together. There is whole notion in the UK about status, it is about training, it is about recognising overridingly that this clinical interface is a major concern. Unless we begin to face this and Dr. Smit Sibinga and I tried to face this about 6 years ago and when you look back what has happened the answer is nothing. There are some big, big issues here that are almost as big as Codabar and goodness knows what and they are much trickier because they involve the medical profession.

F. Canal: I think the topic of quality principles and risk management has indeed been addressed but there are a number of topics that have been put on the table that go beyond or are implicit in the topic. They just are the patient and the importance of processes and the importance of technologies and what we can do together. I would like to thank again for the question around the industry I think it is very important really that we in the future together. There have to be forms to be able to discuss relevant things so we understand where to put our efforts.

VI. TRANSFUSION MEDICINE AT THE BEDSIDE

THE EPIDEMIOLOGY OF BLOOD COMPONENT TRANSFUSION IN SOUTH EASTERN SCOTLAND, 1990 TO 1997

D.B.L. McClelland[1]

Introduction

In October 1997, when the first cases of New Variant CJD were acknowledged, the then UK Chief Medical Officer, Professor Kenneth Calman, sought to reassure patients and the public with a statement that included the line: "Blood products are only given to patients who have a serious and in many cases very urgent need for them ..." [1].

To support this statement, one ideally needs to be able to:

- Quantitate the current use of blood,
- Describe how it is distributed on a population basis,
- Identify the groups of patients for whom it is most important to target blood safety efforts
- Identify for particular case groups best practice [or practice that may need improvement],
- Monitor the effects of interventions intended to change practice.

Numerators

The blood supply service generally has information about units of blood supplied to hospitals and their subunits. The hospital blood bank should record the identities and basic demographic data of the patients for which each unit is dispatched. It may have a positive record of transfusion to the patient, or it may infer that blood that is issued to a patient and not returned has been transfused.

The individual elements of this information can be useful for identifying secular changes in blood use within an area or an institution, but have limited value in identifying prime targets for practice improvement interventions. However, if the information about blood distribution is linked with simple data on the recipients and placed in the context of a relevant population based denominator, it can help to identify priorities for transfusion safety interventions.

Furthermore, if clinically relevant case groups can be defined so as to permit comparison of like with like being treated in different institutions or by different clinicians, important variations in practice can be revealed as a starting point for studies on outcome, clinical trials or quality improvement initiatives.[2-4] In the

1. Edinburgh and South East Scotland Blood Transfusion Service, Edinburgh, Scotland.

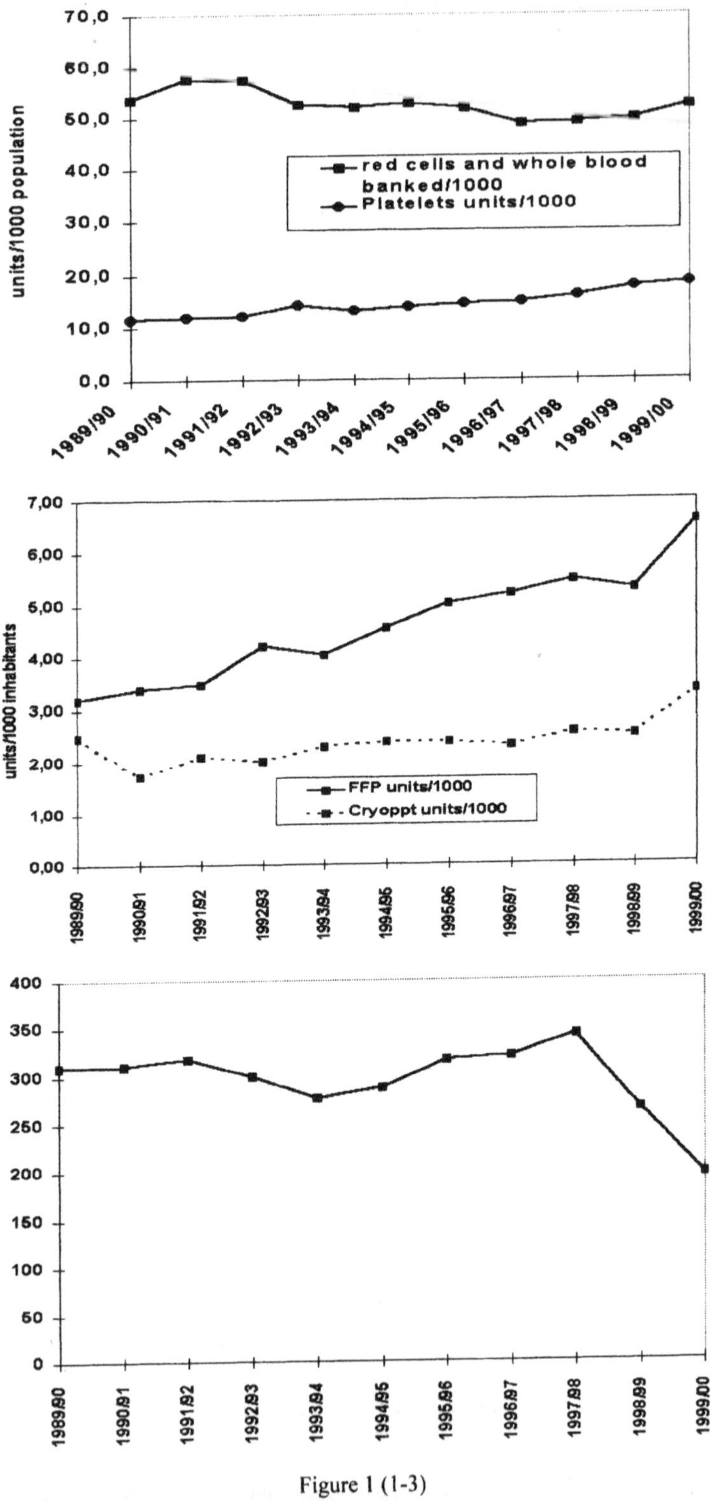
70,0
60,0
50,0
40,0
30,0
20,0
10,0
0,0
units/1000 population
red cells and whole blood banked/1000
Platelets units/1000
1989/90
1990/91
1991/92
1992/93
1993/94
1994/95
1995/96
1996/97
1997/98
1998/99
1999/00
7,00
6,00
5,00
4,00
3,00
2,00
1,00
0,00
units/1000 inhabitants
FFP units/1000
Cryoppt units/1000
400
350
300
250
200
150
100
50
0

Figure 1 (1-3)

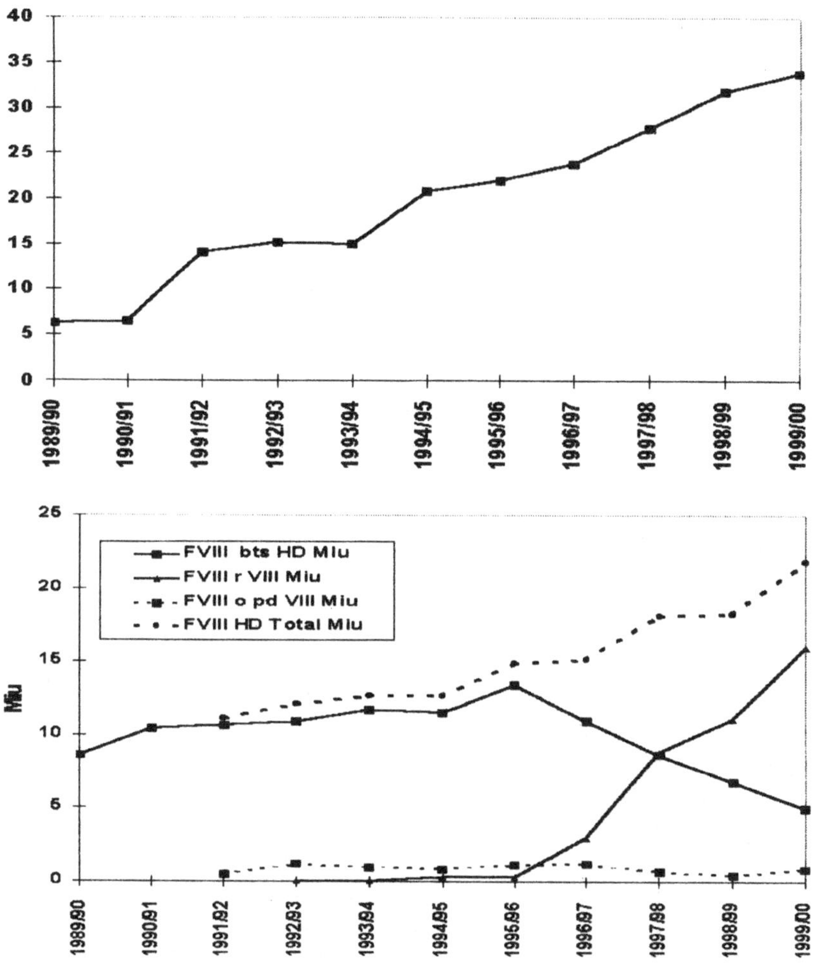

Figure 1 (4-5).

following pages, some examples are shown to illustrate some applications of these different types of data.

Denominators

Blood product use for a whole population

Figure 1 illustrates the 10-year trends in the use of the main blood components and plasma derivatives per million population for Scotland [population 5 million] This shows the contrast between the rather stable use of red cells and the rising use of platelets and plasma and the equally striking contrast between the falling use of albumin and factor VIII and the relentless rise in use of IgG. However, these data in isolation give us no information on the key questions in Table 1.

Table 1. We need to know ...

1.	How much blood is used where, by who, for who and why
2.	Which categories of patient would derive most benefit from an improvement in blood use safety
3.	Do desirable changes in practice occur in response to interventions intended to change clinicians' behaviour

Table 2.

(a) Blood component use per patient transfused:	48,000
Number of patients transfused	5,930
Number of units of blood components transfused whole blood, platelets, plasma and cryoprecipitate	
Average blood component units per patient	8.1
(b) Blood component use per acute hospital episode	
Hospital inpatient episodes/million patients/year	200,000
Patients transfused/year	10,000

Blood component use per patient who is transfused

This figure is an average of all the blood components transfused to all patients transfused during a period – typically a year. An example from the Edinburgh region is given in Table 2.

Although blood use data is often reported as average blood use per patient, the use of a simple average obscures extremely important features and may give a very misleading picture of the use of blood components.

Figure 2 shows, for the Edinburgh region, the distribution, among all red cell recipients, of the number of units received. This emphasises the frequency of the 2-unit transfusion, and reveals a 'tail' of patients who receive more than 10 units.

Figure 3 however shows that the small number of intensively transfused patients account for a high proportion of all blood components transfused. This data, from a large general haematology unit reveals that a mere 5% of the patients account for 63% of all the episodes of transfusion, while 50% of the patients account for only 0.4% of the transfusion episodes.

Blood component use according to patients' age and gender

It might be expected that the population of individuals who are transfused would contain an excess of the elderly. Figure 4 shows the age and gender distribution in a population of red cell recipients, expressed as the number of red cell recipients per thousand in each age band of the population. This illustrates clearly the steeply increasing incidence of transfusion above the age of 50 years, and also highlights subgroups in the younger age bands where incidence of transfusion appears to be high.

Such broad measurements of blood use in a whole population may be useful for purposes such as:

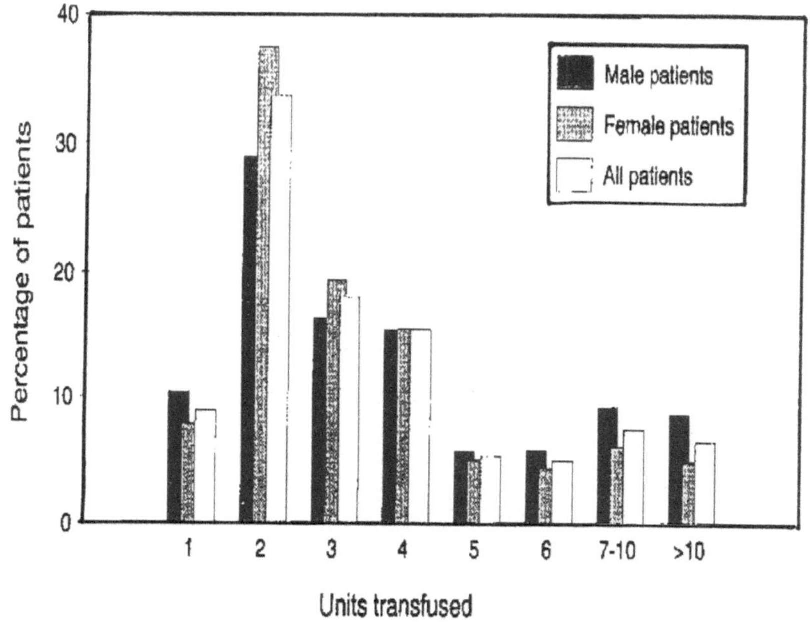

Figure 2. Percentage of transfused patients receiving the specified number of units.

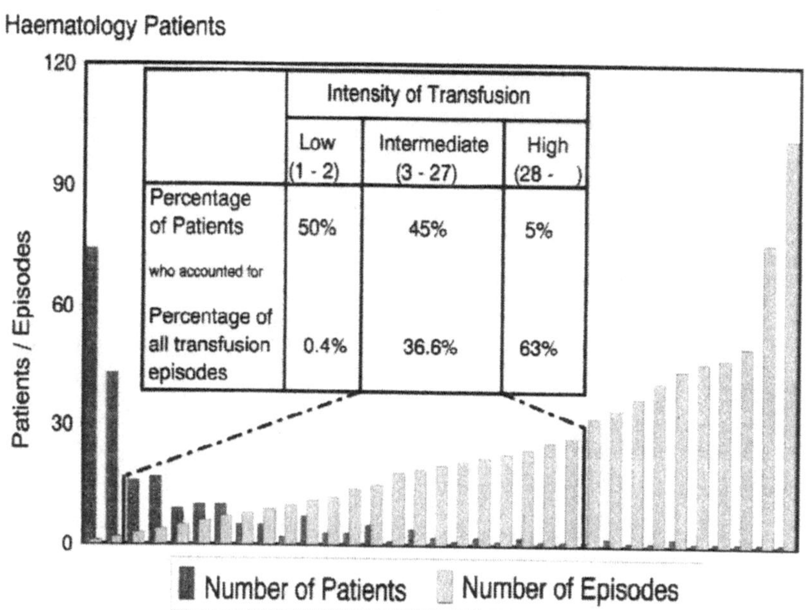

Figure 3.

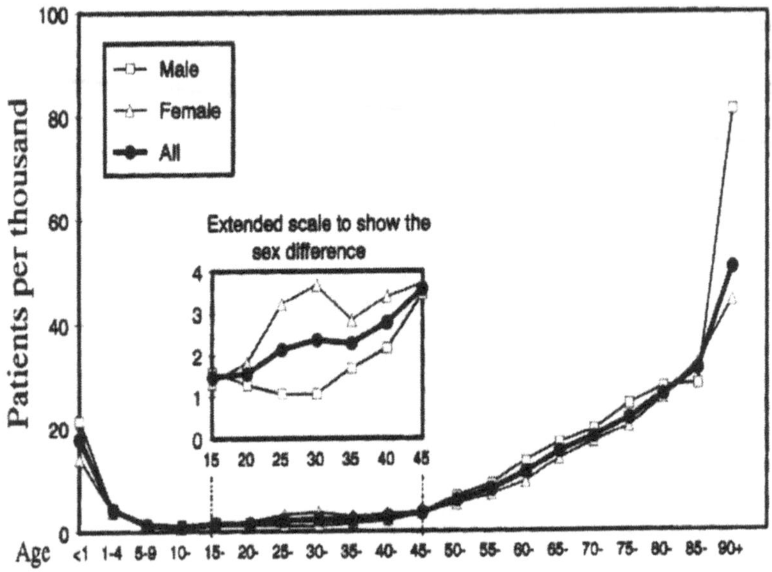

Figure 4. Transfused patients per thousands population in 5 year age bands. South East Regio.

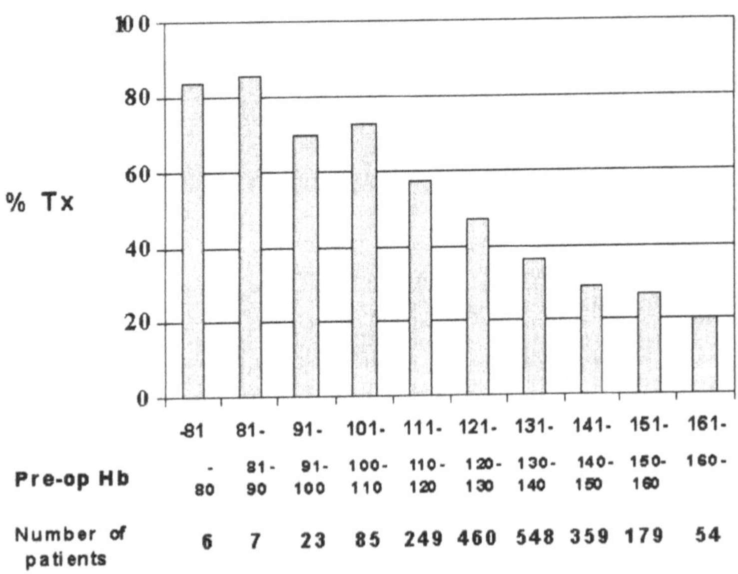

Figure 5. Preoperative hemoglobin vs probability of red cell transfusion.

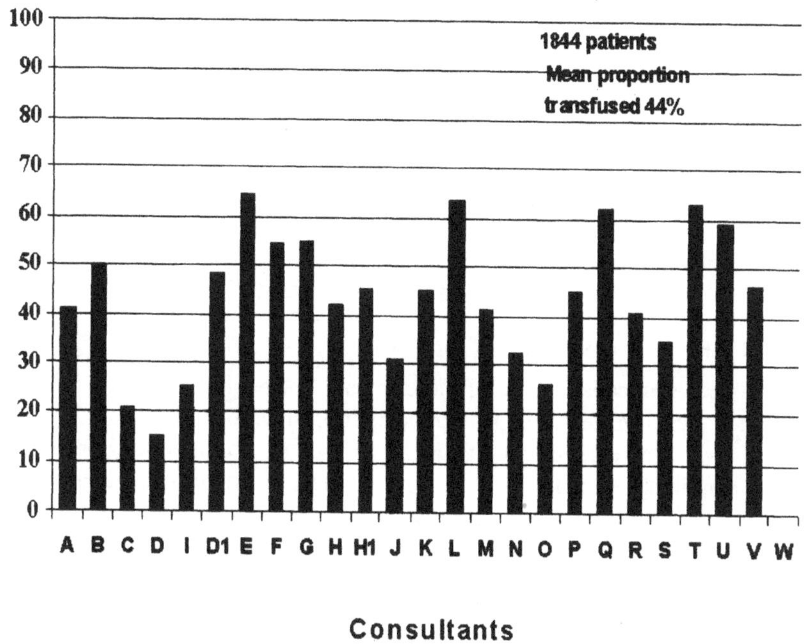

Figure 6. Operator vs probability of transfusion.

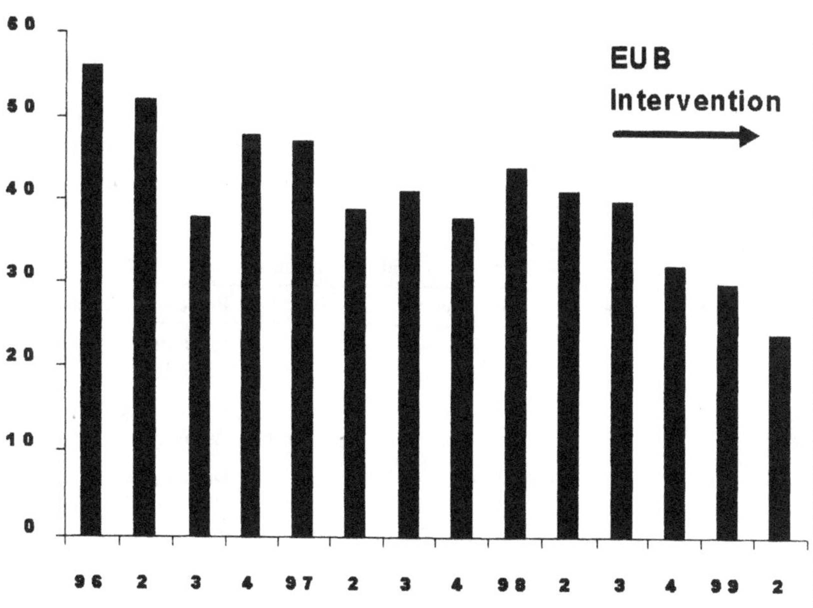

Figure 7. Progressively falling red cell use within a defined clinical category.

- Planning to meet future demand;
- Predicting the likely public health impact of a blood safety intervention such as HTLV-I screening, or measures to reduce any risk of vCJD transmission;
- Interpreting crude data linking transfusion to longevity [5].

However, it has little value as a tool for identifying differences in clinical practice, informing clinical discussion about changing practice or monitoring the effect of interventions intended to change clinical behaviour. For these purposes, some form of clinical categorisation is needed, unless some existing framework, such as Diagnosis Related Groups is thought to be suitable [6].

Blood component use *by clinical category*

Table 3 summarises some of the elements that might be used to construct subcategories of patients that may provide data useful to the clinician. To illustrate how a simple set of classifiers can be used to inform clinical practice, a relatively simple example is taken. That of elective orthopaedic surgery. The patient study group was constructed as shown in table 3b.

By collecting this simple data set routinely on all patients in several hospitals, it is possible to identify, in the local setting, factors that increase a patient's risk of being transfused; Figures 4 and 5 illustrate factors that may be amenable

Table 3a. Example of a patient classification for studying blood use.

Demographic classifiers	Clinical classifiers	Process of care classifiers
Age	Primary diagnosis	Institution
Gender	Main intervention	Operator e.g. surgeon or anaesthesist
Socio-economic status	Severity Apache score, ASH score etc	Discharge arrangements after episode
	Nutritional status	
	Haemoglobin	

Table 3b. Definition of a patient group for study of transfusion.

Demographic classifiers	Clinical classifiers	Process of care classifiers
Age Recorded	Primary diagnosis Osteoarthritis	Institution Recorded
Gender Recorded	Main intervention Primary unilateral hip arthropalsty	Operator e.g. surgeon Recorded
Socio-economic status Not used	Severity Not used Apache score, ASH score, etc.	Discharge arrangements after episode Not used
	Nutritional status Not used	
	Preoperative haemoglobin level Recorded	

to change and improvement if the information can be used effectively to catalyse a sustained quality improvement effort by each team, as shown by a sustained progressive reduction in blood use.

Conclusion

Simple epidemiological data can provide one important basis for a rational and defensible approach to managing patients at risk of transfusion by, for example.

Predicting the impact on the needs for transfusion of:

- Demographic change;
- Change in disease patterns;
- Changes in medical technology.

Assessing the impact of alternative interventions to improve transfusion safety. Demonstrating the extent to which transfusion practice consistent with local and national norms of good practice.

References

1. United Kingdom Department of Health Press Statement October 6, 1997.
2. The SANGUIS Study Group. Use of blood products for elective surgery in 43 European hospitals. Transfusion Medicine 1994;4:351-68.
3. Capraro L. Transfusion prcatices in primary total hip replacements in Finland. Vox Sang 1998;75:1-6.
4. Kytola L, Nuutinen G, Myllyla G. Transfusion policies in coronary artery bypass – a nationwide survey in Finland. Acta Anaesthesiol Scand 1998;42:178-83.
5. Whyte GS. The transfusion population of Canterbury, New Zealand and its mortality. Vox Sang 1988;54:65-70.
6. Whyte GS, Brook CW. Suitability of casemix classifications for output funding of blood services in Victoria. Med J Australia 1998;169:415-18.

CONTRIBUTIONS OF META-ANALYSIS TO TRANSFUSION MEDICINE

E.C. Vamvakas[1]

Introduction

Meta-analysis is the structured and systematic integration of information from different studies of a given problem. It refers to the disciplined synthesis of previous research findings where the results of multiple reports on the efficacy of an intervention are compared, contrasted, and re-analyzed. When the results are discrepant, the purpose of the meta-analysis is to investigate the reasons for disagreements among the studies. When the results are concordant, the goal of the overview is to derive, through the application of a number of quantitative techniques, a measure of the effect of the intervention across the combined investigations. This measure is referred to as the 'average' or 'summary' effect of the treatment under study [1-5].

The term 'meta-analysis' was coined by Glass [6], and is used synonymously with the term 'statistical overview'. An overview differs from the traditional narrative reviews of the literature in that:

1. All completed investigations that meet specific eligibility criteria are retrieved and included in the analysis;
2. The quality of the retrieved studies is assessed systematically;
3. The degree of agreement among the studies is evaluated, both conceptually and based on statistical criteria, and the synthesis of the findings proceeds only if the variation in reported results is sufficiently modest to be attributed to chance; and

Providing that this prerequisite is met, quantitative methods are used to calculate the "average" effect of the intervention across the available studies, and to test that effect for statistical significance [1-5] (Table 1).

If a meta-analysis is conducted in accordance with these guidelines [7-9], it can provide the reader with "an objective view of the research literature, unaffected by the sometimes distorting lens of individual experience and personal preference that can affect a less structured review" [10]. According to Goodman, meta-analysis is possibly the most important health policy research method that has been developed in the past two decades [11]. So far, however, meta-analysis

1. Department of Pathology, New York University School of Medicine, Blood Bank, New York, NY, USA.

Table 1. Sequence of steps to be followed in conducting a meta-analysis.

1.	Retrieval of all completed studies on the effect of the intervention of interest
2.	Determination of the eligibility of the retrieved studies for inclusion in the analysis, based on criteria specified in advance and relating to: – the scope of the hypothesis under study, and – the quality of the retrieved studies
3.	Extraction of data from each study on the effect of the intervention of interest
4.	Assessment of the degree of concordance among the studies (both conceptually and using statistical criteria
5.	If the studies are concordant, calculation of a 'summary' or 'average' estimate of the effect of the intervention across the combined investigations
6.	If the studies are discordant, examination of the reasons for disagreement among the studies

has been used only to a limited extent in the field of transfusion medicine. Randomized controlled trials (RCTs) of the efficacy of white cell (WBC) reduction in preventing human leukocyte antigen (HLA)-alloimmunization and refractoriness to platelet transfusions [12-18] were meta-analyzed by Heddle [19], Andreu and Dewailly [20] and Vamvakas [21]. Other areas addressed have included observational studies of the association of perioperative allogeneic blood transfusion with cancer recurrence [22-26]; RCTs [27-35] of the effect of allogeneic blood transfusion on the incidence of cancer recurrence or postoperative infection [36-38]; RCTs of the effect of paternal WBC immunization in preventing recurrent miscarriage [39-42]; observational studies of the effect of allogeneic blood transfusion on the likelihood of recurrence of Crohn's disease [43]; and studies of the efficacy of therapeutic [44] or prophylactic [45] granulocyte transfusions in adult and neonatal sepsis; and of therapeutic plasma exchange in chronic progressive multiple sclerosis [46].

Moreover, a Canadian team meta-analyzed the studies of the efficacy of intraoperative autotransfusion [47], acute normovolemic hemodilution [48], preoperative autologous blood donation [49], platelet-rich plasmapheresis [50], or erythropoietin [51], in reducing perioperative exposure to allogeneic red cell (RBC) transfusions. Finally, meta-analyses conducted in related fields, such as the overview of studies of the sensitivity and specificity of tests of human immunodeficiency virus (HIV) seropositivity [52], the meta-analyses of the efficacy of erythropoietin in myelodysplastic syndromes [53] or in HIV/zidovudine-related anemia [54], the overviews of the efficacy of interferon-alpha for chronic hepatitis C [55], and of the relative efficacy of bone marrow transplantation versus chemotherapy in acute myelogenous leukemia [56], or the meta-analysis of studies of the efficacy of desmopressin, tranexamic acid, epsilon-aminocaproic acid, or aprotinin in reducing perioperative blood transfusion in cardiac surgery [57], are also of interest to transfusion medicine professionals.

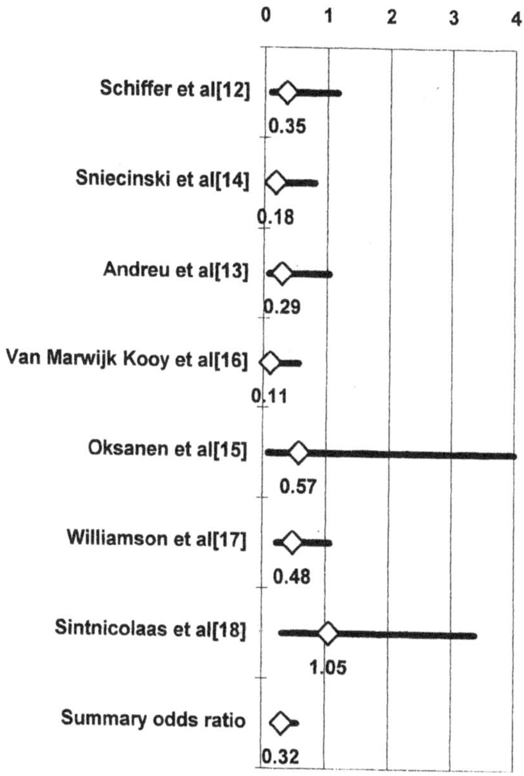

Figure 1. Odds ratio (OR) of HLA-alloimmunization in recipients of WBC-reduced cellular blood components versus controls, as reported in randomized controlled trials (RCTs) of the efficacy of WBC reduction in preventing HLA-alloimmunization published through 1995 [12-18]. Each OR is surrounded by its 95% Confidence Interval (CI). If the CI does not include the null value (1), the calculated OR is statistically significant ($p<0.05$). The figure also shows the summary OR of HLA-alloimmunization in the treatment (as compared with the control) group across the 7 RCTs, as calculated by Vamvakas [21]. Because the hypothesis of homogeneity of effects was rejected across the 7 studies [21] ($p=0.025$ for the Q test statistic), the summary OR is plotted here solely for the purpose of illustration. A legitimate integration of the findings of the 7 studies [12-18] was possible only after the heterogeneity of effects across the studies was explained (Figures 6 and 7 – see text) [21].

Uses of Meta-Analysis

Meta-analysis has three generally accepted applications and one controversial use. It can serve to integrate the findings of studies which report treatment effects operating in the same direction, but varying substantially in size between the reports. The purpose of the synthesis is to provide a more precise estimate of the most likely magnitude of the treatment effect, so that a definitive RCT can be designed, enrolling as many patients as are needed for establishing the existence of this effect [58].

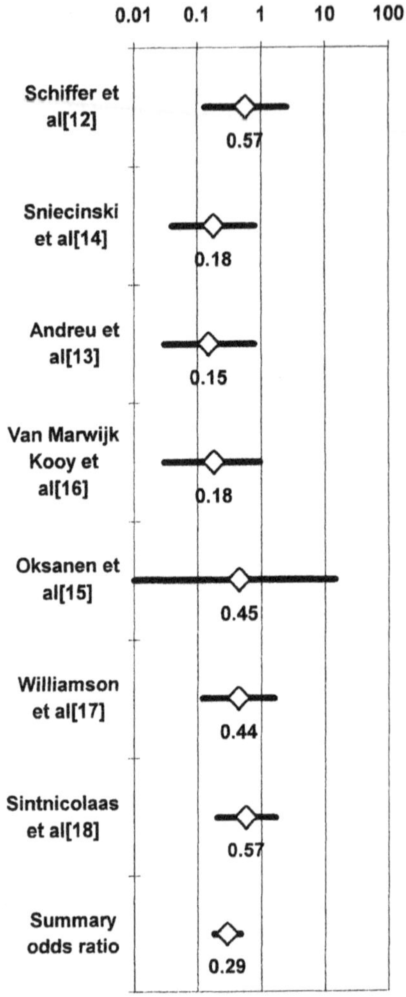

Figure 2. Odds ratio (OR) of refractoriness to random-donor platelet transfusions in recipients of WBC-reduced cellular blood components versus controls, as reported in randomized controlled trials (RCTs) of the efficacy of WBC reduction in preventing platelet refractoriness published through 1995 [12-18]. The data are plotted on a logarithmic scale, and each OR is surrounded by its 95% Confidence Interval (CI). If the CI does not include the null value (1), the calculated OR is statistically significant ($p<0.05$). The figure also shows the summary OR of platelet refractoriness in the treatment (as compared with the control) group across the 7 RCTs, as calculated by Vamvakas [21]. There was a greater than 10% probability that the variation in the reported results [12-18] could have arisen by chance ($p>0.10$ for the Q test statistic), and it was thus appropriate to combine the findings of the studies [12-18] by the techniques of meta-analysis [21].

For example, by the end of 1995, only two [10,12] of seven [12,18] published RCTs had produced a statistically significant ($p<0.05$) finding indicating that WBC reduction could decrease the occurrence of HLA-alloimmunization in patients needing multiple platelet transfusions; three studies [13, 14, 16] had

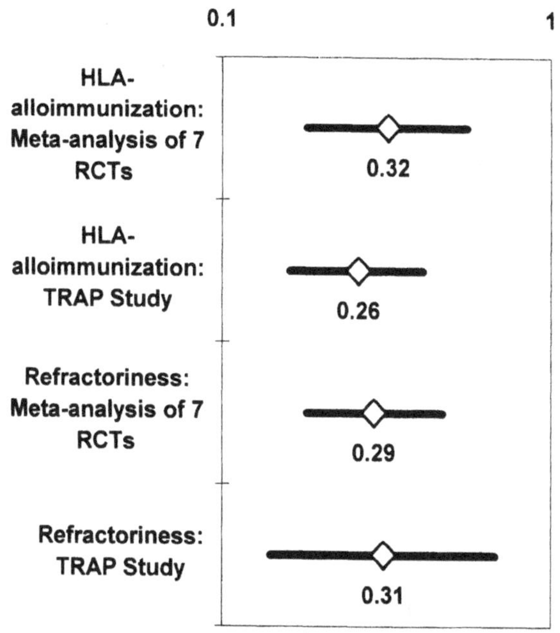

Figure 3. Comparison of the results of the meta-analysis [21] of the 7 randomized controlled trials of WBC reduction in preventing HLA-alloimmunization and platelet refractoriness available through 1995 [12-18], with the results of the definitive Trial to Reduce Alloimmunization to Platelets (TRAP Study) [59]. For the meta-analysis [21], the figure shows the summary odds ratio (OR) of HLA-alloimmunization or platelet refractoriness, surrounded by its 95% Confidence Interval (CI). For the TRAP Study [59], the figure shows the OR of HLA-alloimmunization or platelet refractoriness, also surrounded by its 95% CI. The data are plotted on a logarithmic scale. All summary ORs or ORs shown in this figure are statistically significant ($p<0.05$).

shown that WBC reduction could prevent the development of refractoriness to random-donor platelet transfusions. All but one [18] of the trials had shown a sizable trend toward efficacy, but the use of WBC reduction in preventing HLA-alloimmunization and platelet refractoriness was considered unproven. A large, multicenter RCT – the Trial to Reduce Alloimmunization to Platelets (TRAP Study) – was thus undertaken in the U.S. to determine definitively whether the use of WBC-reduced platelets could prevent the development of anti-HLA antibodies and/or refractoriness to random-donor platelet transfusions [59].

To calculate the sample size needed for the TRAP Study [59], investigators had to know the most likely magnitude of the effect of WBC reduction on the risk of HLA-alloimmunization and refractoriness [58]. As shown in Figure 1, the summary odds ratio (OR) of HLA-alloimmunization in patients receiving

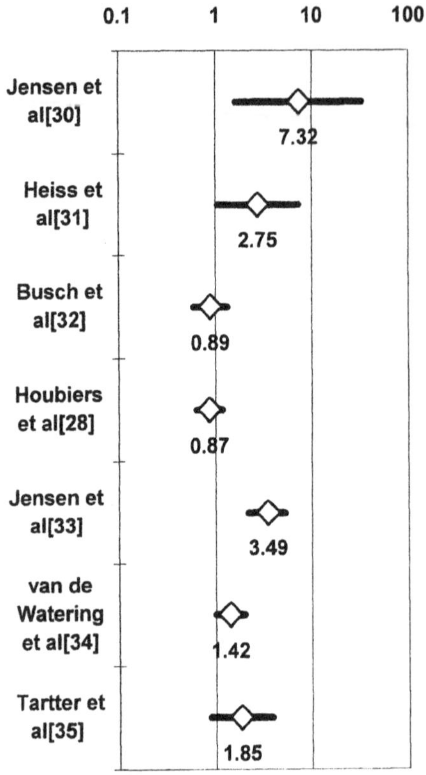

Figure 4. Odds ratio (OR) of postoperative bacterial infection in recipients of buffy-coat-reduced or standard allogeneic RBCs or whole blood, versus recipients of WBC-reduced or autologous RBCs or whole blood, as reported in randomized controlled trials investigating the immunomodulatory (TRIM) effect of allogeneic blood transfusion [29-35]. The data are plotted on a logarithmic scale, and each OR is surrounded by its 95% Confidence Interval (CI). If the CI does not include the null value (1), the calculated OR is statistically significant ($p<0.05$).

WBC-reduced (as compared to non-WBC-reduced) cellular blood components was 0.32 across the 7 RCTs published through 1995 [12-18]. Similarly, the summary OR of platelet refractoriness was 0.29 across the same 7 investigations [12-18]. The findings of the meta-analysis of the studies available through 1995[21] thus indicated a 68% decrease in the risk of HLA-alloimmunization (Figure 1), and a 71% decrease in the risk of platelet refractoriness (Figure 2), attributable to WBC reduction of the transfused cellular blood components. These estimates of the size of the treatment effect [21] could be used to calculate the sample size needed for the TRAP Study [59].

The treatment effect calculated when the TRAP Study [59] was completed was virtually of the same magnitude as the effect calculated by the meta-analysis of the 7 RCTs available through 1995 [21]. The definitive TRAP Study [59] demonstrated a reduction in the risk of alloimmunization by approximately 74% [OR=0.26; 95% Confidence Interval (CI), 0.16-0.41], and a reduction in the risk of refractoriness by approximately 69% (OR=0.31, 95% CI, 0.14-0.68)

(Figure 3). In this RCT [59], 400 patients were used to compare the incidence of HLA-alloimmunization and platelet refractoriness in recipients of WBC-reduced (versus non-WBC-reduced) cellular blood components. This number of subjects was approximately equal to the total number of patients enrolled in the 7 RCTs published between 1983 and 1995 (n=418) [12-18].

Alternatively, meta-analysis can be used to investigate reasons for disagreements among studies which report treatment effects operating in opposite directions or differing markedly in size when they all point in the same direction. The aim of the analysis is to explain discrepancies among published results, based on relevant characteristics of the patients who were included in the available studies, or the treatments that were administered, or differences in the quality of study design and analysis.

Figure 4 shows the 7 RCTs [29-35] investigating the association of perioperative allogeneic blood transfusion with postoperative bacterial infection, which is attributed to a purported immunomodulatory (TRIM) effect of allogeneic blood transfusion. According to these studies [29-35], the allogeneic blood transfusion effect varied from a 7.3-fold increase ($p<0.001$) [30] to a 10% reduction ($p<0.25$) [29,32] in the risk of postoperative infection, in the treatment (allogeneic transfusion) compared with the control group of patients. Subjects in the former group received buffy-coat-reduced or standard allogeneic whole blood or RBCs; patients in the latter group were transfused with autologous [31,32] or WBC-reduced allogeneic whole blood or RBCs.

The intention-to-treat analyses shown in Figure 4 indicate a more than 7-fold variation among the findings of these studies [29-35]. In fact, when the magnitude of the disagreements among the RCTs [29-35] was evaluated by a formal statistical procedure (the Q test statistic), the probability that this degree of variation in reported results could have arisen by chance was smaller than 1 per 10,000 ($p<0.0001$ for the Q test statistic) [1-5]. This magnitude of the disagreements among the 7 RCTs precludes any attempt at integration of these results by the techniques of meta-analysis [1-5]. The findings of available studies can be integrated in an overview only if the variation in reported results is sufficiently modest to be attributed to chance, that is, only if there is a greater than 5% probability that any disagreements among the studies could have arisen by chance. The Q test statistic quantifies the probability that the variation in reported results might have arisen by chance. Usually, meta-analysts consider that there is sufficient agreement among the available studies to permit the undertaking of a meta-analysis if $p>0.05$ for the Q test statistic. Others choose a more stringent threshold (e.g., $p>0.10$, or even $p>0.20$) for the results of the Q test statistic.

The RCTs investigating the association of allogeneic transfusion with postoperative infection differed in the surgical setting where each trial was conducted (i.e., gastrointestinal [29-33,35] versus open-heart [34] surgery), the homogeneity of the enrolled patient population (i.e., patients undergoing elective surgery for any gastrointestinal disease [35] or any disease of the colorectum [30,33] versus patients undergoing elective colorectal cancer resection [29,31,32]), the RBC product transfused to the treatment or the control group, the proportion of transfused patients (which ranged from 26.7% [35] to 94.8%

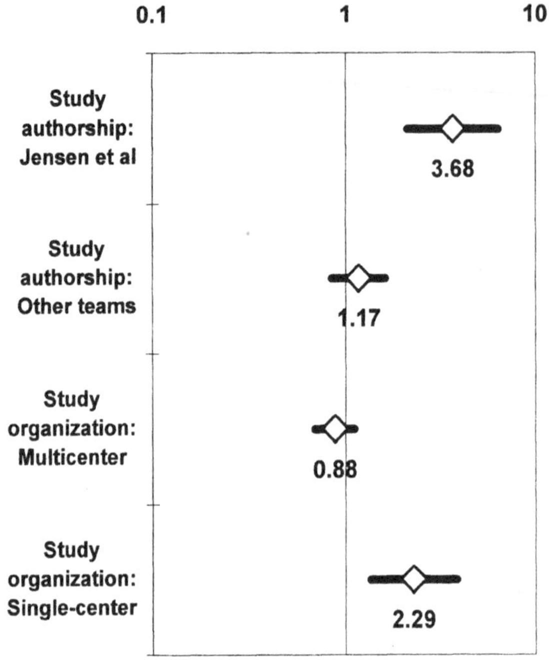

Figure 5. Possible sources of variation in the findings of the 7 randomized controlled trials [29-35] investigating the association between perioperative allogeneic blood transfusion and postoperative bacterial infection [60]. The available RCTs are stratified by study authorship (i.e., conducted by Jensen et al. [30,33] or by other teams of investigators), or by study organization (i.e., multicenter [29,32] versus single-center RCTs), and findings of studies that are homogeneous in terms of study authorship or organization are integrated by the techniques of meta-analysis. For each meta-analysis, the figure shows the summary odds ratio (OR) of postoperative bacterial infection in the treatment (allogeneic transfusion) compared with the control group of patients. The data are plotted on a logarithmic scale, and each summary OR is surrounded by its 95% Confidence Interval (CI). If the CI does not include the null value (1), the calculated summary OR is statistically significant ($p<0.05$).

[34]), and the proportion of patients who developed postoperative infection according to the criteria used by the investigators (8.1% [30] to 33.4% [29]).

McAlister et al. [37] observed that, for the most part, the disagreements among the 7 RCTs [29-35] were due to the results reported in two articles [30, 33]. McAlister et al. [37] observed that, for the most part, the disagreements among the 7 RCTs [29-35] were due to the results reported in two articles [30, 33] published published by the same team of investigators. This team found an implausibly large allogeneic blood transfusion effect, because they observed an extremely low postoperative infection rate among patients who received WBC-reduced RBCs. In their 1996 study [33], Jensen et al detected 0 post-operative wound infections and intra-abdominal abscesses among 118 patients sick enough to need perioperative transfusion with WBC-reduced RBCs. If this finding were not due to the effect(s) of bias and confounding, it would implicate the TRIM effect as the sole cause of postoperative wound infections, because the incidence of postoperative wound infections and intra-abdominal abscesses among the 142 patients who were transfused with buffy-coat-reduced RBCs in that trial [33] was 12%.

Accordingly, McAlister et al. [37] combined the findings of the available RCTs [29-33] before and after excluding the two RCTs of Jensen et al. [30,33] from the analysis. Vamvakas et al. [38] subsequently updated the results of McAlister et al. [37], by including in the analysis the recent RCTs by van de Watering et al. [34] and by Tartter et al. [35]. If the two RCTs of Jensen et al. [30,33] are excluded, the disagreements among the remaining 5 studies [29,31, 32,34,35] are sufficiently modest to be attributed to chance ($p>0.05$ for the Q test statistic). The summary OR of postoperative infection in the treatment (compared with the control) group across the 5 studies [29,31,32,34,35] is 1.17 (95% CI, 0.84-1.62; $p>>0.05$) [38]. The 2 RCTs of Jensen et al. [30,33] are highly homogeneous ($p=0.50$ for the Q-test statistic), and – if the findings of these 2 studies are integrated – the summary OR is 3.68 (95% CI, 2.11-6.43; $p<0.001$) [38].

However, it is also possible to explain the disagreements among the 7 RCTs [29-35] by excluding the 2 multicenter studies[29,32] from the analysis. When the 5 single-center RCTs [30,31,33-35] are integrated, the disagreements among the studies are sufficiently modest to be attributed to chance ($p>0.05$ for the Q test statistic), and the summary OR across the 5 studies is 2.29 (95% CI, 1.35-3.87; $p<0.05$) [38]. The 2 multicenter RCTs [29,32] are highly homogeneous ($p=0.95$ for the Q test statistic), and – if the findings of these 2 studies are integrated – the summary OR is 0.88 (95% CI, 0.69-1.12; $p>>0.05$) [38].

Either approach explains the initial heterogeneity among the 7 studies [29-35] equally well. The former analysis attributes the disagreements among the 7 RCTs to the possible effects of bias and residual, uncontrolled confounding factors in the 2 studies of Jensen et al. [36]. The latter approach ascribes the noted discrepancies to the reduced statistical power of multicenter (compared with single-center) RCTs [60]. Figure 5 summarizes the data on these two possible sources of variation in the findings of the 7 RCTs investigating the association between perioperative allogeneic blood transfusion and postoperative bacterial infection [60].

Establishing the Existence of a Treatment effect

The third, and controversial, application of meta-analysis is to integrate the findings of studies which report a treatment effect operating in the same direction, but not attaining statistical significance in any study, presumably due to the small sample size and inadequate statistical power of each report [61]. The purpose of the synthesis is to establish the existence of a treatment effect, by means of a combination of patient populations enrolled in separate studies. This use of

Table 2. Puplished randomized controlled trials of the efficacy of WBC reduction in preventing HLA-alloimmunization and refractoriness to random-donor platelet transfusion have differed.*

1. Patient polupation enrolled (acute myeloid leukemia versus acute leukemia versus hematologic malignancy and aplastic anemia)
2. Treatment protocol for undelying disease
3. Efficacy of method for WBC reduction used in the treatment arm of the study
4. Laboratory versus bedside WBC reduction and quality control of the process of WBC reduction/prestorage versus poststorage WBC reduction
5. WBC content of blood components administered to the control arm of the study
6. Number of platelet and RBC transfusions given to each arm of the study
7. Freshness of the RBC and platelet components transfused to each arm of the study
8. Definition of platelet alloimmunization
9. Sensitivity of method used to detect anti-HLA antibodies
10. Definition of platelet refractoriness
11. Length of follow-up for the detection of anti-HLA antibodies
12. Proportion of enrolled patients with previous exposure to HLA antigens
13. Statistical/methodologic limitations in the design and analysis of the reports

*Modified from Transf Med Rev 1998;12:261.

meta-analysis makes overviews appear as a possible alternative to RCTs. However, a meta-analysis is observational and retrospective even when the combined studies are experimental. As an observational study, a meta-analysis is subject to all sources of bias which afflict traditional observational investigations. Therefore, a treatment effect, associated with a particular treatment by a meta-analysis, may be either due to the treatment itself, or due to some undetected error or uncontrolled factor that escaped the analysts. Because it is an observational study, a meta-analysis cannot be undertaken to resolve a hypothesis. A hypothesis formulated by a meta-analysis may – or may not – be corroborated when a definitive RCT is eventually conducted.

Overviews should thus be considered a supplement (as opposed to an alternative) to RCTs. Even if a definitive RCT for establishing the efficacy of a therapeutic intervention is – eventually – conducted, its findings may not necessarily apply to all patients. Trialists use highly restrictive inclusion/exclusion criteria for patient enrollment, because they strive to include a patient population as homogeneous as possible, to make it easier to detect a treatment effect untainted by confounding factors. The results of an RCT may thus not apply to patients who do not meet the eligibility criteria of that trial [62,63]. RCTs constitute the gold standard for evaluating the efficacy of therapeutic interventions, but need to be supplemented by meta-analyses in order to broaden the applicability of the findings. A meta-analysis integrates the findings of separate studies, which usually differ in many aspects of their design. This variation in the design attributes of reports included in a meta-analysis results in greater generalizability of the findings of a statistical overview, as compared to the results of an RCT–because – by combing studies with disparate design characteristics – a

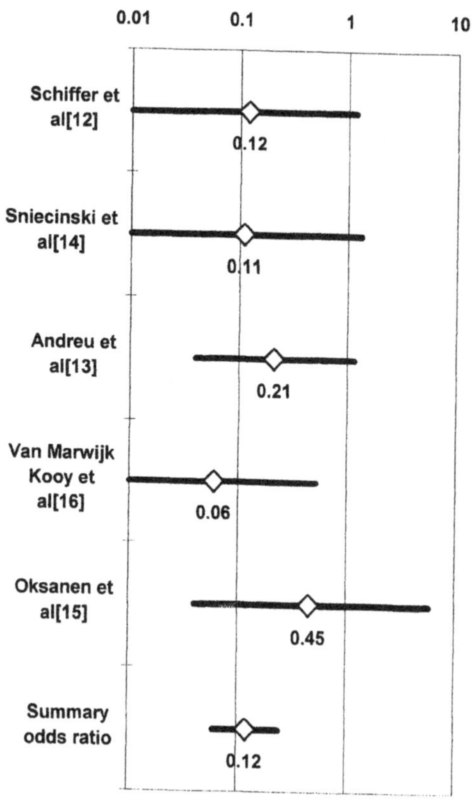

Figure 6. Efficacy of WBC reduction in preventing primary HLA-alloimmunization: subset of patients without history of pregnancy or transfusion enrolled in 5 RCTs [12-16] published between 1983 and 1995. For each RCT, the figure shows the odds ratio (OR) of primary HLA-alloimmunization in recipients of WBC-reduced blood components versus controls. The data are plotted on a logarithmic scale, and each OR is surrounded by its 95% Confidence Interval (CI). If the CI does not include the null value (1), the calculated OR is statistically significant ($p<0.05$). The figure also shows the summary OR of primary HLA-alloimmunization in the treatment (as compared with the control) group across the 5 RCTs, as calculated by Vamvakas [21].

meta-analysis permits examination of the effect of an intervention in many different situations. If the treatment effect is consistent in all studies, this consistency favors a true treatment effect, rather than one due to chance, or some systematic error or uncontrolled factor that may have compromised the results of all completed investigations.

For example, Table 2 shows the variation in the design attributes of the 7 RCTs investigating the efficacy of WBC reduction in reducing the risk of HLA-alloimmunization and platelet refractoriness [12-18]. The 7 RCTs encompassed a great variety of clinical situations (Table 2), and the clinical heterogeneity of the RCTs published between 1983 and 1995 [12-18] resulted in statistical heterogeneity ($p=0.025$ for the Q test statistic). The heterogeneity among studies was explained, however, when the efficacy of WBC reduction in preventing primary, or secondary, HLA-alloimmunization was considered separately [21].

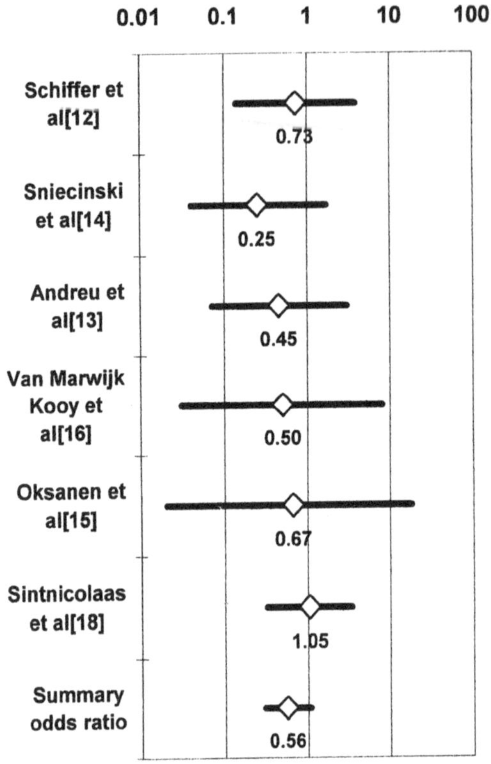

Figure 7 Efficacy of WBC reduction in preventing secondary HLA-alloimmunization: subset of patients with history of pregnancy or transfusion enrolled in 6 RCTs [12-16,18] published between 1983 and 1995. For each RCT, the figure shows the odds ratio (OR) of secondary HLA-alloimmunization in recipients of WBC-reduced blood components versus controls. The data are plotted on a logarithmic scale, and each OR is surrounded by its 95% Confidence Interval (CI). If the CI does not include the null value (1), the calculated OR is statistically significant ($p<0.05$). The figure also shows the summary OR of secondary HLA-alloimmunization in the treatment (as compared with the control) group across the 6 RCTs, as calculated by Vamvakas [21].

Figure 6 shows the findings from 5 RCTs [12-16] for the subset of the enrolled patients who had not been 'presensitized' to HLA antigens before their enrollment in those studies. These patients could be expected to develop a primary immune response to HLA antigens that are present in transfused blood components. A trend toward a benefit from WBC reduction is evident in all of these studies [12-16], but the trend attains statistical significance in only one investigation [16]. When the analysis is limited to patients without prior exposure to HLA antigens, the disagreements among the studies are sufficiently modest to be attributed to chance ($p=0.25$ for the Q test statistic) [21]. Therefore, it is legitimate to combine the results of these studies, and – when the findings of the 5 RCTs [12-16] are integrated – the summary OR of HLA-alloimmunizationin

This finding is in agreement with the result of the TRAP Study 59], and is much more generalizable than the result of that large, multicenter trial [59]. The

TRAP Study used highly restrictive inclusion/exclusion criteria for patient enrollment, a strict working protocol, and specific definitions of HLA-alloimmunization and platelet refractoriness; on the contrary, these 5 studies [12-16] covered a wide gamut of possible clinical situations in patients with hematologic malignancies. Therefore, one can conclude, based on the results of this meta-analysis [21], that WBC reduction is effective in preventing primary HLA-alloimmunization, and that this finding is robust across studies varying with respect to many of the design attributes listed in Table 2.

Figure 7 shows the results from 6 RCTs [12-16,18] for the subset of enrolled patients who had been presensitized to HLA antigens before their enrollment in those studies. No benefit is evident from the use of WBC-reduced blood products in any of the studies. The agreement among these trials is reflected in a $p=0.75$ for the Q test statistic: the noted variation in the reported results could have arisen by chance 75% of the time [21]. When the findings of the 6 RCTs [12-16,18] are integrated, the summary OR of HLA-alloimmunization in 140 patients with history of pregnancy or transfusion is 0.56 (95% CI, 0.30-1.07. $p>0.05$) across the 6 studies (Figure 7).

However, the value of meta-analysis in combining patient populations enrolled in separate studies for the purpose of documenting the existence of a treatment effect has been questioned [64-66]. This recent scrutiny of the value of overviews in the medical literature was in part provoked by three discordant reports [67-69] on the degree of agreement between overviews of small trials and subsequently published large RCTs [70]. Meta-analyses and large trials disagree 10-35% of the time, that is, more often than would be expected by chance [67-69]. Until the reasons for the disagreements are better understood, medical practitioners should not rely on meta-analyses for concluding that the existence of a treatment effect has been established. An overview can be used to demonstrate the generalizability of a treatment effect in many clinical situations that a practitioner can expect to encounter in his/her medical practice. However, the existence of the treatment effect should be established by a double-blind RCT, in accordance with the tenets of evidence-based medicine.

Assessing the Quality of Published Studies

Another application of meta-analysis has been advocated by Jenicek [1], O'Rourke and Detsky 71] and Goodman [10]. According to Jenicek [1], the first phase of a statistical overview should be a "qualitative" meta-analysis, which must precede the "quantitative" phase of the report. An assessment of the quality of all retrieved studies should be made, and studies of unacceptable quality should be excluded from the overview. O'Rourke and Detsky [71] assert that the major contribution of a meta-analysis lies in the attention that it draws to flaws in the design and conduct of previous studies. When all published studies are subjected to a detailed review of the methods – with a focus on the impact of the methods on the validity of the results – inadequacies can be identified and their resolution encouraged. Recognized shortcomings can be avoided in future individual research efforts, so that more valid results are produced. In Goodman's opinion [10], a meta-analysis should "raise research and editorial standards, by calling attention to the strengths and weaknesses of the body of research in an area."

According to this view [1,10,71], the assessment of the quality of the completed studies should be one of the main reasons – if not the primary reason – for conducting a meta-analysis. The assessment of the quality of studies meeting the eligibility criteria for inclusion in an overview was listed as a necessary part of any meta-analysis in the early guidelines for meta-analysis in clinical research [1,2,10,72]. This position was also endorsed by Moher and Olkin [7] in their call for standards for reports of meta-analyses published in the medical literature. Formal instruments for assessing the quality of RCTs have been developed [73-78]. Chalmers et al. [73] developed a detailed list of items to be used for scoring the quality of published RCTs on a scale from 0 to 1. A simple instrument was developed by Jadad et al. [78] for use by all readers of RCTs.

The maximum quality score that can be given to a study [78] based on this instrument is 5. Two points are given to a report for random assignment of subjects to treatment and control groups; 2 points are granted for blinding both investigators and patients; and 1 point is added if the number of patients excluded from the analysis, along with the reasons for all dropouts and withdrawals, are presented in the report of the RCT. With regard to the randomization procedure, 1 point is given if a study is designated as "randomized", but the randomization procedure is not described; 0 point is given if the randomization procedure is described, but is judged to be inappropriate; and 2 points are given if the randomization procedure is described, and is appropriate. One, 0, or 2 points are given, in a similar manner, for the technique used to blind investigators and patients.

Moher et al. [79] used the instrument of Jadad et al. [78] to measure the quality of 127 RCTs from the medical literature. Few RCTs had reported either the method used to generate the randomization sequence (15%), or the method used to conceal this sequence until the point of randomization occurred (14%). RCTs that had not adequately described the measures taken to conceal the treatment allocations exaggerated the effect of the intervention under study by 37% ($p<0.01$), compared to RCTs that had adequately reported the method(s) used for concealment. Furthermore, RCTs receiving a low total quality score exaggerated the estimate of the effect of the intervention by 34%, compared with high-quality trials ($p<0.001$). Moher et al. [79] concluded that the pooling of the findings of low-quality RCTs results in a clinically important and statistically significant exaggeration of the efficacy of an intervention under study.

The main reason for undertaking an RCT is to establish a causal relationship, that is, to show a statistically significant treatment effect that cannot be ascribed to the effects of selection bias, observation bias, or confounding factors. Bias is any systematic error in the design of a study (or execution of the study protocol) that may result in a systematic deviation from the truth when the data are analyzed and reported [80]. Selection (allocation) bias refers to systematic differences between patients who received the treatment under study and those who did not. Observation (ascertainment) bias refers to systematic differences in the investigators' diagnoses of subsequent disease in patients who received the treatment and those who did not. Confounding refers to the situation in which an unrecognized variable is associated with both the outcome of interest and its putative cause, producing a spurious association (or concealing a true relationship) between the treatment and the outcome when the data are analyzed and reported [81].

Bias is introduced into RCTs when the investigators become aware of the next treatment assignment [82,83], and channel participants preferentially to one or the other arm of the study; and when patients and investigators are unblinded (and thus influenced by notions about benefit from the treatment in reporting signs and symptoms or assessing disease activity) [84]. In other words, bias is introduced into an RCT when those responsible for admitting patients into the study decipher the treatment allocation sequence; or when those assessing the occurrence of the outcome of interest become aware of the treatment allocations. Whether the issue is deciphering the treatment allocation sequence or breaking the blind, both situations can occur either inadvertently or deliberately, and they do not appear to represent rare occurrences [82-85].

There is consensus among epidemiologists that meta-analyses should be limited to RCTs [86-88], but experts disagree on the appropriate quality criteria to be used for disqualifying RCTs for inclusion in an overview. Indeed, experts disagree whether any randomized trial, no matter how poorly designed or conducted, should ever be excluded from a meta-analysis [89]. However, if the purpose of an overview is to reach a conclusion about the existence of a treatment effect, the quality of the studies to be included in the overview should be explicitly addressed in the report of the meta-analysis [89]. An overview can be only as good as its component parts, and – if bias and confounding compromise the results of the RCTs included in the overview – the findings of the meta-analysis will be similarly flawed. Therefore, if the issue of study quality is not addressed in the report of the meta-analysis, the overview can be criticized[90,91] as an 'exercise in megasilliness' where 'a mass of reports – good, bad, and indifferent – are fed into the computer in the hope that people will cease caring about the quality of the material on which the conclusions are based,' and where 'garbage in – garbage out, a well-known axiom of computer specialists, applies with equal force'.

Bias in Meta-Analytic Research

An observational study conducted at a single institution and investigating the effect of a treatment on a disease must enroll all patients who are sequentially admitted to that hospital with a specific diagnosis. If subjects are missed or excluded, selection bias may occur [92]. Similarly, the validity of a meta-analysis depends on complete sampling of all studies performed on a particular topic. Validity can be preserved if a representative sample is obtained, but any incomplete sample is a potentially biased one [93]. Unfortunately, meta-analysts may not be able to locate all published studies, because computerized data bases do not cover all periodicals, search algorithms often fail to identify relevant articles, and the indexing of studies is imperfect [94-98]. Even if the literature is optimally searched, studies published as government reports, book chapters, dissertations, conference proceedings, etc, may not be captured, while unpublished studies will not be identified. Published trials differ systematically from unpublished ones, in that they are more likely to have a larger sample, and to have generated statistically significant results [99]. The systematic exclusion of small and negative studies from a meta-analysis that conditions eligibility on achievement of publication status is referred to as publication bias [99-104].

There is ample evidence of publication bias in the medical literature. Easterbrook et al. [105] documented a 3.8-fold increase in the odds of publication (95% CI, 1.5-9.8) for observational studies reporting statistically significant findings, as compared to studies with null results. Multivariate analysis showed that the better odds of publication could not be explained by the quality of study design. On the contrary, there was a trend toward a greater number of statistically significant results with poorer quality studies [105]. Chalmers et al. [106] corroborated the finding of Easterbrook et al. [105] that achievement of publication status does not depend on the quality of study design. They also detected publication bias favoring studies with larger samples, but not studies with statistically significant results [106].

A specific type of publication bias is the language of Babel bias [107] or English language bias[108]. Although differences in quality between English and non-English reports are small [108,109], authors are more likely to publish RCTs in English-language journals if the results are statistically significant [108,109]. Accordingly, if RCTs published in languages other than English are excluded, the findings of meta-analyses may be biased toward the reporting of statistically significant results. Grégoire et al. [107] reported that 72% of the meta-analyses in their survey had restricted the literature search to studies published in English.

Selection bias can arise not only during retrieval of studies from the literature, but also during assessment of the eligibility of the retrieved reports. In evaluating the quality of investigations, analysts may be influenced by knowl-

Table 3. Publication bias in studies evaluating the effect of paternal white cell immunization for recurrent miscarrage.*

Summary estimate of effect	Published reports (n=4)	Unpublished trials (n=4)
Fixed-effects analysis		
– Relative live birth ratio	1.29	1.01
– 95% confidence interval	1.03-1.60**	0.74-1.28
Random-effects analysis		
– Relative live birth ratio	1.38	1.01
– 95% confidence interval	0.89-1.87	0.74-1.28

Abbreviation: n = sample size.

* Based on data from Jeng et al. [42]. Reprinted with permission from Transfusion 1997;37:338. Overviews of published and unpublished randomized controlled trials generated discrepant conclusions wheh a fixed-effects analysis was used; with a random-effects method, the results were concordant [1-5,113].

** Statistically significant finding p <0.05).

edge of the results of a study, or the journal of publication. They may even be inclined to modify eligibility criteria, so as to include in the overview reports from prestigious journals. According to Felson [93], selection bias is the principal reason for discrepant results in meta-analyses. Different teams of analysts may base their conclusions on alternate sets of original reports, generating either statistically significant or null (i.e., statistically insignificant) findings.

The impact of publication bias on the findings of a meta-analysis is illustrated in Table 3, using the data of Jeng et al. [42]. These authors demonstrated that the average effect of paternal WBC immunization in preventing recurrent miscarriage was significant if calculated by a fixed-effects method from a meta-analysis of published studies, but null when based on an overview of unpublished trials. (For a discussion of the assumptions of a fixed- versus random-effects analysis [1-5], and the statistical methods used in overviews [110-112], the reader is referred to the literature [1-5,113].)

Conclusion

Meta-analyses are a supplement to RCTs, which remain the gold standard for evaluating the efficacy of therapeutic interventions, but need to be supplemented by meta-analyses in order to broaden the applicability of the findings. Furthermore, meta-analyses can be an important research tool for the systematic evaluation of the quality of published studies, and for the disciplined investigation of reasons for disagreements among reports. Overviews can identify errors and shortcomings in completed studies, and may be able to explain why trial results differ. In the past, narrative reviews of the literature served these functions in a less formal manner. Meta-analyses are much better suited for these purposes, because of their objective and quantitative nature.

Meta-analyses have also been used to establish the existence of a treatment effect in situations where multiple small RCTs have been conducted, but have not demonstrated a statistically significant effect, perhaps because of their small sample size. The value of meta-analysis in this area has been questioned. However, the controversy over this specific use of meta-analysis should not detract from the value of overviews in assessing the quality of completed studies and the reasons for disagreements among reports. Future meta-analyses will likely find a more suitable role in addressing potential sources of heterogeneity, in lieu of trying to fit a summary estimate of the effect of an intervention among diverse studies. The development of quantitative methods for examining sources of heterogeneity among studies is an active area of research. Formal assessments of the quality of completed studies can also contribute to an investigation of the sources of heterogeneity, and they should be one of the main reasons for conducting meta-analyses in the future.

References

1. Jenicek M. Meta-analysis in medicine: where we are and where we want to go. J Clin Epidemiol 1989; 42:35-44.
2. L'Abbé KA, Detsky AS, O'Rourke K. Meta-analysis in clinical research. Ann Intern Med 1987; 107:224-33.
3. Glass GV, McGraw B, Smith ML. Meta-analysis in social research. Beverly Hills, CA: Sage Publications, 1981.

4. Light RJ, Pillemer DB. Summing up: The science of reviewing research. Cambridge, MA: Harvard University Press, 1984.
5. 18. Cooper H, Hedges LV, eds. The handbook of research synthesis. New York, NY: Russell Sage Foundation, 1994.
6. Glass GV. Primary, secondary, and meta-analysis of research. Educ Res 1976; 5:3-8.
7. Moher D, Olkin I. Meta-analysis of randomized controlled trials: a concern for standards. JAMA 1995; 274:1962-64.
8. Sacks HS, Berrier J, Reitman D, Ancona-Berk VA, Chalmers TC. Meta-analyses of randomized controlled trials. N Engl J Med 1987; 316:450-55.
9. Yusuf S, Simon R, Ellenberg S, eds. Proceedings of "Methodologic Issues in Overviews of Randomized Clinical Trials". Workshop sponsored by the National Heart, Lung and Blood Institute and the National Cancer Institute. Bethesda, MD, 15-16 May, 1986. Stat Med 1987; 6:217-409.
10. Goodman SN. Have you ever met a meta-analysis you didn't like? Am Intern Med 1991; 114:244-46.
11. Goodman SN. Meta-analysis in health services research. In: Armenian HK, Shapiro S, eds. Epidemiology and health services. New York, NY: Oxford University Press, 1998:229-59.
12. Schiffer CA, Dutcher JP, Aisner J, et al. A randomized trial of leukocyte-depleted platelet transfusion to modify alloimmunization in patients with leukemia. Blood 1983; 62:815-20.
13. Andreu G, Dewailly J, Leberre C, et al. Prevention of HLA immunization with leukocyte-poor packed red cells and platelet concentrates obtained by filtration. Blood 1988; 72:964-69.
14. Sniecinski I, O'Donnell MR, Nowicki B, et al. Prevention of refractoriness and HLA alloimmunization using filtered blood products. Blood 1988; 71:1402-07.
15. Oksanen K, Kekomaki R, Ruutu T, et al. Prevention of alloimmunization in patients with acute leukemia by use of white cell-reduced blood components-A randomized trial. Transfusion 1991;31:588-94.
16. van Marwijk Kooy M, van Prooijen HC, Moes M, et al. Use of leukocyte-depleted platelet concentrates for the prevention of refractoriness and primary HLA alloimmunization: A prospective, randomized trial. Blood 1991; 77:201-05.
17. Williamson LM, Wimperis JZ, Williamson P, et al. Bedside filtration of blood products in the prevention of HLA alloimmunization-A prospective, randomized study. Blood 1994; 83:3028-35.
18. Sintnicolaas K, van Marwijk Kooij M, van Prooijen HC, et al. Leukocyte depletion of random single-donor platelet transfusions does not prevent secondary human leukocyte antigen-alloimmunization and refractoriness: A randomized prospective study. Blood 1995; 85:824-28.
19. Heddle NM. The efficacy of leukodepletion to improve platelet transfusion response: A critical appraisal of clinical studies. Transf Med Rev 1994; 8:15-28.
20. Andreu G, Dewailly J. Prevention of HLA alloimmunization by using leukocyte-depleted components. In: Lane TA, Myllyla G, eds. Leukocyte-depleted blood products. Curr Stud Hematol Blood Transf, no. 60. Basel, Switzerland: Karger, 1994: 29-40.
21. Vamvakas EC. Meta-analysis of randomized controlled trials of the efficacy of white cell reduction in preventing HLA-alloimmunization and refractoriness to random-donor platelet transfusions. Transf Med Rev 1998; 12:258-70.
22. Wooley AL, Hogikyan ND, Geates GA, Haughney BH, Schechtman KB, Goldenberg JL. Effect of blood transfusion on recurrence of head and neck carcinoma. Retrospective review and meta-analysis. Ann Otol Rhinol Laryngol 1992; 101:724-30.
23. Chung M, Steinmetz OK, Gordon PH. Perioperative blood transfusion and outcome after resection for colorectal carcinoma. Br J Surg 1993; 80:427-32.
24. Amato A, Pescatori M. Perioperative blood transfusion and outcome after resection for colorectal carcinoma. Br J Surg 1994; 81:313-14.

25. Vamvakas E. Perioperative blood transfusion and cancer recurrence: meta-analysis for explanation. Transfusion 1995; 35:760-68.
26. Brand A, Houbiers JGA. Clinical studies of blood transfusion and cancer. In: Vamvakas EC, Blajchman MA, eds. Immunomodulatory effects of blood transfusion. Bethesda, MD: American Association of Blood Banks Press, 1999: 145-90.
27. Busch ORC, Hop WCJ, Hoynek van Papendrecht MAW, Marquet RL, Jeekel J. Blood transfusions and prognosis in colorectal center. N Engl J Med 1993; 328:1372-76.
28. Heiss MM, Mempel W, Delanoff C, et al. Blood transfusion-modulated tumor recurrence: first results of a randomized study of autologous versus allogeneic blood transfusion in colorectal cancer surgery. J Clin Oncol 1994; 12:1859-67.
29. Houbiers JGA, Brand A, van de Watering LMG, et al. Randomized controlled trial comparing transfusion of leukocyte-depleted or buffy-coat-depleted blood in surgery for colorectal cancer. Lancet 1994; 344:573-78.
30. Jensen LS, Andersen AJ, Christiansen PM, et al. Postoperative infection and natural killer cell function following blood transfusion in patients undergoing elective colorectal surgery. Br J Surg 1992; 79:513-16.
31. Heiss MM, Mempel W, Jauch KW, et al. Beneficial effect of autologous blood transfusion on infectious complications after colorectal cancer surgery. Lancet 1993; 342:1328-33.
32. Busch ORC, Hop WCJ, Marquet RL, et al. Autologous blood and infection after colorectal surgery (letter). Lancet 1994; 343:668-69.
33. Jensen LS, Kissmeyer-Nielsen P, Wolff B, et al. Randomized comparison of leukocyte-depleted versus buffy-coat-poor blood transfusion and complications after colorectal surgery. Lancet 1996; 348:841-45.
34. van de Watering LMG, Hermans J, Houbiers JGA, et al. Beneficial effect of leukocyte depletion of transfused blood on postoperative complications in patients undergoing cardiac surgery: A randomized clinical trial. Circulation 1998; 97:562-68.
35. Tartter PI, Mohandas K, Azar P, et al. Randomized trial comparing packed red blood cell transfusion with and without leukocyte depletion for gastrointestinal surgery. Am J Surg 1998; 176:462-66.
36. Vamvakas E. Transfusion-associated cancer recurrence and infection: meta-analysis of randomized, controlled clinical trials. Transfusion 1996; 36:175-86.
37. McAlister FA, Clark HD, Wells PS, Laupacis A. Perioperative allogeneic blood transfusion does not cause adverse sequelae in patients with cancer: A meta-analysis of unconfounded studies. Br J Surg 1998; 85:71-78.
38. Vamvakas EC, Dzik WH, Blajchman MA. Deleterious effects of transfusion-associated immunomodulation: Appraisal of the evidence and recommendations for prevention. In: Vamvakas EC, Blajchman MA, eds. Immunomodulatory effects of blood transfusion. Bethesda, MD: American Association of Blood Banks Press, 1999:253-85.
39. Cowchock S. What's a mother to do? Analysis of trials evaluating new treatments for unexplained recurrent miscarriages and other complaints. Am J Reprod Immunol 1991; 26:156-59.
40. Fraser EJ, Grimes DA, Schulz KF. Immunization as therapy for recurrent spontaneous abortion: a review and meta-analysis. Obstet Gynecol 1993; 82:854-59.
41. The Recurrent Miscarriage Immunotherapy Trialists Group. Worldwide collaborative observational study and meta-analysis on allogeneic leukocyte immunotherapy for recurrent spontaneous abortion. Am J Reprod Immunol 1994; 32:55-72
42. Jeng FT, Scott JR, Burmeister LF. A comparison of meta-analytic results using literature vs. individual patient data: paternal cell immunization for recurrent miscarriage. JAMA 1995; 274:830-36.
43. Hollaar GL, Gooszen HG, Post S, et al. Perioperative blood transfusion does not prevent recurrence in Crohn's disease. J Clin Gastroenterol 1995; 21:134-38.

44. 57. Vamvakas EC, Pineda AA. Meta-analysis of clinical studies of the efficacy of granulocyte transfusions in the treatment of bacterial sepsis. J Clin Apheresis 1996; 11:1-9.
45. Vamvakas EC, Pineda AA. Determinants of the efficacy of prophylactic granulocyte transfusions: A meta-analysis. J Clin Apheresis 1997; 12:74-81.
46. Vamvakas EC, Pineda AA, Weinshenker BG. Meta-analysis of clinical studies of the efficacy of plasma exchange in the treatment of chronic progressive multiple sclerosis. J Clin Apheresis 1995; 10:163-70.
47. Huet C, Salmi LR, Fergusson D, Koopman-van Gemert AW, Rubens F, Laupacis A. A meta-analysis of the effectiveness of cell salvage to minimize perioperative allogeneic blood transfusion in cardiac and orthopedic surgery. Anesth Analg 1999; 89:861-69.
48. Bryson GL, Laupacis A, Wells GA. Does acute normovolemic hemodilution reduce perioperative allogeneic transfusion? A meta-analysis. Anesth Analg 1998; 86:9-15.
49. Forgie MA, Wells PS, Laupacis A, Fergusson D. Preoperative autologous donation decreases allogeneic transfusion but increases exposure to all red blood cell transfusion: results of a meta-analysis. Arch Intern Med 1998; 158:610-16.
50. Rubens FD, Fergusson D, Wells PS, Huang M, McGowan JL, Laupacis A. Platelet-rich plasmapheresis in cardiac surgery: a meta-analysis of the effect on transfusion requirements. J Thorac Cardiovasc Surg 1998; 116:641-47.
51. Laupacis A, Fergusson D. Erythropoietin to minimize perioperative blood transfusion: a systematic review of randomized trials. Transfus Med 1998; 8:309-17.
52. Phillips K. The use of meta-analysis in technology assessment: a meta-analysis of the enzyme immunosorbent assay human immunodeficiency virus antibody test. J Clin Epidemiol 1991; 44:925-31.
53. Hellstrom-Lindberg E. Efficacy of erythropoietin in the myelodysplastic syndromes: a meta-analysis of 205 patients from 17 studies. Br J Haematol 1995; 89:67-71.
54. Henry DH, Beall GN, Benson CA, et al. Recombinant human erythropoietin in the treatment of anemia associated with human immunodeficiency virus (HIV) infection and zidovudine therapy. Overview of four clinical trials. Ann Intern Med 1992; 117:739-48.
55. Pagliaro L, Crazi A, Cammaa C, et al. Interferon-alpha for chronic hepatitis C: an analysis of pretreatment clinical predictors of response. Hepatology 1994; 19:820-28.
56. Begg CB, Pilotte L, McGlave PB. Bone marrow transplantation versus chemotherapy in acute non-lymphocytic leukemia: a meta-analytic review. Eur J Cancer Clin Oncol 1989; 25:1519-23.
57. Laupacis A, Fergusson D. Drugs to minimize perioperative blood loss in cardiac surgery: meta-analyses using perioperative blood transfusion as the outcome. Anesth Analg 1997; 85:1258-67.
58. Fleiss JL, Tytum A, Ury HK. A simple approximation for calculating sample sizes for comparing independent proportions. Biometrics 1980; 36:343-46.
59. The Trial to Reduce Alloimmunization to Platelets Study Group. Leukocyte reduction and ultraviolet B irradiation of platelets to prevent alloimmunization and refractoriness to platelet transfusions. N Engl J Med 1997; 337:1681-89.
60. Vamvakas EC. Multicenter randomized controlled trials in transfusion medicine. Trans Med Rev 2000; 14:137-50.
61. Freiman JA, Chalmers RC, Smith H Jr, et al. The importance of beta, the type II error and sample size in the design and interpretation of the randomized controlled trial: Survey of 71 "negative" trials. N Engl J Med 1978; 299:690-94.
62. Passamani E. Clinical trials: are they ethical? N Engl J Med 1991; 324:1589-91.
63. Hellman S, Hellman DS. Of mice but not men: problems of the randomized clinical trial. N Engl J Med 324:1585-89.
64. Borzak S, Ridker PM. Discordance between meta-analyses and large-scale randomized controlled trials: examples from the management of acute myocardial infarction. Ann Intern Med 1995; 123:873-77.

65. Bailar JC III. The promise and problems of meta-analysis. N Engl J Med 1997; 337:559-61.
66. Meta-analysis under scrutiny. Lancet 1997; 350:675.
67. Villar J, Carrolli G, Belizan JM. Predictive ability of meta-analyses of randomized controlled trials. Lancet 1995; 345:772-76.
68. Cappelleri JC, Ioannidis JPA, Schmid CH, et al. Large trials versus meta-analyses of small trials: How do their results compare? JAMA 1996; 276:1332-38.
69. LeLorier J, Grégoire B, Benhaddad A, et al. Discrepancies between meta-analyses and subsequent large randomized, controlled trials. N Engl J Med 1997; 337:536-42.
70. Ioannidis JPA, Cappelleri JC, Lau J. Issues in comparisons between meta-analyses and large trials. JAMA 1998; 279:1089-93.
71. O'Rourke K, Detsky AS. Meta-analysis in medical research: strong encouragement for higher quality in individual research efforts. J Clin Epidemiol 1989; 42:1021-24.
72. Gerbarg ZB, Horowitz RI. Resolving conflicting clinical trials: guidelines for meta-analysis. J Clin Epidemiol 1988; 41:503-09.
73. Chalmers TC, Smith H Jr, Blackburn B, et al. A method for assessing the quality of a randomized controlled trial. Control Clin Trials 1981; 2:31-49.
74. Detsky AS, Naylor CD, O'Rourke K, McGeer AJ, L'Abbé KA. Incorporating variations in the quality of individual randomized trials into meta-analysis. J Clin Epidemiol 1992; 45:255-65.
75. Zelen M. Guidelines for publishing papers on cancer clinical trials: responsibilities of editors and authors. J Clin Oncol 1983; 1:164-69.
76. Moher D, Jadad AR, Nichol G, Penman M, Tugwell P, Walsh S. Assessing the quality of randomized controlled trials: An annotated bibliography of scales and checklists. Control Clin Trials 1995; 16:62-73.
77. Moher D, Jadad AR, Tugwell P. Assessing the quality of reports of randomized trials. Int J Technol Assess Health Care 1996; 12:195-208.
78. Jadad AR, Moore RA, Carroll D, et al. Assessing the quality of reports of randomized trials: Is blinding necessary? Control Clin Trials 1996; 17:1-12.
79. Moher D, Jones BA, Cook DJ, et al. Does quality of reports of randomized trials affect estimates of intervention efficacy reported in meta-analyses? Lancet 1998; 352:609-13.
80. Sackett DL. Bias in analytic research. J Chron Dis 1979; 32:51-63.
81. Miettinen OS, Cook EF. Confounding: Essence and detection. Am J Epidemiol 1981; 114: 593-603.
82. Schultz KF, Chalmers I, Hayes RJ, et al. Empirical evidence of bias: Dimensions of methodological quality associated with estimates of treatment effects in controlled trials. JAMA 1995; 273:408-12.
83. Huskisson EC, Scott J. How blind is double-blind? And does it matter? Br J Clin Pharmacol 1976; 3:331-32.
84. Pocock SJ, Lagakos SW. Practical experience of randomization in cancer trials: An international survey. Br J Cancer 1982; 46:368-75.
85. Chalmers TC, Celano P, Sacks HS, et al. Bias in treatment assignment in controlled clinical trials. N Engl J Med 1983; 309:1358-61.
86. Chalmers TC, Levin H, Sacks HS, Reitman D, Berrier J, Nagalingam R. Meta-analysis of clinical trials as a scientific discipline. I. Control of bias and comparison with large co-operative trials. Stat Med 1987; 6:315-25.
87. Peto R. Why do we need systematic overviews of randomized trials? Stat Med 1987; 6:233-40.
88. Yusuf S. Obtaining medically meaningful answers from an overview of randomized clinical trials. Stat Med 1987; 6:281-86.
89. Fleiss JL, Gross AJ. Meta-analysis in epidemiology, with special reference to studies of the association between exposure to environmental tobacco smoke and lung cancer: a critique. J Clin Epidemiol 1991; 44:127-39.
90. Eysenck HJ. An exercise in megasilliness. Am Psycol 1978; 35:517.

91. Wachter KW. Disturbed by meta-analysis? Science 1988; 241:1407-08.
92. Kleinbaum DG, Kupper LL, Morgenstern H. Epidemiologic research. New York, NY: Van Nostrand Reinhold Co, 1982: 194-219.
93. Felson DT. Bias in meta-analytic research. J Clin Epidemiol 1992; 45:885-92.
94. Hewitt P, Chalmers TC. Using MEDLINE to peruse the literature. Control Clin Trials 1985; 6:75-83.
95. Hewitt P, Chalmers TC. Perusing the literature: methods of accessing MEDLINE and related data bases. Control Clin Trials 1985; 6:168-77.
96. Poynard T, Conn HO. The retrieval or randomized clinical trials in liver disease from the medical literature: a comparison of MEDLARS and manual methods. Control Clin Trials 1985; 6:271-79.
97. Dickersin K, Kewitt P, Mutch L, Chalmers I, Chalmers TC. Perusing the literature: comparison of MEDLINE searching with a perinatal database. Control Clin Trials 1985; 6:306-17.
98. Haynes RB, McKibbon KA, Walker CJ, et al. Computer searching of the medical literature: an evaluation of MEDLINE search systems. Ann Intern Med 1985; 103:812-16.
99. Begg CB, Berlin JA. Publication bias and dissemination of clinical research. J Natl Cancer Inst 1989; 81:107-14.
100. Begg CB, Berlin JA. Publication bias: a problem in interpreting medical data. J Royal Stat Soc A 1988; 151:419-63.
101. Dickersin K, Chan S, Chalmers TC, et al. Publication bias and clinical trials. Control Clin Trials 1987; 8:343-53.
102. Simes RJ. Confronting publication bias: a cohort design for meta-analysis. Stat Med 1987; 6:11-29.
103. Simes RJ. Publication bias: the case for an international registry of trials. J Clin Oncol 1986; 4:1529-41.
104. Dickersin K, Min YI, Meinert CL. Factors influencing publication of research results: follow-up of applications submitted to two institutional review boards. JAMA 1992; 267:374-78.
105. Easterbrook PJ, Berlin JA, Copalan R, Matthews DR. Publication bias in clinical research. Lancet 1991; 337:867-72.
106. Chalmers I, Adams M, Dickersin K, et al. A cohort study of summary reports of controlled trials. JAMA 1990; 263:1401-05.
107. Grégoire G, Derderian F, LeLorier J. Selecting the language of publication included in a meta-analysis: Is there a Tower of Babel bias? J Clin Epidemiol 1995; 48:159-63.
108. Egger M, Zellweger-Zatner T, Schneider M, Junker C, Lengeler C, Antes G. Language bias in randomized controlled trials published in English and German. Lancet 1997; 350:326-29.
109. Moher D, Fortin P, Jadad AR, et al. Completeness of reporting of trials published in languages other than English: Implications for conduct and reporting of systemic reviews. Lancet 1996; 347:363-66.
110. Yusuf S, Peto R, Lewis J, Collins R, Sleight P. Beta blockade during and after myocardial infarction: an overview of the randomized trials. Prog Cardiovasc Dis 1985; 27:335-71.
111. DerSimonian R, Laird N. Meta-analysis in clinical trials. Control Clin Trials 1986; 7:177-88.
112. Cochran WG. The combination of estimates from different experiments. Biometrics 1954; 10:101-29.
113. Vamvakas EC. Meta-analysis in transfusion medicine. Transfusion 1997; 37:329-45.

IMMUNOMODULATION: FACTS AND INTERPRETATIONS

A.Brand[1]

Introduction

Blood transfusions expose the recipient to multiple antigens and immunisation against a particular antigen occurs simultaneously with suppression towards other antigens. Moreover, transfusions can stimulate or suppress the host immunity against environmental antigens.

- The immune effects of blood transfusions can be separated into:
- MHC (Major Histocompatibility Complex)-specific;
- non-MHC antigen-specific and;
- non-antigen specific interactions affecting the innate immune response.

The immune response against HLA-antigens can follow two pathways. Donor cells can directly present MHC-antigens to recipient CD4 helper cells. This direct presentation is unique for donor MHC-class II bearing cells (and microbial superantigens). Mouse experiments suggest that not only antigen presenting cells (APCs) that constitutionally express MHC class II antigens, but also donor CD4 T cells which express class II upon activation by recipient MHC can directly activate recipient CD4 cells [1]. Activated CD4 recipient cells produce cytokines, which activate cytotoxic CD8 cells (CTLs) and B cells. This Th1 response is presumably the major mechanism leading to rejection of transfused donor cells and the formation of HLA-antibodies.

Allo-MHC and non-MHC allo-antigens are also processed by recipient APCs, who indirectly present these allo-peptides in their MHC groove to T cells. If a Th1 response is activated, generating interleukin (IL)-12 and Interferon (IFN)-γ, CTLs and antibodies will emerge as described above. Indirect presentation accounts for the residual primary HLA-immunisation after leukocyte-depleted blood transfusions, and for antibodies against erythrocyte and platelet-specific antigens evoked by transfusion and pregnancy. Antigen presentation can also result in a Th 2 response, with production of IL-4, IL-5 and IL-10, and formation of non-complement activating antibodies against cell-derived and soluble proteins.

1. Blood Bank Leiden-Haaglanden and Dept. of Immunohaematology and Blood Transfusion, Leiden University Medical Centre, Leiden, NL.

Table 1A. Immunomodulation by blood products with intended aim.

Intended effect	Target in recipient	Effector(s) in blood product	Mechanism
Passive immunity	HAV, HBV, CMV, RSV	– Neutralizing/ opsonising anti-bodies – Other?	– Virus kill – Blocking cellular receptors
Graft versus cancer	– Malignant cells – Minor MHC anti-gens	CD4, CD8, NK cells	Unknown
Rh D immuno-prophylaxis	Prevention of Rh D antigen presentation	Anti-Rh D with potent ADCC	Unknown
Transient suppression of auto-immunity	– B, T, NK cells – Cytokines – Proliferating cells – Auto-antibodies – Fc-receptors – Complement	– Soluble HLA – Anti-idiotypic Ab – Receptor Ab – Dimers/ monomeric IgG	– Catabolism of IgG – Fc receptor blocking – Anticomplementary – Modulation of cell surface receptors – Intra-cellular signal-ling
Condition trans-fusion prior to solid organ transplantation	Alloreactive T cells	– Viable HLA-DR shared APCs and lymphocytes – Non-viable cells lacking co-stim-ulatory signals	Unknown
Prevention of (primary) HLA immunisation	Alloreactive T helper cells, stimulating B cells	Removal of (viable) donor APCs	Abscence of direct APC/T cell interaction
Habitual abortion	Unknown	– Partner/donor PBL – IvIg	Unknown

Table 1B. Immunomodulation by blood products with unintended effects.

Unintended effect	Effector recipient	Causal factor in blood product	Mechanism
HLA-antibodies	CD4 T cells recipient	Viable donor APCs	Direct presentation
Non-HLA/HLA antibodies	APCs presenting processed peptides to CD4 T cells	Allo-antigens	Indirect presentation
Postoperative bacterial infections	NK cells, macrophages	– Non-viable red cells – Leukocyte aggregates	Blocking of leuko-cyte functions and phagocytosis?
Cancer surveillance	– Cytotoxic cells – Angiogenesis	Unknown	Unknown
Organ damage	Unknown	Unknown	Inappropriate cytokine cascade
GvHD	Minor MHC antigens	Immunocompetent T cells	Recipient can not reject donor T cells

HAV: hepatitis A; HBV: hepatitis B; CMV: cytomegalovirus; RSV: respiratory syncytium virus: Ab: antibodies; PBL: peripheral blood leukocytes; GvHD: graft-versus-host disease.

Third, transfusion influences the non-antigen specific innate immune system of natural killer (NK) cells and macrophages.

Transfusion, transplantation and pregnancy introduce allogeneic cells. In case of transfusions the effect in the recipient is determined to a large extend by apoptotic cells and activated cells administered with blood products. Processing and storage of blood components (and organs) can have profound effects on the immunogenicity.

Single factors obtained from purified blood derived components may be the ultimate aim of deliberate transfusion induced immunomodulation. However the unravelling of transfusion induced immunomodulation is extremely complicated and only a few strong messages can be discriminated from noise.

Immunomodulation is also a confusing term as it covers a wide range of immune events from immunisation to immune suppression. Immunisation and immune suppression are often the clinical or in-vitro defined endpoints, which both require *activation* of either a T helper (Th type 1 or 2) or a regulatory T cell circuit.

At one side of the spectrum of *intended* immunomodulation by blood (derived) products we find passive vaccination and graft versus leukaemia (GVL) by donor lymphocyte infusions (DLI), while at the other side of the spectrum immune suppressive treatments such as Rh(D) immunoprophylaxis, amelioration of auto-immune diseases by high dose intravenous immunoglobulin (IVIg) and conditioning by pre-transplantation blood transfusion can be categorised (Table 1A).

Unintended transfusion induced immunomodulation similarly ranges from undesired allo-antibody formation with obvious side effects such as transfusion reactions, platelet transfusion refractoriness or graft versus host disease (GVHD) to presumed suppression of the host defence against infections and cancer. Furthermore there seems to exist, unclassified with respect to stimulation or suppression, transfusion effects playing a role in the systemic inflammatory response leading to organ failure (Table 1B).

Symptomatic transfusion reactions are almost exclusively caused by allo-antibodies, which are the result of a Th 1 response. The transfusion induced changes in the host *cellular* immunity is often referred to as immunomodulation. The clinical consequences of changes in the host cellular immune system are either unknown or, if obvious such as the improvement of outcome of organ transplantation after blood transfusion or donor lymphocyte infusions for leukaemia, not understood.

Progress of clinical treatment is often not designed in the laboratory, but based on bedside observations, serendipity, retrospective multivariate analysis and well designed clinical trials. In fact a large part of fundamental research tries to offer explanations for clinical observations. Transfusion induced immunomodulation is no exception to this rule. Therefore this paper is based on clinical observations and speculates about causal factors in blood products and the mechanism of their effects.

Intended Immunomodulation

Pre-transplantation blood transfusion: clinical observations

The recognition of a protective effect of pre-transplantation blood transfusion(s) on subsequent rejection of a kidney graft is based on multivariate analysis of factors contributing to graft survival [2 ,3]. Two transfusion strategies seem, presumably by different mechanisms, to protect against organ graft rejection. The eldest strategy to establish pre- transplantation immune suppression is mediated by transfusion of (stored) blood or red cells from random donors. This effect is dose-related and increases with the number of transfusions [4].

The second strategy is to give a single blood transfusion, containing viable mononuclear cells, from a donor who shares a HLA-DR antigen with the patient and who is mismatched for the other haplotype [5]. These DR- shared blood transfusions induce less often HLA-antibodies [5] and the transfused nucleated cells are less readily rejected [6].

Pre-transplantation blood transfusions: causal factors and mechanism

The mechanism of the beneficial effect of blood transfusions ameliorating graft rejection is still unknown. The immune suppressive effect exerted by multiple blood transfusions may result from lack of co-stimulatory signals on HLA-expressing red cells, platelets and leukocytes and/or repeat infusion of high concentrations of soluble HLA molecules or cytokines, which suppress Th 1 [7 , 8]. Although this effect is transient, repetitive exposure to red cells or impure Factor VIII preparations may cause prolonged suppression of Th 1 responses [9, 10].

The immunoregulatory effect of a single DR-shared transfusion seems dependent on antigen presentation by viable MHC-bearing donor cells. It is suggested by animal studies that foreign peptides, which may be shared between organ and transfusion donor and which are presented by the DR sharing 'self' APCs from the transfusion donor are recognised as 'self' antigens and induce regulatory cells in the recipient. Such regulatory cells subsequently down-regulate an (anti-'self') immune response of T cells activated by passenger cells in the graft and involved in graft rejection [11]. The mechanism how such regulatory T cells down-regulate the induction of allo-reactive T cells against the organ donor is unknown. Despite it has been shown that these regulatory cells produce Interleukin-10 in-vitro, also lysis of target cells occurs. The induction of CD8 cells, which kill donor cells when these proliferate upon stimulation with recipient class II antigens, was observed as a common effect after blood transfusions in humans and may be the major mechanism that prohibits transfusion associated graft versus host disease (TA-GVHD) [12]. It is unknown however, whether a similar mechanism is involved in killing the autologous allo-proliferative cells, stimulated by the organ donor.

Chimaerism: clinical effects and mechanisms

Mononuclear cells from a bone marrow or peripheral blood stem cell donor can, post transplantation, cure relapsed leukaemia by graft versus leukaemia (GVL), if the leukaemia cells express costimulatory antigens [13,14]. For GVL a complete chimaerism of donor haematopoietic cells is not required. Which donor cells recognise, respond to and eliminate host leukaemia cells is unknown . The target antigen on leukaemia cells, recognised by donor lymphocytes can be a minor transplantation antigen predominantly expressed on haematopoietic cells or a leukaemia specific antigen. Because GVL is associated in approximately 40-60% of the cases with graft versus host disease there are hopeful expectations that these two effector mechanisms can be separated [15].

Pregnancy, blood transfusion, solid organ transplantation and stem cell transfusions can all establish various degrees of chimaerism without GVHD. Micro-chimaerism, with a frequency of chimaeric cells of 1 in 104 or 105 cells is observed more than 20 years after pregnancy in up to 60% of females [16, 17] and in adult recipients of intra-uterine transfusions [18]. Long-term (>1 year) intermediate-levels of chimaerism with 5-50% of persisting donor cells has been shown after neonatal blood transfusions [19, 20] and in immune competent transfused female trauma patients [21]. Macro-chimaerism (>50%) after (mini)stem cell transplantation tolerizes for immunocompetent donor lymphocytes and enables leukaemia and even solid cancer treatment in the future. The characterisation of the chimaeric cells under these various circumstances, why some cells escape from rejection and lack aggressiveness towards the recipient and do not cause GVHD and why chimaerism is not necessarily associated with non-responsiveness will improve our understanding of immunomodulation by blood transfusion.

Immunomodulation by antibodies

Coating of a potentially immunising antigen with specific antibodies, such as in Rh-D immunoprophylaxis prohibits CD4 T cell activation and antibody formation.

In auto-immune diseases the target antigens are often unknown. In auto-immune disease the destruction of autologous tissues is mediated by antibodies and/or by a cell mediated inflammatory reaction. High dose polyvalent intravenous immunoglobulin (IVIg) contains, besides natural and immune antibodies, a large variety of soluble factors transported by immunoglobulins. IVIg can ameliorate antibody- as well as cell-mediated auto-immune diseases [22]. Although it is recognised that IVIg has multiple immunomodulatory effects, the mechanism which effect is dominant in a particular auto-immune disease is unknown.

IVIg inhibits cell proliferation and enhances a Th 2 response [23]. Furthermore increase of IgG concentration enforces catabolism of (also pathogenic) IgG [24], while monomeric and dimeric IgG block and down-regulate different Fc-receptors [25]. In contrast to immunomodulation by donor cells, the potent and clinically established immunoregulatory effect of polyvalent immunoglobulins, as present in IVIg, is often transient and does not harbour the risks of uncontrollable effects. Improvement of immune mediated chronic inflammatory neuropathy or auto-immune thrombocytopenia can not only be obtained by IVIg but also by multiple units of donorplasma [26]. Plasma may thus result in unintended immunomodulatory effects comparable with the intended IVIg effect in auto-immune diseases [27].

Unintended Immunomodulation

Allo-antibodies: clinical results and mechanism

Leukocyte depletion prevents HLA-antibody formation by direct presentation. Meta-analysis of randomised trials calculate a more than 70% reduction in HLA-antibodies after leukocyte depleted platelet transfusions [28, 29]. Residual HLA-antibodies and antibodies against non-HLA antigens expressed by blood cells and proteins result from indirect presentation and from boostering of a memory response e.g. after pregnancy [30]. Indirect immunisation can be prevented by immunoprophylaxis using specific antibodies against the offending antigens, comparable to prevention of Rh-D immunisation. Although it has been shown that this is effective in animal models [31] and foetomaternal transfusions this approach is not practicable in the transfusion setting. Secondary boosting of a memory response to HLA-antibodies is not always prevented by leukocyte removal and once strong and broad-reactive antibodies are present there are no proven concepts to reverse the immune response.

Cancer immunosurveillance

Whether the beneficial effect of blood transfusions on kidney graft survival might have consequences for other transfusion recipients was first questioned by Gantt in 1981: "..is it possible that patients with malignant tumours who receive transfusions of whole blood are suppressed to the point where the malignant tumour has a better chance to survive?"

Since, more than hundred retrospective studies including more than 25,000 patients could not answer this question [32]. Three prospective randomised trials have been conducted in colorectal cancer surgery. In all three studies buffy-coat depleted red blood cells (RBC) were administered in the control arms. Two trials studied the possible beneficial effect of autologous buffy-coat depleted RBC [33, 34] and one the effect of pre-storage filtered red cells [35]. In none of these 3 studies increased cancer recurrence in the control arm compared to the study arm was found. A meta-analysis of the prospective studies excluded a deleterious effect larger than a 1.3 increase in relative risk in cancer recurrence after standard buffy-coat depleted red cell transfusions compared to filtered leukocyte reduced or autologous RBC [36]. However, the results from these randomised studies cannot be extrapolated to other types of cancer. Even it cannot be concluded that there is no deleterious effect of blood transfusions on cancer surveillance, because at the point where tumours are removed often (allele) specific down regulation of HLA antigens has already occurred and tumour cells escape from HLA-restricted cytotoxicity [37].

Blood transfusions and postoperative infections: Clinical results

In observational studies the occurrence of postoperative infections is increased by approximately 20% in per-operative transfused patients compared to non-transfused patients, but it is unknown whether transfusions play a causal role. The role of allogeneic leukocytes as a possible causal factor for the susceptibility for postoperative infections was investigated in eight randomised controlled trials (RCTs), seven in colorectal surgery and one in cardiac surgery.

Two RCTs compared autologous with allogeneic red blood cell (RBC) products, all these RBCs were buffy-coat depleted. In a large Dutch multicenter trial, in which 475 patients were randomised, no difference in infections (25% versus 27%, p 0.64) was found between the allogeneic and the autologous trial arms respectively [34]. In a smaller study from Germany 12% of the 58 patients in the autologous group and 27% of the 62 patients in the allogeneic group developed postoperative infections (p 0.04). In the latter study there were, however, imbalances between the trial arms. In the autologous group none of the non-transfused patients and 8% of the patients who received 1-2 units of homologous RBC suffered from an infection. In comparison 8% in the non-transfused patients in the homologous trial arm and 35% of the patients who received 1-2 homologous units developed postoperative infections. From this it must be concluded that the study group and not the actual transfusion of homologous blood was a risk factor for infection [33]. There is thus no convincing clinical evidence that homologous leukocytes in RBC enhance postoperative infections compared to autologous leukocytes in red cell products.

Six studies investigated filtered leukocyte reduced RBCs [35, 37, 38-42].

In two studies whole blood or red cells containing buffy-coat was used in the control arms [38, 41], the four other studies used RBC without buffy-coat as control. One of the latter studies is only published as poster-abstract [42]. The results are shown in Table 2 . Analysis according to randomisation was given by three studies and none of these yielded a significant difference between the study and control arm (Table 2).

When only transfused patient groups are compared, three studies [38, 39, 41] find less infections in patients who received filtered RBC. Only one of these used buffy-coat depleted RBC in the control arm [39]. In a fourth study that used buffy-coat depleted RBC in the control arm a significant increase in postoperative infections was observed in a subgroup of patients who received 4 or more transfusions [42]. Two studies found no significant differences between transfused trial arms.

The low level of evidence of filtered red blood cells to reduce postoperative infections was extensively discussed, in particular the role of partial leukocyte reduction by buffy-coat depletion in many of the control arms [43].

Causal fsactors and mechanism

The observation that studies with more postoperative infections in the control group did not use buffy-coat depleted RBC and our findings in cardiac surgery patients showing an increased infection rate only in patients who received four or more transfusions , suggest a deleterious dose-dependent effect of leukocytes in RBC contributing to postoperative infections. This effect is determined by the amount of leukocytes per transfusion and number of units transfused. It is unknown whether below a threshold of leukocytes , there is absence of an effect or whether this dose-dependency is linear but at low dosages the effect is so small that it can only be revealed by studies comparing even larger number of patients. Cytokines produced by leukocytes during storage of blood may not play a major role. We compared the effect of post storage filtered red cells, which still contain cytokines a with pre-storage filtered red cells and observed no difference in postoperative infections in cardiac surgery patients [40].

Table 2. Postoperative infection and leukoreduction of peri-operative RBC transfusions.

Author	Jensen '92	Houbiers '94	Jensen '96	v.d. Watering '98	Tartter '98	Litlestad 2000
Type of surgery	abdominal	colorectal	abdominal	cardiac	abdominal	colorectal
Number of patients	197	679	586	909	221	279
Control arm	WB	RBC-bcd	RBC-bcd	RBC-bcd	RBC	RBC-bcd
Study arm	SF-RBC	SF-RBC	SF-RBC	FF/ SF-RBC	SF-RBC	FF-RBC
Analysis according to randomisation						
Infections	10%	33%	17.5%	20%	16%	30%
All patients:						
in controls	NA	32	NA	23	NA	32
in study arm	NA	36	NA	17/18	NA	28
Significance	NA	p.42	NA	p.13	NA	p>.05
Analysis according to transfusion						
Transfused %/N patients	53%/104	64%/446	44%/258	92%/861	27%/59	45%/112
Infections						
in control arm	23%	36%	17%	>4 units 31%	44%	45%
in study arm	2%	42%	3.5%	>4 units 24%/21%	16%	38%
Significance	p.0033	p>.75	<.0001	p.04	p<.063	0.525

WB: whole blood; RBC: red blood cells; bcd: buffy-coat depleted; FF: fresh filtered; SF: stored filtered; NA: not available.

Postoperative infections observed are wound infections, lower urinary tract infections often associated with indwelling catheters and lower respiratory infections associated with artificial ventilation introducing nosocomial micro-organisms during and after surgery. An effective host defence against microbial invasion requires recruitment of leukocytes to the extra-vascular sites, needing rolling, sticking and diapedesis. The intruding micro-organisms are then cleared by macrophages and NK cells with the help of antibodies and complement. Blood transfusions may compromise leukocyte locomotion and phagocyte functions. Several lines of evidence are available that sub-lethally damaged red cells and leukocyte aggregates block phagocytosis [45]. Storage of blood enhancing micro-aggregate formation and increasing the number of non-viable erythrocytes may aggravate these deleterious effects. Modest reduction of leukocytes below 90% should prevent micro-aggregate formation (45).

(Multi) Organ failure and blood transfusions: clinical results

Massive transfusion is life-saving in bleeding, but mortality increases with the amount transfused and is after two or more exchanges of the blood volume still 30-60%. Multiple transfusions are often needed in critical situations and it is difficult to estimate the contribution of transfusions in addition to re-perfusion injury after tissue damage or shock from bleeding. In particular ARDS (acute respiratory distress syndrome) as a consequence from micro-aggregates in heavily transfused trauma patients was suspected [46] but may be of minor importance compared to the role of sepsis or lipid emboli [47]. In our study in cardiac surgery patients we found an increase of mortality in patients transfused with buffy-coat depleted RBC compared to patients transfused with pre- or post-storage filtered erythrocytes (Table 3). When the number of transfusions was analysed the increase in mortality was only present in patients who received four or more RBC. This group also suffered from more complicated surgery.

Table 3. Cause of death in a randomised study in 914 patients comparing three RBC products.

Patient number	**Total no 914**	**PC no 306**	**FF no 305**	**SF no 303**	**P**
Cardiac causes of death	Total 12	14	10	9	.53
Infarction	11	4	4	3	
Heart failure	13	6	3	4	
Arrhythmia	9	4	3	2	
Non-cardiac death	Total 12	10	1	1	.001
Multiorgan failure	9	7	1	1	
Anastomotic dehiscence	3	3	0	0	

PC: RBC buffy-coat depleted; FF: prestorage filtered RBC; SF: RBC filtered after storage.

Causal factors and possible mechanism

Although there is preliminary evidence that allogeneic transfusions, and in particular leukocytes, can contribute to multi-organ dysfunction (MODS) the pathophysiology is far from clear. Tissue damage and repair cause profound alterations in cellular immunity, which are of short duration for a few weeks after surgery. NK function [38] and delayed type hypersensitivity [49], both Th type 1 functions, are decreased after surgical interventions . In line with this, decrease of interleukin (IL)-12, a crucial cytokine for dendritic cells to induce the Th1 helper response has been found in critical ill patients [49]. Surgery thus induces a Th2 type response and peri-operative transfusions further skew the immune response towards the Th2 type with increase of IL-4 and IL-10 [50]. It was postulated that a Th2 type response is a normal stress reaction in absence of a specific antigenic stimulus in order to protect an individual against a systemic inflammatory response reaction [51]. Major surgery and transfusions elicit such a Th2 type stress reaction, which enhances susceptibility for infection [49].

How does MODS and the role of transfused leukocytes fit into this Th2 model? MODS is the result of a dys-balanced inflammatory response reaction. In animal models MODS requires neutrophils and Tumour Necrosis Factor-alfa (TNF-α), which are induced by a Th1 response [53]. We presume that for MODS a (relative) increase of Th1 cytokines is required, while the Th2 system is already activated. This relative increase of Th1 can be the result of an allogeneic effect, but in addition, recipient genetic and environmental factors such as cardiovascular bypass or endotoxins, contribute to the disbalance.

Conclusion

Any blood transfusion modulates the immune system of the recipient. For intended immunomodulation of MHC-restricted responses increase in knowledge of regulatory circuits will ultimately allow specific modulation with purified cells. Unintended immunomodulation by blood transfusion remains. The clinical consequences on the host adoptive and innate cellular immune response are largely unknown and precise measurements for more appropriate donor and product selection are not available. Future clinical and fundamental studies should focus on effects of MHC-sharing or mismatch, micro-aggregates, activation of leukocytes and platelets during processing and on non-viable erythrocytes and other residual cells during storage.

References

1. Fast L.D. Recipient elimination of allogeneic lymphoid cells: donor CD4+ cells. are effective alloantigen-presenting cells. Blood, 2000;96:1144-48.
2. Opelz G, Sengar DFP, Mickey MR, Terasaki PI. Effect of blood transfusions on subsequent kidney transplants. Transplant Proc 1971;5:253-59.
3. Opelz G, Vanrenterhem Y, Kirste G, Gray DW, et al. Prospective evaluation of pretransplant blood transfusion in cadaver kidney recipients. Transplantation 1997, 63:964-6.
4. Opelz G, Terasaki PI. Improvement of kidney-graft survival with increased numbers of transfusions. N Engl J Med 1978;299:799-803.
5. Lagaaij EL, Henneman IP, Ruigrok M, et al. Effect of one-HLA-DR antigen matched and completely HLA-DR mismatched blood transfusions on survival of heart and kidney allografts. New Eng J Med 1989;321:701-05.
6. Vervoordeldonck SF, Doumaid K, Remmerswaal M et al. Long-term detection of microchimaerism in peripheral blood after pretransplantation blood transfusion. Br J Haematol 1998;102:1004-09.
7. Mincheff MS, Meryman HT, Kapoor V, Alsop P, Wotzel M. Blood Transfusion and immunomodulation a possible mechanism. Vox Sang 1993:65:18-24.
8. Mc Donald JC, Adamashvili I. Soluble HLA. Human Immunology 1998;59:387-403.
9. Hodge G, Lloyd JV, Hodge S, Story C, Han P. Functional lymphocyte immunophenotypes observed in thalassaemia and haemophilia patients receiving current blood product preparations. Br J Haematol 1999,105:817-25.
10. Hay CRM, Mc Evoy P, Duggan-Keen M. Inhibition of lymphocyte IL-3 receptor expression by factor VIII concentrate: A possible cause of immunosuppression in haemophiliacs. Br J Haematol 1990;75:278-81.
11. Young NT, Roelen DL, Iggo N, et al. Effect of one HLA-haptotype matched and HLA mismatched blood transfusions on recipient T lymphocyte allorepertoires. Transplantation 1997;63:1160-65.

12. van der Mast BJ, Hornstra N, Ruigrok MB, Claas FJH, van Rood JJ, Lagaaij EL. Transfusion-associated graft-versus-host disease in immunocompetent patients: a self protective mechanism. Lancet 1994;343:753.
13. Kolb HJ, Schattenberg A, Goldman JM, et al. Graft-versus leukemia effect of donor lymphocyte transfusions in marrow grafted patients. Blood 1995;86:2041-50.
14. Hirano N, Takanashi T. Ohtake S et al. Expression of costimulatory molecules in human leukemias. Leukemia 1996;10:1168-76.
15. Mackinnon S, Papadopoulos EB, Carabasi MH, et al. Adoptive immunotherapy evaluating escalating doses of donor leukocytes for relaps of chronic myeloid leukemia after bone marrow transplantation: Separation of graft-versus-leukemia responses from graft-versus-host disease. Blood 1995;86:1261-68.
16. Turner JH, Hutchinson DL, Petricciani JC. Chimerism following fetal transfusion: report of leukocyte hybridization and infant with acute lymphocytic leukaemia. Scand J Haematol 1973;10:358-60.
17. Bianchi DW, Zickwolf GK, Weil GJ, Sylvester S, DeMaria MA. Male fetal progenitor cells persist in maternal blood for as long as 27 years postpartum. Proc Natl Acad Sci USA 1996;93:705.
18. Viëtor HE, Hallensleben E, van Bree SPMJ, et al. Survival of donor cells 25 years after intrauterine transfusion. Blood 2000;95:2709-14.
19. Jones WR. Immunological aspects of intrauteriene transfusion. BMJ 1968;3:280.
20. Fowler R, Schubert WK, West CD. Acquired partial tolerance to homologous skin grafts in the human infant at birth. Ann NY Acad Sci 1960;87:403.
21. Lee TH, Paglieroni T, Ohto H, Holland PV, Busch MP. Survival of donor leukocyte subpopulations in immunocompetent transfusion recipients: frequent long-term microchimerism in severe trauma patients. Blood 1999;93:3127-39.
22. Jungi TW, Nydegger UE. Proposed mechanisms of action of IVIg in autoimmune diseases. Transfus Sci 1992;13:267-300.
23. Brand A, Vuist WM, van Schaik IN, Vermeulen M. In vitro investigation of immunoglobulin treatment mechanisms in autoimmune diseases. Clin Exper Rheumatol 1996;14 (suppl. 15):27-30.
24. Ghetie V, Ward SE: FcRn: the MHC cluss I-related receptor that is more than an IgG transporter. Immunol Today 1997:592-95.
25. Fehr J, Hofmann V, Kappeler U. Transient reversal of thrombocytopenia in idiopathic thrombocytopenic ipurpura by high-dose intravenous gammaglobulin. N Engl J Med 1982;306:1254-58.
26. Vermeulen M, van der Meché FGA, Speelman JD, Weber A, Busch HFM. Plasma and gamma-globulin infusion in chronic inflammatory polyneuropathy. J Neurol Sci 1985;70:317-26.
27. Blumberg N, Heal JM, Evidence for plasma-mediated immunomodulation transfusions of plasma-rich blood components are associated with a greater risk of acquired immunodeficiency syndrome than transfusions of red blood cells alone. Transplant Proc 1988;20:1138-42.
28. Vamvakas EC, Meta-analysis of randomized controlled trials of the efficacy of white cell reduction in preventing HLA-Alloimmunization and refractoriness to random-donor platelet transfusions. Transf Med Rev 1998;12:258-70.
29. Co-operative study group. Leukocyte Reduction and ultraviolet B irradiation of platelets to prevent alloimmunization and refractoriness to platelet transfusions. N Engl J Med 1997;337:1861-69.
30. Sintnicolaas K, van Marwijk Kooij M, van Prooijen HC, et al. Leukocyte depletion of random single-donor platelet transfusions does not prevent secondary human leukocyte antigen-alloimmunisation and refractoriness: a randomized prospective study. Blood 1995;85:824-28.
31. Lazarus AH, Crow AR. Semple JW, et al. Induction of a secundary human anti-HLA alloimmune response in severe combined immunodeficient mice engrafted with human lymphocytes. Transfusion 1997;37:1192-99.

32. Brand A, Houbiers JGA. Clinical Studies of Blood Transfusion and Cancer. In: Vamvakas EC, Blajchman MA, eds Immunomodulatory Effects of Blood Transfusion. AABB Press, 1999:145-90.
33. Heis MM, Jauch KW, Delanoff C, et al. Blood transfusion modulated tumor recurrence: A randomized study of autologous versus homologous blood transfusion in colorectal cancer. J Clin Oncol 1994;12:1859-67.
34. Busch ORC, Hop WJC, van Papendrecht MAWH, et al. Blood transfusions and prognosis in colorectal cancer. N Engl J Med 1993;328:1372-76.
35. Houbiers JGA, Brand A, van de Watering LMG, et al. Randomized controlled trial comparing transfusion of leukocyte-depleted or buffy-coat-depleted blood in surgery for colorectal cancer. Lancet 1994;344:573-78.
36. Vamvakas E. Transfusion-associated cancer recurrence and infection: Meta-analysis of the randomized controlled clinical trials. Transfusion 1996;36:175-86.
37. Smith MEF, Bodmer WF, Bodmer JG, Selective loss of HLA- A,B and C locus products in colorectal adenocarcinoma. Proc Natl Acad Sci 1989;86:5557-61.
38. Jensen LS, Andersen AJ, Christiansen PM, et al. Postoperative infection and natural killer cell fucntion following blood transfusion in patients undergoing elective colerectal surgery. Br J Surg. 1992;79:513-16.
39. Jensen LS, Kissmeyer-Nielsen P, Wolff B, et al. Randomized comparison of leukocyte-depleted verus buffy-coat-poor blood transfusion and complications after colorectal surgery. Lancet 1996;348:841-45..
40. van de Watering LMG, Hermans J, Houbiers JGA et al. Beneficial effects of leukocyte depletion of transfused blood on postoperative complications in patients undergoing cardiac surgery. Am Heart Assoc 1998:562-68.
41. Tartter PI, Mohandas K, Azar P, Endres J, Kaplan J, Spivack M. Randomized trial comparing packed red cell blood transfusion with and without leukocyte depletion for gastrointestinal surgery. Am J Surg 1998;176:462-66.
42. Titlestad IL, Ebbesen LE, Ainsworth A, Lillevang ST, Qvist N, Georgsen J. Leukocyte depletion and complications to colorectal surgery. Vox Sang 2000. (Abstract ISBT).
43. Blajchman MA. Allogeneic blood transfusions, immunomodulation and postoperative bacterial infection: Do we have the answers yet? Editorial. Transfusion 1997; 37:121-25.
44. Editorial. Block the phagocytes. Lancet 1993:342:199.
45. Swank RL, Seaman GVF. Microfiltration and microemboli: a history. Transfusion 2000;40:114-19.
46. International Forum. Does a relationship exist between massive blood transfusions and the adult repiratory distress syndrome? If so, what are the best preventive measures? Vox Sang 1977;32:311-20.
47. Ware LB, Matthay MA. The acute respiratory distress syndrome. N Engl J Med 2000;342:1334-48.
48. Nielsen HJ, Hammer JH, Moesgaard F, Kehlet H. Ranitidine prevents postoperative transfusion-induced depression of delayed hypersensitivity. Surgery 1989;105:711-19.
49. Ertel W, Keel M, Neidhardt R, Steckholzer U, Kremer JP, Ungethuem U, Trentz O. Inhibition of the defense system stimulating interleukin-12 interferon-(pathway during critical illness. Blood 1997;89:1612-20.
50. Kirkley SA. Cowles J, Pellegrini VD, Harris CM. Boyd AD. Blumberg N. Blood transfusion and total joint replacement surgery: T helper 2 (TH2) cytokine secretion and clinical outcome. Transplant Med 1998:8:195-204.
51. Matzinger P. Tolerance, danger and the extended family. Annu Rev Immunol 1994; 12:991-1045.

DEVELOPMENT AND IMPLEMENTATION OF NEW CELLULAR THERAPIES

J. McCullough[1]

Introduction

The original concept of blood component therapy involved separating a standard unit (approximately 450 mL) of whole blood into red cells, plasma, and platelets in order to store each component under ideal conditions and to make the different components of whole blood available for different kinds of patients. This revolutionized transfusion therapy. However, the number and kind of components that can be prepared are limited by the volume and composition of the whole blood collected. The next advance in the production of blood components and blood component therapy was the development of blood cell separators and apheresis. This made it possible to process a larger volume of donor blood and selectively remove one component to produce a much larger blood component from an individual donor. Developments in science and technology are now making it possible to produce new, even more complex blood components.

Hematopoietic Stem Cells as a Blood Component

Bone Marrow

During the last 20 years, hematopoietic cell transplantation has become a widely used therapy [1] and hematopoietic stem cells can be considered a third generation of blood component therapy. There are several reasons to consider hematopoietic stem cells a blood component [2]. Bone marrow looks like blood, has a cellular composition similar to peripheral blood, is usually contained and manipulated in the same kind of plastic bag systems as whole blood, and is administered to patients as a transfusion, even though this is called a transplant procedure. Although bone marrow is obtained by bone puncture and in the operating room, the issues involved in stem cell 'banking' are similar to blood banking [3] (Table 1). Thus, the expertise of those involved in transfusion medicine is needed for effective conduct of these processes and procedures.

---

1. Department of Lab Med and Pathol, Univ of Minnesota, Minneapolis, MN, USA.

Table 1. General areas of stem cell 'banking'.

Donor evaluation
Collection
Processing
Preservation
Transportation
Thawing
Transfusion

As hematopoietic cell transplantation has become more widely used, the source of cells for transplantation has become more diverse. In addition to marrow, peripheral blood stem cells, umbilical cord blood, unrelated marrow donors, partially matched related donors, and women who have recently delivered a baby (cord blood) are all potential sources of hematopoietic stem cells for transplantation. As stem cell transplantation has increased in complexity, a variety of procedures have been developed for manipulating the stem cells in order to improve the results of transplantation. These manipulations range from simple reduction of the volume of marrow to be transplanted by removing plasma in order to avoid fluid overload in the recipient to depletion of T-lymphocytes or malignant cells from the marrow; cryopreservation of marrow, peripheral blood stem cells, or cord blood for long-term storage; selection of primitive progenitor cells; and expansion in culture systems of different populations of primitive cells (Table 2). This increased the number of different methods used to manipulate hematopoietic stem cells and the different starting products result in a wide variety of different final blood cellular components, each with different characteristics and prepared for a particular therapeutic strategy.

Peripheral Blood Stem Cells (PBSCs)

Hematopoietic progenitor cells circulate in the peripheral blood although in relatively smaller numbers than in the bone marrow. These peripheral blood stem cells (PBSCs) can be collected by apheresis [4, 5]. The growth factor G-CSF is used to increase in the level of circulating PBSCs from 0.05% pretreatment to about 1.5% after 5 days [6-9]. This results in a yield of CD34+ cells of about 4.5×10^{8} from a single apheresis which is adequate for a transplant for most adult's transplants [10]. The use of PBSCs began with autologous but has been extended to allogeneic transplantation. Transplants using PBSCs are successful and the time to engraftment is shorter than with marrow. The larger dose of T-cells contained does not cause an increase in acute graft-versus-host disease. This new hematopoietic progenitor component for stem cell transplantation eliminates marrow collection in the operating suite, the attendant risks of anesthesia, and the marrow collection process. The extent to which PBSCs will replace marrow remains to be determined but the advantage of more rapid engraftment makes this transplant strategy very attractive. Most of the issues involved in the production of traditional blood components apply to PBSCs. There

Table 2. General stem cell processing procedures.

Volume reduction
RBC depletion
Bone marrow
Cord blood
Buffy-coat preparation
Purging marrow of malignant cells
Immunotoxins
4HC
Antibody-complement
T-cell depletion of bone marrow
Elutriation
Immunotoxin
Antibody-complement
Positive stem cell (CD34+) selection
Magnetic beads
Antibody coated flasks
Antibody coated colums
Transduction-genes using viral vectors
Peripheral blood lymphocytes
Bone marrow stem cells
Peripheral blood stem cells
Cord blood stem cells
Expansion
Stem cells
Myeloid
Lymphocytes
Freezing and storing
Bone marrow
Peripheral blood stem cells
Cord blood

is an even greater donor safety issue due to the administration of G-CSF. Thus, PBSCs are very much a blood component.

Stem Cell and Myeloid Ex Vivo Cell Expansion

Developments in the understanding of hematopoiesis and the discovery of many hematopoietic growth factors and cytokines have now made possible an even more sophisticated production of blood components. Combinations of cytokines and growth factors can be used with different selected populations of hematopoietic cells to activate or expand the number of those cells ex vivo to develop a new therapeutic blood product [2, 11]. Many investigators are attempting to increase the number of hematopoietic stem cells without inducing maturation. In this way, very small amounts of marrow or small numbers of primordial cells could be multiplied ex vivo in the laboratory to generate a dose suitable for transplantation. Unfortunately, this has not yet been successful. However, successful culture systems have been developed to expand ex vivo the number of progenitors and this results in a blood product with a mixture of different degrees of maturation from very primitive to relatively mature hematopoietic progenitors [12-16]. These ex vivo cell expansion systems can increase the number of CD34+ cells or CFU-GM colonies by up to 60 fold. It was hoped that transfusion of these components along with the stem cell transplant would greatly reduce the period of neutropenia and/or thrombocytopenia since partially mature cells would be transfused. In general this strategy has not proven to be effective in shortening the period of neutropenia, possibly due to the increasing use of peripheral blood stem cells, autologous marrow transplants, and other patient management strategies.

Adoptive Immunotherapy

Subsets of peripheral blood mononuclear cells can be isolated and expanded ex vivo and these components are proving to be useful clinically. Transfusion of these mononuclear cell blood components induces particular types of immunity and has been called adoptive immunotherapy.

Adjunct to Hematopoietic Progenitor Transplantation

During the past decade, it has become clear that hematopoietic stem cell transplantation provides a graft versus leukemia (GVL) effect. This observation led to the use of supplemental transfusions of donor lymphocytes to patients who experienced relapse of chronic myelogenous leukemia (CML) following transplantation [17-19]. This adoptive immunotherapy induces remission in these patients and is being used to prevent relapse [20]. The lymphocytes are obtained by routine apheresis techniques and transfused to the patients without extensive manipulation. This adoptive immunotherapy of transfusing donor mononuclear cells following marrow transplantation is now being used to treat some solid tumors [21].

Cancer Immunotherapy

Initial attempts at cancer immunotherapy involved the activation of peripheral blood lymphocytes with cytokines in order to enhance their anti-tumor activity (lymphokine-activated killer or LAK cells) and the large-scale expansion of lymphocytes infiltrating tumors (tumor infiltrating lymphocytes or TIL cells) [22-25]. The transfusion of large numbers of LAK cells along with cytokines provided some modest clinical benefit [22], but because this was a rather general immunotherapy approach these cells were not specific for the patient's particular tumor. The use of TIL cells improved the immunotherapy approach in that these cells were more specific for the patient's own tumor, but this strategy also had limited success [23-25].

Recently this cancer immunotherapy has become more specific. For instance, isolation of patients' T-cells with ability to inhibit growth of their own malignant cells, ex vivo expansion of the clone, and transfusion of these cells has induced remission in CML [26]. The recognition that cancer immunotherapy must be more individualized to particular tumors has led to the use of dendritic cells.

Dendritic Cells

Dendritic cells (DC) develop from bone marrow precursors, enter the circulation and migrate to tissues where after exposure to antigens or other soluble inflammatory mediators such as cytokines, and they process antigen for presentation in a complex with the major histocompatibility complex (MHC) molecules. As the dendritic cell presents the complex of antigen and the MHC molecule to T-lymphocytes, the lymphocytes become primed and activate T-cells with cytotoxic specificity for the particular antigen. Cytokines and growth factors also produced in this process result in proliferation of these cytotoxic T-cells to produce a clone of cytotoxic cells specific for the antigen originally processed by the dendritic cell [27]. This antigen processing and subsequent selection of a specific cytotoxic T-cell clone can be carried out ex vivo to generate large numbers of cytotoxic T-cells for therapy. Presently a number of trials of tumor immunotherapy transfusing cytotoxic T-lymphocytes generated ex vivo by dendritic cell antigen presentation are underway [27]. Diseases being studied include melanoma, renal cell carcinoma, B-cell lymphoma, CML, and carcinoma of the prostate [28-33]. This is an exciting strategy for cancer immunotherapy which has proven to be successful in laboratory animals and shows promise in patients.

Immunotherapy for Infectious Disease

Lymphocytes with cytotoxicity against cytomegalovirus (CMV) can be isolated and increased by number by ex vivo culture. When cells are obtained from the hematopoietic stem cell donor and transfused to the recipient, immunity to CMV is promptly restored and, thus, posttransplant CMV infections are minimized [34]. Similarly, T-cells with cytotoxicity for Epstein-Barr virus can be isolated and increased in number ex vivo and used as a transfusion blood component to treat posttransplant lymphoproliferative disease which is due to EBV [35, 36].

A similar approach could be taken for the treatment of some autoimmune diseases. The patient's lymphocytes could be collected by apheresis, the clone with the desired immunologic activity isolated and increased by ex vivo culture with appropriate cytokines, then transfused as a temporary treatment of the autoimmune disease.

Thus, peripheral blood mononuclear cells are a rich source of new blood components for provision of adoptive immunotherapy in several situations. The cells may undergo general activation and expansion for anti-tumor effect, clones of these cells can be isolated for an anti-viral or anti-tumor effect, or dendritic cells can be isolated and used to present antigen to prime cytotoxic lymphocytes to develop clones of cells with specific anti-tumor or anti-viral activity.

Gene Therapy

Inherited Disease

Although gene therapy is exciting, its potential has not yet been realized. Some of the first gene therapy treatments involved the use of peripheral blood lymphocytes from the patient and ex vivo culture, expansion, and transduction of those cells to insert a normal copy of the defective gene [37] and we have carried out a similar protocol [38]. These transduced lymphocytes were then transfused to the patients in an effort to provide temporary gene replacement. These efforts have met with very limited success. Initial hopes to transduce the primitive hematopoietic stem cell so that a cure of genetic disease could be obtained by transplantation of cells containing normal genes has proven to be extremely difficult because of the inability to obtain stable transduction of a large percentage of primitive hematopoietic stem cells. However, as efforts to develop gene therapy continue, it seems likely that in the future suspensions of cells containing a normal gene will be prepared ex vivo and administered either as a transfusion for temporary treatment or permanent transplant to correct inherited disease. This will represent an even more complex and sophisticated blood component.

Malignant Disease

Another form of gene therapy is being developed as a potential treatment for cancer. By inserting genes such as tumor necrosis factor (TNF), interleukin-2, or others into tumor cells, it is possible to increase the immune recognition of the tumor and, thus, deliver toxic agents directly to the tumor [22]. In separate studies, a marker gene was inserted into lymphocytes in order to determine the survival of the activated anti-cancer cells [22]. More recently a 'suicide gene' has been inserted into T-cells given to facilitate engraftment of hematopoietic stem cells [39]. If graft-versus-host disease occurs, medication can be administered to the patient to kill the genetically transduced T-cells and reduce the graft-versus-host disease. Thus, it is possible that peripheral blood cells will become used as part of a broad anticancer gene therapy and, thus, become another blood component.

Regulation of New Blood Components

The development of a regulatory approach to these new blood components is complex. The components are still undergoing refinement – none is anywhere near the present standardized blood component. Virtually all of these new components are used as experimental therapeutic agents in clinical trials. None is yet produced in very large quantity, and it can be expected that this phase of multiple products undergoing further development will continue. However, it seems clear that these products will be regulated as biologics in a manner similar to blood components [40].

Conclusion

Scientific and technologic developments are making possible the development of many new blood cell components. These are being used to treat a variety of malignant, viral, and immune diseases. Several organizations are collaborating to develop standards for hematopoietic progenitor cells. In addition, it seems appropriate to begin to prepare these new blood components using well thought out quality assurance systems. This will provide the most consistency in these new blood components, and provide the best opportunity to relate the benefits observed to the component itself. Transfusion medicine professionals can make valuable contributions to these developments and should actively participate in the further development, refinement, and production of these exciting new therapeutic agents.

References

1. Sobocinski KA, Horowitz MM, Rowlings PA, et al. Bone marrow transplantation--1994: A report from the International Bone Marrow Transplant Registry and the North American Autologous Bone Marrow Transplant Registry. J Hematotherapy 1994;3:95-102.
2. McCullough, J. The new generation of blood components. Transfusion 1995;35:374-77.
3. McCullough J, Lasky LC, Warkentin PI. Role of the blood bank in bone marrow transplantation, in Advances in Immunobiology: Blood Cell Antigens and Bone Marrow Transplantation, New York, Alan R. Liss, Inc., 1984:379-412.
4. Hillyer CE, Lackey DA, Hart KK, et al. CD34+ progenitors and colony-forming units--granulocyte macrophage are recruited during large-volume leukapheresis and concentrated by counterflow centrifugal elutriation. Transfusion 1993;33:316-21.
5. Snyder EL, Baril L, Min K, et al. In vitro collection and posttransfusion engraftment characteristics of MNCs obtained using a new separator for autologous PBPC transplantation. Transfusion 2000; 40:961-67.
6. Stroncek DF, Clay ME, Petzoldt ML, et al. Treatment of normal individuals with granulocyte-colony-stimulating factor: donor experiences and the effects on peripheral blood CD34+ cell counts and on the collection of peripheral blood stem cells. Transfusion 1996;36:601-10.
7. Stroncek DF, Clay ME, Herr G, et al. The kinetics of G-CSF mobilization of CD34+ cells in healthy people. Transf Med 1997;7:19-24.
8. Anderlini P, Przepiorka D, Champlin R, Korbling M. Biologic and clinical effects of granulocyte colony-stimulating factor in normal individuals. Blood 1996;88:2819-25.
9. Lane TA, Law P, Maruyama M, et al. Harvesting and enrichment of hematopoietic progenitor cells mobilized into the peripheral blood of normal donors by granulocyte-macrophage colony-stimulating factor (GM-CSF) or G-CSF: potential role in allogeneic marrow transplantation. Blood 1995;85:275-82.
10. Pettengell R, Morgenstern GR, Woll PJ, et al. Peripheral blood progenitor cell transplantation in lymphoma and leukemia using a single apheresis. Transfusion 1993; 82:3770-77.
11. Emerson SG. Ex vivo expansion of hematopoietic precursors, progenitors, and stem cells: the next generation of cellular therapeutics. Blood 1996;87:3082-88.
12. Koller MR, Emerson SG, Palsson BO. Large-scale expansion of human stem and progenitor cells from bone marrow mononuclear cells in continuous perfusion cultures. Blood 1993;82:378-84.

13. Haylock DN, To LB, Dowse TL, Juttner CA, Simmons PJ. Ex vivo expansion and maturation of peripheral blood CD34+ cells into the myeloid lineage. Blood 1992; 80:1405-12.
14. Lee WJ, Loudovaris MF, Oiao X, et al. Large scale selection of CD34+ cells and expansion of neutrophil precursors in PIXY321 for clinical application. Blood 1994; 84; 542a (abstract).
15. Muench MO, Firpo MT, Moore MAS. Bone marrow transplantation with interleukin-1 plus kit-ligand ex vivo expanding bone marrow accelerates hematopoietic reconstitution in mice without the loss of stem cell lineage and proliferative potential. Blood 1993;81:3463-73.
16. Williams S, Lee W, Bender JG, et al. Selection and expansion of peripheral blood CD34+ cells in autologous stem cell transplantation for breast cancer. Blood 1996; 86:1687-91.
17. Porter D, Roth M, McGarigle C, Ferrara J, Antin J. Adoptive immunotherapy induces molecular remission in relapsed CML following allogeneic bone marrow transplantation (BMT). Proc Am Soc Clin Oncol 1993;12:303.
18. Kolb HJ, Mittermuller J, Clemm CH. Donor leukocyte transfusions for treatment of recurrent chronic myelogenous leukemia in marrow transplatn patients. Blood 1990;76; 2462-65.
19. Drobyski WR, Keever CA, Roth MS, et al. Salvage immunotherapy using donor leukocyte infusions as treatment for relapsed chronic myelogenous leukemia after allogeneic bone marrow transplantation: Efficacy and toxicity of a defined T cell dose. Blood 1993; 82:2310-18.
20. van Rhee F, Lin F, Cullis JO, et al. Relapse of chronic myeloid leukemia after allogeneic bone marrow transplant: The case for giving donor leukocyte transfusions before the onset of hematologic relapse. Blood 1994;83:3377-83.
21. Childs R, Chernoff A, Contentin N, et al. Regression of metastatic renal-cell carcinoma after nonmyeloablative allogeneic peripheral-blood stem-cell transplantation. N Engl J Med 2000;343:750-58.
22. Rosenberg SA. Gene therapy for cancer. JAMA 1992;268; 2416-19.
23. Mitropoulos D, Kooi S, Rodriguez-Villanueva J, et al. Characterization of fresh (uncultured) tumor-infiltrating lymphocytes (TIL) and TIL-derived T cell lines from patients with renal cell carcinoma. Clin Exp Immunol 1994;97:321-27.
24. Goedegebuure PS, Douville LM, Li H, et al. Adoptive immunotherapy with tumor-infiltrating lymphocytes and interleukin-2 in patients with metastic malignant melanoma and renal cell carcinoma: a pilot study. J Clin Oncol 1995; 3:1939-49.
25. Belldegrun A, Pierce W, Kaboo R, et al. Interferon-a primed tumor-infiltrating lymphocytes combined with interleukin-2 and interferon-a as therapy for metastatic renal cell carcinoma. Urol 1993;150:1384-90.
26. Falkenberg JHF, Wafelman AR, Joosten P, et al. Complete remission of accelerated phase chronic myeloid leukemia by treatment with leukemia-reactive cytotoxic T lymphocytes. Blood 1999;94:1201-08.
27. Troy AJ, Hart DNJ. Dendritic cells and cancer: progress toward a new cellular therapy. J Hematotherapy 1997;6:523-33.
28. Hsu FJ, Benike C, Fagnoni F, et al. Vaccination of patients with B-cell lymphoma using autologous antigen-pulsed dendritic cells. Nat Med 1996;2:52-58.
29. Murphy G, Tjoa B, Ragde H, et al. Phase I clinical trial: T-cell therapy for prostate cancer using autologous dendritic cells pulsed with HLA-A0201-specific peptides from prostate-specific membrane antigen. Prostate 1996;29:371-80.
30. Nestle FO, Gilliet M, Alljagic S, et al. Vaccination of melanoma patients with peptide-pulsed dendritic cells. Melanoma Res 1997;7:S14.
31. Mayordoma JI, Zorina T, Storkus WJ, et al. Bone marrow-derived dendritic cells pulsed with synthetic tumor peptides elicit protective and therapeutic antitumor immunity. Nat Med 1995;1:1297-302.

32. Karanikas V, Hwang L, Pearson J, et al. Antibody and T cell responses of patients with adenocarcinoma immunized with mannan-MUC1 fusion protein. J Clin Invest 1997;100:2783-92.
33. Choudhury A, Gajewski JL, Liang J, et al. Use of leukemic dendritic cells for the generation of antileukemic cellular cytotoxicity against Philadelphia chromosome-positive chronic myelogenous leukemia. Blood 1997;89;1133-42.
34. Walter EA, Greenberg PD, Gilbert MJ. Reconstitution of cellular immunity against cytomegalovirus in recipients of allogeneic bone marrow by transfer of T-cell clones from the donor. N Engl J Med 1995;333:1038-44.
35. Papadopoulos EB, Ladanyi M, Emanuel D, et al. Infusions of donor leukocytes to treat Epstein-Barr virus-associated lymphoproliferative disorders after allogeneic bone marrow transplantation. N Engl J Med 1994;330:1185-91.
36. Subklewe M, Chahroudi A, Schmalijohn A, Kurilla M, Bhardwaj N, Steinman RM. Induction of Epstein-Barr virus-specific cytotoxic T-lymphocyte responses using dendritic cells pulsed with EBNA-3A peptides or UV-inactivated, recombinant EBNA-3A vaccinia virus. Blood 1999;94:1372-81.
37. Blaese RM, Anderson WF, Culver KW. The ADA human gene therapy clinical protocol. Hum Gene Ther 1990;1:327-62.
38. Stroncek DF, Hubel A, Shankar RA, et al. Retroviral transduction and expansion of peripheral blood lymphocytes for the treatment of mucopolysaccharidosis II, Hunter syndrome. Transfusion 1999;39:343-50.
39. Cohen JL, Boyer O, Salomon B, et al. Prevention of graft-versus-host disease in mice using a suicide gene expressed in T lymphocytes. Blood 1997;89:4636-45.
40. Kessler DA, Siegel JP, Noguchi PD, Zoon KC, Feiden KL, Woodcock J. Regulation of somatic-cell therapy and gene therapy by the Food and Drug Administration. N Engl J Med 1993; 329:1169-73.

TRANSFUSION MEDICINE AND THE DEVELOPMENT OF GENE THERAPY

M.L. Turner[1]

Introduction

For many years it has been proposed that genetic modification of human cells could be undertaken for therapeutic purposes. The first human experimentation was initiated in 1980 when Cline and colleagues treated two patients with end stage thalassaemia. The study was regarded at the time as premature and based on insufficient pre-clinical data [1]. There was a subsequent gap of some ten years before the first approved gene marking protocol was initiated in 1989. In this study, tumour infiltrating lymphocytes were obtained from a patient with malignant melanoma. Part of the tumour was resected, a tumour cell suspension created and the cells cultured in Interleukin 2 (IL-2). The T lymphocytes were subjected to retroviral transduction with a transgene encoding for neomycin resistance. No adverse effects were observed and the genetically marked T lymphocytes were found to persist in the patient for several weeks following transfusion [2]. The first gene therapy protocol was initiated in 1990 in two patients with adenosine deaminase (ADA) deficiency, which gives rise to severe combined immunodeficiency (SCID). These children underwent retroviral transduction of IL-2 expanded autologous peripheral blood T lymphocytes with a transgene encoding the ADA gene. Post infusion it was found that the patients had 20-25% circulating gene-corrected T cells, some improvement in immune function and resolution of clinical symptoms. Both patients however remained on PEG-ADA replacement therapy [3].

From these fairly humble beginnings, there has been a marked increase in the number of approved clinical protocols. As of August 2000, there were 431 clinical protocols awaiting initiation or in progress, 393 in the United States and 38 in other countries [4]. Although almost all the initial gene therapy protocols involved ex vivo cellular manipulation, the picture now is more balanced, with 242 clinical protocols involving direct in vivo administration of the transgene and 189 involving ex vivo cellular engineering. The breakdown of indications is summarised in Table 1. Clinical studies in cardiovascular disease and cystic fibrosis largely involve in vivo gene therapy, those involving lysosomal storage

1. Univ of Edinburgh and Leukaemia Research Fund John Hughes Bennett Laboratories, Western General Hospital, Edinburgh, Scotland.

Table 1. Current clinical gene therapy protocols.

	in vivo	*ex vivo*	Total
Cancer	164	152	316
Cystic fibrosis	22		22
Cardiovascular disease	25		25
HIV	9	9	18
Single gene disorders	10	16	26
Others	12	12	24
Total	242	189	431

diseases involve ex vivo cellular manipulation, and those in cancer, HIV and haemophilia are split between the two approaches.

Overall it can be said that the safety/tolerability of gene therapy has been found to be reasonably good. Over 4,000 patients have now being treated on clinical protocol with some 40 'long-term' survivors, the 2 initially treated patients with ADA SCID, 5 patients with familiar hypercholesterolaemia and 30 patients with cystic fibrosis. Thus far there has been no evidence of the increased risk of tumour formation and no evidence of germline transmission. However in September 1999, gene therapy reached something of a watershed with the first death [5]. Jesse Gelsinger, an 18 year old patient with partial ornithine transcarbamylase deficiency, received an E1B deleted adenovirus direct into the hepatic artery as part of a phase I clinical trial. Within hours he suffered a fatal immunological reaction. The University of Pennsylvania was subject to significant criticism to the effect that it had failed to report previous adverse reactions and that supervision of the study was inadequate, and its Institute for Human Gene Therapy was forced to suspend all clinical studies.

Despite this setback the year 2000 has brought the first modest gene therapy successes and, with completion of the first draft of the human genome project, promises exiting progress to come.

Vectors for Cellular Transfection and Transduction

The ideal gene transfection vector should be capable of easy and sustained production, should be immunologically inert, capable of targetting to specific cells or tissues, should have an high transgene carrying capacity, allow efficient site specific chromosomal integration and be capable of transfecting non-dividing as well as dividing cells. No current vector display all these features, though different groups of vectors display different combinations of features.

Physical gene transfection vectors have been in use in laboratory research for many years (Table 2a). These include calcium phosphate precipitation, electroporation, various forms of liposomes including cationic lipsomes and non-ionic surfactant vesicles, DNA-ligand complexes and cell microinjection. Overall, these reagents and devices are relatively easy to produce, present few toxicity and immunological problems and can incorporate large amounts of DNA

(>30kb). However, whilst some of these approaches give satisfactory transient transfection efficiencies, stable transfection efficiencies are low due to poor integration of the transgene into the host genome. The transgene therefore fails to replicate during cell division and genetic material is diluted out. Also the introduced DNA is often present in a coneatemeric form which means that the copy number and physical orientation is uncontrolled and the regulation of expression difficult. Finally, in the majority of cells, the introduced genetic material is degraded and lost. Physical vectors have not been widely used in clinical gene therapy and where used, tend to be confined to conditions in which transient expression of the transgene in a large number of cells is likely to be helpful eg. modulation of host immunity [6].

Viral vectors are much more widely used in clinical gene therapy protocols because they can provide sustained and high level expression of the transgene. They are derived from viruses by replacing the genetic elements essential for replication with the transgene. Examples include the retroviruses, adenovirus and adeno-associated virus (Table 2b).

Table 2. Vectors used for cellular gene transfection and transduction.

a. Physical gene transfer
–Naked DNA
–Calcium phosphate precipitation
–Electroporation
–Liposomes
–DNA – Ligand complexes
–Cellular microinjection
b. Viral gene transduction vectors
– Retroviral vectors
–Adenoviral vectors
–Adeno-associated viral vectors
–Lentivirus
–Vaccinia
–Herpes viruses

Retrovirus mediated gene transfer systems have been widely used, particularly those based on the Moloney murine-leukaemia virus. Some important functions are provided in cis by the LTRs and Psi sequence, but the gag, pol and env elements can be removed from the single-stranded RNA virus and replaced by a promoter and the gene of interest. A packaging cell line engineered to contain the gag, pol and env sequences provides these functions in trans. Thus the retroviral vector with its transgene can infect a target cell but no further replication can occur. Random insertion into the host genome occurs, allowing stable transduction and retention of the transgene during cellular replication. However, there are a number of limitations, the maximum insert size is around 7kb and stable integration only occurs in replicating cells. Concerns exist that the random genomic integration could give rise to insertional mutagenesis, or that recombination events could lead to the generation of replication competent retrovirus. The Moloney murine-leukaemia virus is rapidly destroyed by human complement in vivo and has been mainly used in the context of ex vivo cell transduction.

Adenoviral vectors are able to encompass larger transgenes (up to 20 kb) and can be produced at high titres, can be used for gene delivery in vivo and will transduce a wide variety of human cell types. Genome integration does not occur and the transgene is maintained as an episome. Concerns relate to the possibility of recombination with wild-type adenoviruses resulting in new infectious adenovirus containing the transgene. Additionally the existing human immune response to adenovirus can limit efficacy and give rise to significant toxicity as demonstrated by the Gelsinger case.

Adeno-associated virus (AVV) is a small parvovirus which requires a helper virus (usually adenovirus or herpes virus) to replicate. It can transduce non-replicating cells, integrates into the genome at a specific site on chromosome 19 and is non pathogenic in man. Its limitations are related to its small transgene carrying capacity (of around 2.5kb) and the difficulty of generating high titre virus. Clinically AAV have been used since 1994 to transduce haematopoietic and pulmonary epithelial cells. Concerns include the difficulty of ensuring that clinical grade preparations are free of contamination with wild-type helper virus and the immune response to AAV which may reduce efficacy and increase toxicity.

There is considerable work ongoing with other viral vectors including lentiviruses (such as modified HIV), vaccinia, herpes viruses (such as herpes simplex and Epstein Barr virus), rabies, Semliki forest virus, hepatitis B, polio and influenza.

Several chimaeric methods of gene transfer combining physical and viral vectors are also under investigation. Examples include inactivated adenovirus with DNA bound by polylysine which uses the biological properties of the adenovirus to improve cellular uptake and lysosomal release of the transgene.

Regulation of Transgene Expression

Transgene expression remains problematic even in those cells in which stable transduction occurs. The major focus of researchers at present is on maximising the level of expression and on achieving persistence of expression. Even in the presence of stable transduction, silencing of transgenes tends to occur, probably due to inhibitory transcriptional factors, methylation of cytosine bases in the long-terminal repeats and inaccessible chromatin conformation. Ideally, researchers would wish to achieve tight regulation over transgene expression, including control over the integration site and copy number (to minimise the risk of insertional mutagenesis), control over the level of expression (particularly where excessively high expression may cause toxicity), control over the duration of expression (inducible promotors or repressors), lineage and differentiation specific expression (cell / tissue specific promotors) and transduction of multiple genes to afford control over complex or multigenic disorders (using internal ribosomal entry systems). Advances in this field depend both on improvements in the vectors – particularly in their carrying capacity and ability to achieve stable transduction in non-replicating cells, and on our developing a better understanding of gene regulation.

Cellular Engineering

Developing the potential for ex vivo gene therapy is partially dependent upon advances in ex vivo cellular engineering. Issues include access to appropriate tissue, enrichment of target cell populations, optimising ex vivo cellular manipulation including transfection/transduction conditions, evaluation of transduction efficiency and the impact on cellular phenotype and assessing the presence of adventitious agents such as residual reagents, bacterial contamination etc.

- Cellular engineering approaches fall into three categories.
- Genetic modification of cells as delivery vehicles e.g. haemophilia
- Genetic modification of cells for correction of single gene disorders e.g. severe combined immune deficiency, lysosomal storage diseases or thalassaemia.
- Genetic modification of cells to treat multi-factorial disease, e.g. cancer, HIV.

Haemophilia

Haemophilia represents an attractive target for gene therapy. It represents a single gene disorder, Factors VIII and IX can be delivered to the circulation from a variety of cell types and low levels of expression may suffice to ameliorate the clinical disease. It is unlikely that tightly regulated expression will be required and murine and canine models have demonstrated the feasibility of partial persistent correction of the haemophilic phenotype [7]. Several clinical gene therapy studies have been initiated, some involving ex vivo cellular manipulation, for example fibroblasts have been transduced with a retroviral vector containing Factor VIII cDNA. Recently 3 patients with severe Factor IX deficiency were treated with an adeno-associated viral vector containing Factor IX cDNA administered by intramuscular injection [8]. The transgene was found to be present by PCR and Factor IX was demonstrated in the extracellular space by immuno-histochemistry. There was no evidence of muscle injury or inflammation. One patient demonstrated elevated levels of Factor IX at 2-3%, with shortening of the APTT and a reduction in clinical clotting factor consumption at 100 days. A second patient had no detectable elevation in Factor IX but did demonstrate a reduction in clotting factor consumption at 100 days, suggesting that even very small increases in factor expression could have some clinical benefits. The third patient experienced no elevation of Factor IX and no obvious clinical benefit. This represents the first evidence that gene therapy for single genes disorders can have clinically beneficial effects.

Haematopoietic Stem Cells

There are a considerable number of single gene disorders affecting the haematopoietic and immune systems including haemoglobinopathies, defects in leucocyte production and function, congenital immunodeficiencies, lysosomal storage diseases and stem cell defects. Transduction of haematopoietic stem cells represents an attractive approach to these disorders because it could result in permanent long-term correction. However there are significant problems, haematopoietic stem cells represent a rare cell population perhaps 1 in 10^5 to 1 in 10^6 of nucleated cells in the bone marrow. Stable transfection would be required because of the high levels of proliferation required to generate cells of the haematopoietic and immune systems. However 95% of HSC are quiescent at any one time and induction of proliferation without differentiation is problematic [9].

However, 2 patients with X linked form of SCID have currently been treated using this approach. This disorder is caused by a mutation in the gene encoding the γC subunit of the cytokine receptor for IL-2, IL-4, IL-7, IL-9 and IL-15. This leads to an early block in T and NK differentiation and severe immunodeficiency which cannot be ameliorated by replacement therapy. 2 children were treated one of eight months of age and one of eleven months of age with 5 to 10×10^6 CD34 positive cells/kg, retroviral transduced with cDNA for the γC subunit. The haematopoietic stem cells were cultured in stem cell factor, IL-3 and FLT-3 ligand on CH296 recombinant fragment of fibronectin which has been shown to augment stem cell transduction efficiency. The genetically manipulated cells were reinfused intravenously without a conditioning regimen. The patients showed 20-40% transgene expression in their peripheral blood lymphocytes and, between 15 days and nine months, normalisation of T, B and NK cell numbers, normalisation of antigen specific responses and full resolution of the disease phenotype [10]. This therefore represents significant clinical improvement and these children who were previously confined to protective isolation have now been able to be discharged home.

Gene Therapy for Cancer

More than 70% of gene therapy clinical trials now in progress involve cancer management [11]. A number of different approaches have been adopted, including direct replacement of abnormal genes, blocking oncogene expression through antisense oligonucleotides or ribozymes, gene directed enzyme prodrug therapy or the delivery of 'gain of function' genes which seek to alter the malignant phenotype by immune potentiation, stromal reorganisation, or interference with angiogenesis. In addition, there has been considerable interest in altering the immune system in patients with cancer through, for example, transduction of dendritic cells with tumour-derived RNA, tumour-specific fusion genes, or monoclonal immunoglobulin or TCR gene rearrangements. Studies have also been carried out looking at altering the specificity of T cells and of gene-directed enzyme producing therapy for control of graft versus host disease.

Anderson et al. have recently used an adenovirus with a 55kDa E1B gene deletion called ONYX-015, which has been engineered to selectively replicate in and lyse p53 deficient cancer cells whilst sparing normal cells. A phase II study involving intra-tumoural administration of ONYX-015 in patients with squamous cell carcinoma of the head and neck resulted in substantial objective responses in 25 out of 30 cases with only grade I and II toxicities reported [12].

Concluding Remarks

The past decade has seen significant progress in the development of gene therapy with a large number of ongoing clinical trials and the first evidence that these approaches can induce significant morbidity and mortality, but also evidence of clinical efficacy in a number of different settings. Continuing technical advance in vector design and transgene regulation can be expected [13]. At the same time, completion of the human genome project and advances in our understanding of functional genomics is likely to shift the focus from single gene disorders and interventions to more subtle multigenetic interventions in cellular phenotype. The development of genetic medicines for in vivo use is likely to involve pharmaceutical manufacturing. However, ex vivo genetic cellular engineering is a bespoke process and likely to require the expertise of the Blood Transfusion Services in donor selection and screening, harvesting, ex vivo cellular separation, manipulation and storage, good manufacturing practices and quality control, recipient follow up and regulatory affairs. If the Transfusion Services want to involve themselves in this exciting field in the future, then they need to invest now in the development of appropriate expertise and facilities [14].

References

1. Wade N. Gene therapy pioneer draws Mikadoesque rap. Science 1981;212:253.
2. Rosenberg SA, Aebersold P, Cornetta K, et al. Gene transfer into humans – immunotherapy of patients with advanced melanoma using tumour infiltrating lymphocytes modified by retroviral gene transfection. N Engl J Med 1990;323:570-78.
3. Blaese RM, Culver KW, Miller AD, et al. T lymphocyte directed gene therapy for ADA – SCID: initial trial results after 4 years. Science 1995;270 475-80.
4. Human Gene Marker/Therapy Clinical protocols. Hum Gene Ther 2000;11:1745-816.
5. Balter M. Gene therapy on trial. Science 2000;288:951-57.
6. Prince HM. Gene transfer: a review of methods and applications. Pathology 1998;30: 335-47.
7. Kaufman R J. Advances toward gene therapy for hemophilia of the millenium. Hum Gene Ther 1999;10:2091-107.
8. Kay MA, Manno CS, Ragni MV, et al. Evidence for gene transfer and expression of factor IX in haemophilia B patients treated with an AAV vector. Nat Genetics 2000;24:257-61.
9. Halene S, Kohn DB. Gene therapy using hematopoietic stem cells: sisyphus approaches the crest. Hum Gene Ther 2000;11:1259-67.
10. Caveazzana-Calvo M, Hacien-Bey S, de Saint Basile G, et al. Gene therapy of human severe combined immunodeficiency (SCID)-X1 disease. Science 2000;288:669-71.
11. Curiel DT, Gerritsen WR, Krul MR. Progress in cancer gene therapy. Cancer Gene Therapy 2000;7:1197-99.
12. Khuri FR, Nemunaitis J, Ganly I, et al. A controlled trial of intratumoral ONYX-015, a selectively replicating adenovirus, in combination with cisplatin and 5-fluorouracil in patients with head and neck cancer. Nat Medicine 2000;6:879-85.
13. Somia N, Verma IM. Gene therapy: trials and tribulations. Nat Reviews 2000;1:91-99.

14. Islam KB, Blomberg P, Wikstrom K, Edvard Smith CI. An academic centre for gene therapy research with clinical grade manufacturing capability. Ann Med 1997;29:5 79- 83.

MAKING POLICY IN THE 2000s

J.C. Emmanuel[1]

Background

The World Health Organization (WHO) is the United Nations agency responsible for health issues, with 191 Member States. WHO has global responsibility for health.

Ministers of Health of WHO's Member States meet annually in Geneva at the World Health Assembly (WHA). As a governing body, the Health Assembly has the authority to make recommendations to Members with respect to any matter within the competence of the Organization.

The role of WHO has become increasingly crucial to the attainment of the goal of health for all and the reduction in the gap between the health status of the people of developed and developing countries, as well as between the developing and least developed areas. This role has never been important than it is today in 2000. There is a need for global and national policies for the improvement in the safety of blood and blood products. WHO can provide this normative role at global level for national health authorities who seek information on 'Policy formation' as a tool to implement evidence based technologies as a guide to decision-making. Thus international decisions should be considered when making decisions at national level.

The Twenty-eighth World Health Assembly in May 1975 addressed the issue of utilization and supply of human blood and blood products and urged Member States:

- to promote the development of national blood transfusion services based on voluntary non-remunerated donation of blood;
- to enact effective legislation governing the operation of blood services and to take other actions necessary to protect and promote the health of blood donors and of recipients of blood and blood products ..."(Resolution WHA28.72)

The WHO Executive Board, at its 79th session in January 1987 reiterated its support to resolution WHA28.72 whilst recognizing the technical, managerial, financial and ethical complexities of the situation, particularly in developing

1. Director, Blood Safety and Clinical Technology World Health Organization, Geneva, CH.

countries. The importance for Member States to develop national policies in order to ensure timely and adequate supply of safe blood and blood products and to use them rationally as appropriate to their country situations was emphasized (Resolution EB79.R1). A national blood policy should stipulate the commitment and support from the Government to the national blood programme which should have the required legislative or regulatory support. This policy should clearly define the roles and responsibilities for the blood programme/ transfusion service and ensure that it has appropriate legislative/regulatory support and is sustainable. Transfusion medicine, with the exception of the pharmaceutically prepared blood products, has remained largely unregulated or controlled by national blood transfusion services/blood banks, especially in developing countries.

Politics and influence

The human immunodeficiency virus (HIV) transformed the beliefs of the community that the blood supply had never been safer through the improvements in diagnostic testing. HIV brought a new wave of ethical consciousness on donor and recipient care and at the same time made the public less trusting. Injuries became perceived as grievances and affected groups such as the haemophiliac community, seen as the chief sufferers, organized themselves into groups with a clear public identity and political strategy. A new era of medical politics was born. Thus influential social movements became able to mobilize public policy and expectations.

Commitment and support by governments to ensure the correct organizational and management structure with adequate funding has to be in place. There cannot be a country where there are unlimited resources for health care and for the blood transfusion services (BTSs) within this framework. The available resources for safe and adequate blood and blood products will determine what can and cannot be done. Choices will have to be made and where these do not involve policy-makers when responding to known or potential threats there is a real risk of apportioning fault. Where there is public perception of fault then justice will be sought. It has been stated that "Justice is an intuitive response rationalized through a legal system". The politics of justice will vary from one country to another but as has been seen in the variations of legal liability that have occurred this can lead to compensation which may be followed by apology. The question will always be "Is blood a special case for justice claims?" The comparison between blood and vaccination illustrates the different perceptions which lead to legal rationalization. In the case of vaccination, it is considered as a 'public (health) good case' – vaccination benefits other people more than it benefits the vaccinee and therefore the risk is justifiable. This does not apply in the case of liability for injury due to blood transfusion. Public perception is fueled by 'Bad news coverage'. Policy-making should be shared so that there is a clear understanding of whether justice is fault-based or negligence base or even because of need!

Politics and influence are thus linked in decision-making. Evidence-based decisions, cost-effectiveness analyses may suggest that safety measures may be marginal, or even made in the face of no evidence, but on the 'precautionary principle' basis. What is unquestionable is that policy-makers require a tool on how decisions are being made in other countries. There is a need to have a tool for 'formulating policies' and a mechanism to compare how decisions are made to ensure that they are not "too far in front or too far behind" and to be able to respond to the consequences of actions taken!

Collaboration and co-ordination is now recognized as essential for information sharing, coordination of actions, synergies of efforts at global and national level. Global Collaboration for Blood Safety (GCBS) was proposed and supported at the Paris AIDS Summit in 1994 and endorsed at the Forty-eighth World Health Assembly (1995) through resolution WHA48.27.

Blood Policy has thus been identified as an issue of international concern with a common need for risk assessments, exchange of policy issues and state-of-the-art knowledge. The importance in scientific and political terms of knowing the decision-making processes that each country takes will ensure that policy-makers are aware of actions taken, whether they are as a result of a precautionary principle or based on scientific consensus. Developed and developing countries need to have clearly defined minimum standards for product preparation and manufacture. This means recognition of specific quality and safety requirements for plasma-derived pharmaceutical products and for labile blood products (components).

While there is a need to work towards a goal of 'zero-risk' – questions are raised as to the sense of the seeking the unattainable – "no sense, nonsense or no nonsense" was suggested as the title for this presentation. Working toward a goal will, however, lead to a better product but should be in the context of an integrated health care system. Decisions to improve blood safety will need to address all the issues involved and not only those of a scientific nature. Although in the past decisions were made only when there was evidence-based and scientifically proven data endorsed by scientific consensus, because of new and emerging diseases and past experience with HIV 'scandals', a cocktail of principles need to be considered when developing blood policies including the acceptance of reviewing existing policies and the implementation of new interventions.

Guidance on policy formulation should assist developing as well as developed countries. Organizations such as WHO play a key role in providing a mechanism for exchanging information and promoting collaboration on a global scale. The declaration developed at the Paris AIDS Summit of 1994 and endorsed by the Forty-eighth World Health Assembly in 1995 for the establishment of the Global Collaboration for Blood Safety, included the following text:

- "...undertake in our national policies to ensure the safety of blood and blood products..."
- "...resolved to step up international co-operation through the following measures and initiatives..."
- "...strengthen international collaboration for blood safety with a view to coordinating technical information..."
- "...proposing standards for good manufacturing practices for all blood products..."

- "...and fostering the establishment and implementation of co-operative partnerships to ensure blood safety in all countries."

The objectives of the GCBS are:
- to promote international consensus on essential principles of global blood safety;
- to promote the improvement of global blood safety and encourage governments to recognize and establish national blood programmes;
- to assist countries, upon request, to identify national blood safety priorities and prevent transfusion transmitted disease;
- to assist countries, upon request, in the implementation of appropriate and recognized transfusion practices to ensure donor and recipient safety and freedom from discrimination;
- to promote effective recruitment of safe donors through the use of appropriate selection criteria;
- to promote the appropriate preparation and utilization of blood and blood products;
- to encourage safe international practices for the collection, storage and transport of plasma and the preparation and distribution of its derivatives;
- to promote bi-directional traceability of blood products between donor and recipient whether in-country or across national borders; and
- to facilitate the exchange and use of information by encouraging data collection, management and dissemination.

The Global Database for Blood Safety (GDBS), using a checklist and questionnaire is a direct result of the GCBS, and the analysis on the available data will be used to identify areas that require urgent attention and develop intervention strategies, especially in priority countries.

An internationally recognised number of organizations and experts meet as Members of the GCBS with WHO as the Secretariat. Issues of global and national concern will be identified and considered and when there is a need for special attention, specialized working groups will be formed to address these issues as part of the work of the GCBS. One of these issues is that of 'policy formulation' as a tool for assisting policy-makers.

Evidence-based policy making will be key in 2000 using available science and working on theoretical risk – the risks as they relate to what can be done and what cannot be done. The public and the politicians will need to be informed – and consulted – communication will be the key.

Meaningful and *effective* global collaboration will lead to blood transfusions that are as safe and effective as possible through agreed policy formulation mechanisms based on global concerns, national health care systems and available resources.

DISCUSSION

H.J.C. de Wit (Amsterdam, NL): Dr. McCullough, you focused merely with the expansion of the white cell population, but how far - thinking of quo vadis - are we from expanding for red cells, say a factor 1,000 or 10,000 times so that the expanded red cell suspension can be used for routine transfusion.

J. McCullough (Minneapolis, MN, USA): I do not know how far we are from red cells and the other component of great interest would be platelets. As you know the key growth factors for both red cells and platelets are cloned and available. I know that a number of groups are focusing on platelets to attempt to generate large numbers of platelets through cultured systems. As far as I know they have not made a great deal of progress so I would imagine that while this may develop it is still a decade away.

C.Th. Smit Sibinga (Groningen, NL): Dr. McCullough, the dendritic cells are really the great potential for the near future. The question arises what behaviour do they show to your knowledge when storing them instead of immediately manipulating them. Because they are kind of sensitive cells and may lose some of their capacity if you store them under various conditions. Could you give some idea about that?

J. McCullough: We have only a small amount of work with dendritic cells in our laboratory and they have not really been stored to any great extent. Cells have been obtained from marrow and then isolated through selection procedures, a short term culture and then have been used very soon. We have tried not to store them so that we would not get into those kinds of difficulties. So, I am not sure that I can answer your question

C.Th. Smit Sibinga: No, I understand. If you look ahead in time to set up a mechanism or logistic for handling the manoeuvring of the engineering of dendritic cells, conditioning them and so forth, there might come a point in time in which you need to have a certain lapse time from the collection on the one hand up till the moment that you start the real stimulation.

J. McCullough: So, you mean you might want to collect them and then freeze them for later exposure to the tumour?

C.Th. Smit Sibinga: That probably might come up in the future.

J. McCullough: Yes, because there is not really time to go. You need different strategies to isolate the tumour molecules that are going to be used to prime the dendritic cells. There may be a time depending on how and when one wants to process the tumour in order to get the tumour specific antigen to use to prime the dendritic cells. So, maybe you are right it may be necessary to store the cells for a period of time.

J.D. Cash (Edinburgh, Scotland): When I think of cell engineering now in a generic sense, I no longer think exclusively of the haematopoietic stem cells. However - this is hugely important I think for the blood transfusion and blood banking community - I really would ask the question if we can make the intellectual and operational move away from the traditional red cell into the new. Does the new include not only haematopoietic stem cells, but liver stem cells and for instance neurological brain stem cells that are developing very, very rapidly in terms of therapeutic potential. I certainly would hope so.

J. McCullough: I could not agree with you more. You may notice that I am listed in the programme as coming from the centre for molecular and cellular therapy, a centre that the University of Minnesota asked me to establish for the very purpose you describe. The idea is to apply the systems and the thinking and the approaches that we used to manipulate blood cells to the processing of other tissues such as pancreatic islet cells, tumour vaccines but also it includes the collection of embryonic stem cells and the expansion of those cells into nerve tissue or cartilage or other sorts of tissues like that. Actually I was kind of pleased with the way of thinking of the university vice-presidents because they came to the idea that they should have the structure and the systems, the quality and everything else that applies to the way we manipulate blood cells to apply to those other tissues. This is not really the last question.

B.G. Solheim (Oslo, N): Two very short comments. Dendritic cells need not to be stored, because you can drive CD34 cells to dendritic cells with the tissue culture traditions today.

Dr. Cash commented on liver cells. This summer there was a very interesting article in Hepatology[1] describing that patients transplanted with stem cells had regenerated up to 40% of their liver cells if they had active hepatitis by donor liver cells, which only could be generated from bone marrow stem cells, that way. Women were transplanted with male bone marrow.

M.K. Elias (Groningen, NL): To the best of your knowledge is there any preference for the source of dendritic cells, whether they are monocyte derived or CD34 positive cells derived as far as the liability for loading with antigen?

---

1. Theise ND, Nimmakayalu M, Gardner R, et al. Liver from bone marrow in humans. Hepatology 2000; 32: 11-16.

J. McCullough: Again, I am sorry that I have not had enough experience with dendritic cells to know for preference.

A. Brand (Leiden, NL): As far as I know, CD34 derived dendritic cells have a better stimulatory capacity than the monocyte derived dendritic cells from the peripheral blood. But as far as we know now there are four or five different populations of dendritic cells which may be dependent on the purpose you want to establish. You may use in the future different types of dendritic cells for a particular purpose, let us say for the regulation of auto-immunity and for having an allo-response against cancer or other targets.

M.K. Elias: Dr. Brand, you are absolutely right about the term immunemodulation being a confusing and non-specific term. You mentioned the immune defectors that affect the immune modulatory response of blood transfusion. Among those the immune competence of the host and the HLA relationship between the donor and recipient. One of the prerequisites for induction of tolerance is the exposure of the host to foreign MHC antigens and you mentioned that sharing MHC too, between donor recipients facilitates this process probably through establishment of micro-chimeras which renders the patient tolerance to subsequent transplant. My question is which cell in the blood transfusion do you think is or plays the key-role in induction of tolerance. Is it the mature MHC bearing leukocyte or the haematopoietic cell with its self-renewing persistently providing those allo-MHC antigens.

A. Brand: I think that is impossible to answer. Again we have a wide view on tolerance and I think the aim of tolerance is important. But if you look now to the data that even with completely different donor recipient MHC combinations you can establish tolerance once you use a huge amount of antigen with a low expression of class II antigens. For instance, the CD34 stem cell transplantation against an MHC barrier can establish tolerance even when they are a complete mismatch. So, that is an extremely important factor that once you have a huge amount of antigens you can establish tolerance even in mismatch combinations when you delay the appearance of class II expressing molecules. This is only part of the answer. There are several other ways to establish tolerance and we have different kinds of tolerance; central tolerance, peripheral tolerance. There are several regulatory circuits which can establish tolerance. It is very intriguing because we know now that maybe every pregnancy and maybe even every blood transfusion is able to establish a kind of tolerance in which if you use very sensitive methods for instance to detect one in a thousand or 1 in 100,000 or 1 in a million donor cells. You are able to detect these cells and it is very important to know the nature of these cells whether they establish tolerance yes or no. Why do these cells circulate, why do they not cause graft versus host, why do they not proliferate. These are all questions to investigate before I can give you a simple answer. What is the major cell inducing tolerance.

J. Aluoch (Nairobi, Kenya): I have two small questions to dr. Turner and dr. Emmanuel.

There was a reference to haemoglobinopathies and in particular you were mentioning sickle cell disease. I have the impression that we are failing and perhaps even in the 21st century we will not succeed to find a way to put glutamic acid back to the 6th sequence, where it had been replaced by valine. Maybe the problem will be that if one manages to engineer glutamic acid back to where valine is, that the problem will be that wherever else valine is in the betaglobin chain it will be replaced where it should not be. Yet, this is a disease which although it is not quite a problem in Europe it is really affecting some countries in the world. Maybe this is not the forum, I mean blood transfusion is probably not the forum where the problem should be dealt with. I do not know if you can comment a little further on what prospects there are. It seems to be working out in haemophilia for example.

M.L. Turner (Edinburgh, UK): I take your point, I did not speak very much about thalassaemia and sickle cell disease. Not because there is actually quite a lot of work in the area, but we do not tend to be involved. To my knowledge we have one patient with sickle cell anaemia in Edinburgh so you can understand it is not a particularly burning issue for us anyway. But nevertheless clearly on a global basis it is an extremely important issue. There are various devices you can use for transfuses to correct particular point mutations in genes. In general what you have to do is have a strand which obviously binds very selectively to the basis on either side of that particular point mutation. Otherwise, as you frankly said, you will be correcting point mutation all over the place. Most approaches that people are trying for betaglobin disorders is to replace the whole gene and preferentially to replace it by homologous recombination rather than add in a normal betaglobin gene. The problems are that it is not actually easy to do; the approach which probably will work is to transfuse haematopoietic stem cells from the patient, but then you need to get it right. You need to get it expressed in the right lineage at the right level and so on. So, there are quite a lot of technical problems within the issue and there are groups that are working on that. So, I guess we would hope that in the next five or ten years people will start to really deliver in that area. The next issue I think then is, can those countries who have very high proportions of patients with this kind of disease, actually, enforce infrastructure of the technology to implement this kind of policy. I think that is an extremely important issue.

J.R. Aluoch: Thank you. Dr. Emmanuel, a small concern and that is with regard to press releases. Last week I was chairing a session in a haematology and oncology symposium in Nairobi. At least I felt embarrassed when someone came up to announce that when we have blood donors from the UK who may offer to give blood that we should not accept them because of the possibility of vCJD. This person had missed our professional literature released on this type of thing and perhaps picked up some misguided press. Really it might have been picked up by some journalist from somewhere. Am I trying to create an elephant out of a fly, if I say that maybe we should hug the machinery to relay this type of information to government so that the national presses can pick it up and convey the right information?

J.C. Emmanuel (Geneva, Ch): I think it is a very good question. It is one that we are addressing at the moment and giving a short statement in the world how to record epidemiology. You raised a number of fundamental problems. One is that if there was a nationally organised and co-ordinated or responsible body for blood transfusion in your country and a number of other countries, the decision would be made in conjunction with the government on the sort of residual risk of transmission of infection. So, the question might arise if those donors that come from a potentially TSE transmission or variant CJD country are more of a risk than the other donors who are family replacement and carrier (residual risk) of hepatitis B, hepatitis C and HIV, because there does not seem to exist a donor system. So, making decisions under those circumstances of an absence of government commitment and support to a nationally co-ordinated run and responsible body is extremely difficult as there is no-one to talk to. So, there are a number of difficulties, but the country still has to make that decision. Are those donors less safe than the donors that you find in the ordinary population from the statistics that you have. So, you are right. But the fundamental question is governmental support set up the body that could make that decision in light of the facts at hand and the residual risk that it has also. But WHO can be asked that question, sure.

C. Jersild (Arhus, DK): A comment to Dr.McClelland's presentation. In Denmark we decided some three years ago to establish a transfusion database and this collects data from all the blood transfusion services or blood given to patients and combines that with the demographic data from the hospital IT systems and the laboratory databases on haematology and clinical chemistry. Now, my colleague in Arhus dr. Janson just analysed blood usage in total hip replacement and he found that a number of patients were not receiving any blood at all[1] Even second operations for hip replacements which is rather unusual. Looking into the database there were no answers whatsoever what could be the reason for this and the actual fact of importance was the type of anaesthesia - spinal anaesthesia combined with controlled hypotension was actually able to reduce blood usage quite dramatic. I wonder if that kind of information is included in the analysis presented by McClelland.

A. Brand: Dr. Emmanuel, do you think that the blood transfusion community, because it is highly internationalised, has a special responsibility if you compare it with other physicians world-wide like surgeons and internal medicine. Do you think that we have a special responsibility to create something of improvement in the poor countries in relation to the rich countries, because if we cannot make it then it will not be made by other physicians. Can you comment on that?

J. Emmanuel: I think that blood transfusionists are a very special community of people; they are responsible for running as I was saying before a businesslike operation under non-profit conditions. They have to deal with a public much

1. Personal communication from Dr Jan Jørgensen, Medical Director, Dept of Clinical Immunology and Blood Transfusion Service, Århus University Hospital, Skejby, DK.

more than in general terms at a wider public. They have to deal with public opinion because blood has this much greater emotional response, it has this legality involved in it. It deals with all the functions of laboratory and science as was mentioned by dr. Turner. How far does one get involved that has responsibility trust upon them, which has not been clearly defined as to who's responsibility this is. They have this clinical interface with the doctors whom you talk about. So, I think the first responsibility is that they should get their house in order and sort that out which I think is evidenced by what is happening here in the Netherlands.

In addition to that you are quite right; they can help and they do help. Now, individuals going to a place in say China help an individual institution; it is not sustainable. That is why we want a global collaboration to co-ordinate everybody who is doing anything: Council of Europe, WHO, the International Consortium for Blood Safety. Draw to the attention of the funding agencies to give a lot of money to WHO for extra budgetary sources to identify whether there is a problem and pull together people to do defined projects in a co-ordinated and concerted way that leads to full development of that project with WHO asking for government commitment and support. Going and helping with governments themselves will not support, it is not sustainable. It just lasts a lifetime of that particular intervention which could be weeks, it could be a month, it could be a year and it goes back to zero again, which leads to a lot of disillusion and frustration amongst people when another group comes and wants to do something. So, you are right but what we are trying to do is draw the attention to people who are available, people who are retiring and have skills should be made available within the framework of the right countries to work together with WHO and other organisations in a concerted and co-ordinated way and that will make a difference.

S. Poppema (Groningen, NL): Thank you, I think it is time to finish. Prof. John Cash will now come on stage and perform a miracle. He will sum up what we have learnt I think in not too much time.

J.D. Cash: Mr. Chairman, may I first thank Dr. Cees Smit Sibinga for the invitation to contribute to this year's Groningen Symposium? It has been an honour and great pleasure. As Chairman of the Symposium I would like to thank the Dean and all the speakers and chairpersons for their many contributions. I am astonished at the number of distinguished colleagues who, over the last 25 years, have been prepared to come to the Groningen Symposium and share their knowledge and skills. The benefits of these international efforts have been considerable and a great tribute to the Smit Sibinga Team. The team deserves our thanks and congratulations on their 25th anniversary.

One of the many pleasures of retirement is you have more time to think and reflect. In the months preceding this Symposium I have been haunted by a book I read last Spring. The author, Douglas Starr, is an Associate Professor of Journalism and Science from Boston University[1]. The title of the book is **Blood, an epic history of medicine and commerce**. It is extensively and authoritatively researched and starts with leaches and finishes with prions. But a large middle section addresses the way those responsible for all aspects of transfusion medicine, in many parts of the world, dealt with the problem of transfusion transmitted diseases in the preceding two decades. However, a significant part of the epic is a tale of courage, individual tenacity and outstanding scientific, technical and managerial achievements.

There have been many contributions in this Symposium, which testify to continued courage, tenacity and scientific innovation, so well described in Starr's historical treatise. In this context we will all depart with our own examples. Time does not permit me to summarise all aspects of this excellent Symposium. I was profoundly impressed with the contribution of Dr Corash, and could not help but conclude that his group's work on the killing of microbes in therapeutic preparations of red cells and platelets is work of major clinical and economic importance to those concerned with transfusion medicine in all parts of the world.

Once again I enjoyed Dr AuBuchon's updated rallying cry for the need to consider value for money in the practice of transfusion medicine. There are no unlimited supplies of money for health care, even in the USA. It follows that sooner or later we must rejoin our colleagues in other parts of the health care business and look much more carefully at the cost benefits of transfusion therapies. Dr. AuBuchon did much more than beat a philosophical drum. He has pioneered the development of specific but generic methodology by which evidence-based value for money considerations can be developed in each country.

I was particularly delighted with the contribution made by Mr. Kavanagh on Regulation. This topic is of major importance and when in a moment I reflect on the darker side of Douglas Starr's book you will understand why I commend it to you. Some might argue that the Directives coming out of Brussels on this topic are bureaucratic development stoppers. In fact, they are at the heart of a movement forward in transfusion medicine that is centred on safety, efficacy, accountability and transparency. I confess I get a little irritated when I hear too many cries that we are now over regulated. That will, ofcourse, always be a real danger, though I would prefer to call it inappropriate regulation.

The session on Quality Assurance was, in my view, quite outstanding. I reflected, as it went on, that in a previous Groningen Symposium, we had sought to develop the idea that transfusion medicine was a bridge, which linked on the one side the donor and the other the patient[2]. Our session on quality assurance seemed to indicate to me that despite some fascinating problems, which are being vigorously addressed, one side of the bridge (the donor and donation testing and processing) is in good order. But the other side, where the patient lies, this is not so well endowed. The fact is that quality assurance in the clinical

---

1. Douglas Starr. Blood, an epic history of medicine and commerce. Alfred A. Knopf, New York, 1998.
2. Cash JD. Transfusion medicine today and tomorrow: The facts and the fictions. In: Smit Sibinga CTh, Das PC, Cash JD, eds. Transfusion Medicine: Fact and Fiction. Kluwer Academic Publ. Dordrecht, Boston, London 1992:191-94.

setting in general is poorly developed and in the clinical practice of transfusion medicine it is almost non existent. I had hoped that during the Symposium we would have had some reference to the development of evidenced based clinical guidelines. This did not emerge and it is my hope that this topic will find a place in a forthcoming Groningen Symposium.

I sometimes get weary of bumping into people who tell me that transfusion medicine is all played out, that it has no future and donors will soon be as dinosaurs. If we remained even half awake during the fascinating contributions of Drs Turner, McCullough and Brand these views would have been dispelled as we caught sight of the potential of future cellular therapies and the need to embed them into an environment where regulated good manufacturing practice is the norm. What we need to be doing now for tomorrow, is recruiting and training cell biologists and molecular biologists. Of no less importance is the need for managers with courage, vision and energy.

I have previously referred to the fact that as I prepared for this Symposium I was haunted by Douglas Starr's historical treatise. You might ask why, in the certain expectation of so much good scientific news, did I need to feel haunted? This book reveals that the history of blood transfusion has been greatly enriched by individuals showing courage, energy, determination, tenacity and compassion. But when Starr examines the way Blood Services and associated pharmaceutical enterprises responded to problems of the transmission of infectious agents in blood and blood products we witness a dark and sinister side. It reveals frightening human frailty, professional incompetence, greed, bribery, lying, cheating, corruption, denial, and callous systematic individual and corporate disregard for the well-being of patients, which led to thousands of deaths.

I guess as a doctor the most difficult part of this book came when Starr concluded that all the evidence points to the fact that during this period doctors repeatedly testified in support of pharmaceutical companies or the commercial interests of their Blood Banks and against the interests of their patients. Moreover, commercial interests infiltrated some specialised patient support groups and when called to support they responded in favour of these commercial interests rather than their members. We should not conclude that all this darkness resided in the USA, or that it was confined to commercial companies. Many politicians and government officials were involved and, by remaining silent, the International Society of Blood Transfusion, AABB and National Blood Transfusion Services made their contribution too.

Looking back over the last two days I would have to conclude that the most important features of this 25th Groningen Symposium are that it has been organised from within a national blood transfusion service, which is subject to the demands of public accountability and transparency, and has put regulation and quality assurance on a par with scientific innovation. We have also been repeatedly reminded that 80% of the world's population are sitting on the outside unable to enjoy many of the fruits of all this innovative science. And we have been advised that the vast majority of patients, even in developed countries, don't need blood transfusions, but are caught up in shortages of health care resources - for nursing care, home/day care and the management of disabilities.

This has been an excellent Symposium. Once again Pandora's box has been opened and from our deliberations should come many more such occasions.

Congratulations and thanks.

INDEX

DEVELOPMENTS IN HEMATOLOGY AND IMMUNOLOGY

1. H.R. Lijnen, D. Collen and M. Verstraete (eds.): *Synthetic Substrates in Clinical Blood Coagulation Assays.* 1980 ISBN 90-247-2409-0
2. C.Th. Smit Sibinga, P.C. Das and J.O. Forfar (eds.): *Paediatrics and Blood Transfusion.* Proceedings of the 5th Annual Symposium on Blood Transfusion, organized by the Red Cross Blood Bank Groningen-Drenthe, The Netherlands (1980). 1982 ISBN 90-247-2619-0
3. N. Fabris (ed.): *Immunology and Ageing.* 1982 ISBN 90-247-2640-9
4. G. Hornstra: *Dietary Fats, Prostanoids and Arterial Thrombosis.* With an Introductory Chapter by A. Bleakley Chandler. 1982 ISBN 90-247-2667-0
5. C.Th. Smit Sibinga, P.C. Das and J.J. van Loghem (eds.): *Blood Transfusion and Problems of Bleeding.* Proceedings of the 6th Annual Symposium on Blood Transfusion, organized by the Red Cross Blood Bank Groningen-Drenthe (1981). 1982 ISBN 90-247-3058-9
6. J. Dormandy (ed.): *Red Cell Deformability and Filterability.* 1983 ISBN 0-89838-578-4
7. C.Th. Smit Sibinga, P.C. Das and H.F. Taswell (eds.): *Quality Assurance in Blood Banking and Its Clinical Impact.* Proceedings of the 7th Annual Symposium on Blood Transfusion, organized by the Red Cross Blood Bank Groningen-Drenthe (1982). 1984 ISBN 0-89838-618-7
8. A.M.H.P. van den Besselaar, H.R. Gralnick and S.M. Lewis (eds.): *Thromboplastin Calibration and Oral Anticoagulant Control.* 1984 ISBN 0-89838-637-3
9. P. Fondu and O. Thijs (eds.): *Haemostatic Failure in Liver Disease.* 1984 ISBN 0-89838-640-3
10. C.Th. Smit Sibinga, P.C. Das and G. Opelz (eds.): *Transplantation and Blood Transfusion.* Proceedings of the 8th Annual Symposium on Blood Transfusion, organized by the Red Cross Blood Bank Groningen-Drenthe (1983). 1984 ISBN 0-89838-686-1
11. H. Schmid-Schönbein, L.J. Wurzinger and R.E. Zimmerman (eds.): *Enzyme Activation in Blood-perfused Artificial Organs.* 1985 ISBN 0-89838-704-3
12. J. Dormandy (ed.): *Blood Filtration and Blood Cell Deformability.* 1985 ISBN 0-89838-714-0
13. C.Th. Smit Sibinga, P.C. Das and E. Seidl (eds.): *Plasma Fractionation and Blood Transfusion.* Proceedings of the 9th Annual Symposium on Blood Transfusion, organized by the Red Cross Blood Bank Groningen-Drenthe (1984). 1985 ISBN 0-89838-761-2
14. S. Dawids and A. Bantjes (eds.): *Blood Compatible Materials and their Testing.* 1986 ISBN 0-89838-813-9
15. C.Th. Smit Sibinga, P.C. Das and T.J. Greenwalt (eds.): *Future Developments in Blood Banking.* Proceedings of the 10th Annual Symposium on Blood Transfusion, organized by the Red Cross Blood Bank Groningen-Drenthe (1985). 1986 ISBN 0-89838-824-4
16. A. Berlin, J. Dean, M.H. Draper, E.M.B. Smith and F. Spreafico (eds.): *Immunotoxicology.* Proceedings of the International Seminar on the Immunological System as a Target for Toxic Damage – Present Status, Open Problems and Future Perspectives, in collaboration with the UNEP-ILO-WHO IPCS and the Commission of the European Communities. 1987 ISBN 0-89838-843-0
17. T. Ottenhoff and R. de Vries: *Recognition of M. leprae Antigens.* 1987 ISBN 0-89838-887-2
18. J.-L. Touraine, R.P. Gale and V. Kochupillai (eds.): *Fetal Liver Transplantation.* 1987 ISBN 0-89838-975-5
19. C.Th. Smit Sibinga P.C. Das and C.P. Engelfriet (eds.): *White Cells and Platelets in Blood Transfusion.* Proceedings of the 11th Annual Symposium on Blood Transfusion, organized by the Red Cross Blood Bank Groningen-Drenthe (1986). 1987 ISBN 0-89838-976-3
20. C.F.M. Hendriksen: *Laboratory Animals in Vaccine Production and Control.* 1988 ISBN 0-89838-398-6

21. C.Th. Smit Sibinga, P.C. Das and L.R. Overby (eds.): *Biotechnology in Blood Transfusion.* Proceedings of the 12th Annual Symposium on Blood Transfusion, organized by the Red Cross Blood Bank Groningen-Drenthe (1987). 1988 ISBN 0-89838-404-4
22. C.Th. Smit Sibinga, P.C. Das and C.F. Högman (eds.): *Automation in Blood Transfusion.* Proceedings of the 13th Annual Symposium on Blood Transfusion, organized by the Red Cross Blood Bank Groningen-Drenthe (1988). 1989 ISBN 0-7923-0488-8
23. S. Dawids (ed.): *Polymers: Their Properties and Blood Compatibility.* 1989 ISBN 0-7923-0491-8
24. C.Th. Smit Sibinga, P.C. Das and H.T. Meryman (eds.): *Cryopreservation and Low Temperature Biology in Blood Transfusion.* Proceedings of the 14th Annual Symposium on Blood Transfusion, organized by the Red Cross Blood Bank Groningen-Drenthe (1989). 1990 ISBN 0-7923-0908-1
25. C.Th. Smit Sibinga and L. Kater (eds.): *Advances in Haemapheresis.* Proceedings of the 3rd International Congress of the World Apheresis Association (Amsterdam, The Netherlands, 1990). 1991 ISBN 0-7923-1312-7
26. C.Th. Smit Sibinga, P.C. Das and P.M. Mannucci (eds.): *Coagulation and Blood Transfusion.* Proceedings of the 15th Annual Symposium on Blood Transfusion, organized by the Red Cross Blood Bank Groningen-Drenthe (1990). 1991 ISBN 0-7923-1331-3
27. C.Th. Smit Sibinga, P.C. Das and J.D. Cash (eds.): *Transfusion Medicine: Fact and Fiction.* Proceedings of the 16th International Symposium on Blood Transfusion, organized by the Red Cross Blood Bank Groningen-Drenthe (1991). 1992 ISBN 0-7923-1732-7
28. C.Th. Smit Sibinga, P.C. Das and T.H. The (eds.): *Immunology and Blood Transfusion.* Proceedings of the 17th International Symposium on Blood Transfusion, organized by the Red Cross Blood Bank Groningen-Drenthe (1992). 1993 ISBN 0-7923-2380-7
29. C.Th. Smit Sibinga, P.C. Das and H.J. Heiniger (eds.): *Good Manufacturing Practice in Transfusion Medicine.* Proceedings of the 18th International Symposium on Blood Transfusion, organized by the Red Cross Blood Bank Groningen-Drenthe (1993). 1994 ISBN 0-7923-3009-9
30. C.Th. Smit Sibinga, P.C. Das and E. Briët (eds.): *Hereditary Diseases and Blood Transfusion.* Proceedings of the 19th International Symposium on Blood Transfusion, organized by the Red Cross Blood Bank Groningen-Drenthe (1994). 1995 ISBN 0-7923-3694-1
31. C.Th. Smit Sibinga, P.C. Das and E.L. Snyder (eds.): *Trigger Factors in Transfusion Medicine.* Proceedings of the 20th International Symposium on Blood Transfusion, organized by the Red Cross Blood Bank Noord-Nederland (1995). 1996 ISBN 0-7923-4225-0
32. C.Th. Smit Sibinga, P.C. Das and B. Löwenberg (eds.): *Cytokines and Growth Factors in Blood Transfusion.* Proceedings of the 21th International Symposium on Blood Transfusion, organized by the Red Cross Blood Bank Noord-Nederland (1996). 1997 ISBN 0-7923-4787-0
33. C.Th. Smit Sibinga, P.C. Das and J.C. Fratantoni (eds.): *Alternative Approaches to Human Blood Resources in Clinical Practice.* Proceedings of the 22nd International Symposium on Blood Transfusion, organized by the Red Cross Blood Bank Noord Nederland (1997). 1998 ISBN 0-7923-8305-2
34. C.Th. Smit Sibinga and H J. Alter (eds.): *Risk Management in Blood Transfusion: The Virtue of Reality.* Proceedings of the 23rd International Symposium on Blood Transfusion, organized by the Blood Bank Noord Nederland (1998).1999 ISBN 0-7923-6054-0
35. C.Th. Smit Sibinga and H.G. Klein (eds.): *Molecular Biology in Blood Transfusion.* Proceedings of the 24th International Symposium on Blood Transfusion, organized by the Blood Bank Noord Nederland (1999). 2000 ISBN 0-7923-6534-8

KLUWER ACADEMIC PUBLISHERS – DORDRECHT / BOSTON / LONDON

FSC
www.fsc.org
MIX
Papier | Fördert gute Waldnutzung
FSC® C083411

Kolibri 360 GmbH
Ferdinand-Jühlke-Straße 7
99095 Erfurt, Deutschland
produktsicherheit@kolibri360.de